Vascular and Endovascular Controversies

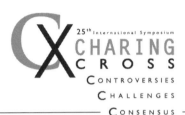

Vascular and Endovascular Controversies

Edited by

Roger M Greenhalgh MA, MD, MChir, FRCS

Jean-Pierre Becquemin MD
Alun Davies DM FRCS
Peter Gaines MRCP FRCR
Peter Harris MD FRCS
Krassi Ivancev MD PhD
Adam Mitchell MB BS FRCAS FRCR
Dieter Raithel MD PhD

BIBA Publishing
A division of BIBA Medical Ltd

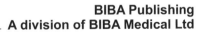

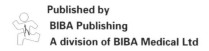

Published by
BIBA Publishing
A division of BIBA Medical Ltd

First published 2003

ISBN 0-9544687-0-8

British Library Cataloguing in Publication Data
A catalogue reserved for this book is available from the British Library

Note
Medical knowledge is constantly changing. As new information becomes available, changes in treatment, procedures, equipment and the use of drugs become necessary. The editors, contributors and the publishers have taken care to ensure that the information given in this text is accurate and up to date. However, readers are strongly advised to confirm that information, especially with regard to drug usage, complies with legislation and standards of practice.

Editorial and Production Services:
Jane Duncan
10 Barley Mow Passage, Chiswick, London W4 4PH, UK

Typeset by Phoenix Photosetting, Chatham, Kent, UK
Printed and bound by MPG Books Ltd, Bodmin, Cornwall, UK

Contents

CAROTID CONTROVERSIES

AORTIC ENDOVASCULAR CONTROVERSIES

THORACIC AORTIC CONTROVERSIES

ABDOMINAL AND RENAL CONTROVERSIES

LOWER LIMB ARTERIAL CONTROVERSIES

VENOUS CONTROVERSIES

Contributors

Amabile P, MD
Department of Vascular Surgery
Hôpital Sainte Marguerite
Marseille, France

Baird RN, ChM FRCS
Department of Vascular Surgery
Royal Infirmary
Bristol, UK

Bartoli J-M, MD
Department of Vascular Surgery
Hôpital Sainte Marguerite
Marseille, France

Baxter S, FCS
Consultant Vascular Surgeon
Department of Vascular Surgery
Southampton General Hospital
Southampton, UK

Beard J, MBBS BSc ChM FRCS
Consultant Vascular Surgeon
Sheffield Vascular Institute
Northern General Hospital
Sheffield, UK

Bell PRF, MBChB MD FRCS
Professor of Surgery
Leicester Royal Infirmary
Leicester, UK

Bell RE, MBBS FRCS
Clinical Research Fellow
Guy's & St Thomas' Hospital
London, UK

Belli A-M, MBBS FRCR
Consultant Radiologist
Department of Radiology
St George's Hospital
London, UK

Bergeron P, MD
Foundation Saint-Joseph Hospital
Department of Thoracic & Cardiovascular Surgery
Marseille, France

Bergqvist D, MD PhD
Professor of Surgery
Department of Surgery
University Hospital
Uppsala, Sweden

Biasi GM, MD FACS FRCS
Professor of Vascular Surgery
Head of Department of Surgical Sciences and
    Intensive Care
Bassini/San Gerardo Teaching Hospital
Cinisello Balsamo (Milan), Italy

Björck M, MD PhD
Department of Surgery
University Hospital
Uppsala, Sweden

Bleyn J, MD
Antwerp Blood-Vessel Centre
Antwerp, Belgium

Bolia A, MBChB DMRD FRCR
Consultant Radiologist
Department of Radiology
Leicester Royal Infirmary
Leicester, UK

Bradbury A, BSc MD FRCSEd
Professor of Vascular Surgery
University Department of Vascular Surgery
Lincoln House Research Institute
Birmingham Heartlands Hospital
Birmingham, UK

Bradley MD, BSc MBBS MRCP
Specialist Registrar in Radiology
Bristol Royal Infirmary
Bristol, UK

Campbell B
Consultant Surgeon
Royal Devon and Exeter Hospital (Wonford)
Exeter, UK

Cohen S, MD
Department of Vascular Surgery
Hôpital Sainte Marguerite
Marseille, France

Chong PL
Specialist Registrar in Vascular Surgery
Sheffield Vascular Institute
Northern General Hospital
Sheffield, UK

Cleveland T, FRCS FRCR
Consultant Vascular Radiologist
Sheffield Vascular Institute
Northern General Hospital
Sheffield, UK

Davey P, MRCS
Research Registrar in Vascular Surgery
Freeman Hospital
Newcastle upon Tyne, UK

Davies AH, MA DM FRCS
Reader and Honorary Consultant in Surgery
Charing Cross Hospital
London, UK

Deleo G, MD
Resident in Vascular Surgery
Bassini/San Gerardo Teaching Hospital
Cinisello Balsamo (Milan), Italy

Dias N, MD
Department of Radiology
Malmo University Hospital
Malmo, Sweden

Diethrich EB, MD
Medical Director
Arizona Heart Institute and Arizona Heart Hospital
Phoenix, Arizona, USA

Dix F, BSc MBBS FRCS
Venous Research Fellow
South Manchester University Hospitals NHS Trust
Wythenshawe Hospital
Manchester, UK

Domenig C, MD
Department of Surgery, Division of Vascular Surgery
AKH Vienna,
Vienna
Austria

Douillez V, MD
Foundation Saint-Joseph Hospital
Department of Thoracic & Cardiovascular Surgery
Marseille, France

Duddy M, FRCR Consultant Radiologist
Department of Radiology
University Hospital
Birmingham NHS Trust
Selly Oak Hospital.
Birmingham, UK

Fay D, FRCR
Clinical Fellow in Interventional Radiology
Freeman Hospital
Newcastle upon Tyne, UK

Franklin I
Department of Surgery
Charing Cross Hospital
London, UK

Froio A, MD
Resident in Vascular Surgery
Bassini/San Gerardo Teaching Hospital
Cinisello Balsamo (Milan), Italy

Fourneau I MD PhD
Department of Vascular Surgery
University Hospital Gasthuisberg
Leuven, Belgium

Gaines PA, MRCP FRCR
Sheffield Vascular Institute
Northern General Hospital
Sheffield, UK

Gay J
Foundation Saint-Joseph Hospital
Department of Thoracic & Cardiovascular Surgery
Marseille, France

Georgopoulos D-SG, MD
Visiting Vascular Surgeon
Heinrich-Heine-University
Dusseldorf, Germany

Gibbs R, MD FRCS
Specialist Registrar in Surgery
Charing Cross Hospital
London, UK

Grabitz K, MD
Professor of Vascular Surgery
Heinrich-Heine-University
Dusseldorf, Germany

Halliday AW, MS FRCS
Consultant Vascular Surgeon
St George's Hospital
London, UK

Hamilton G, MBChB FRCS
Consultant Vascular Surgeon
Royal Free University Hospital
London, UK

Harris P, MD FRCS
Director of Vascular Services
Royal Liverpool University Hospital
Liverpool, UK

Henry I
Polyclinique D'Essay
Essay-les-Nancy
Nancy, France

Henry M
Polyclinique D'Essay
Essay-les-Nancy
Nancy, France

Hinchliffe RJ
Department of Vascular and Endovascular Surgery
University Hospital
Nottingham, UK

Hölzenbein T, MD
Department of Surgery, Division of Vascular Surgery
AKH Vienna,
Vienna, Austria

Hopkinson BR, ChM FRCS
Professor, Department of Vascular and Endovascular
   Surgery
Division of Vascular Surgery
Faculty of Medicine & Health Sciences
University of Nottingham
Queen's Medical Centre
Nottingham, UK

Horrocks M, MS FRCS
Professor of Surgery
Royal United Hospital
Bath, UK

Hugel M
Polyclinique D'Essay
Essay-les-Nancy
Nancy, France

Ivancev K, MD PhD
Department of Radiology
Malmo University Hospital
Malmo, Sweden

Katzen BT, MD
Miami Cardiac & Vascular Institute
Miami, Florida, USA

Khanoyan P, MD
Foundation Saint-Joseph Hospital
Department of Thoracic & Cardiovascular Surgery
Marseille, France

Kieffer E, MD
Department of Vascular Surgery
Pitié-Salpêtrière University Hospital
Paris, France

Klonaris C
Polyclinique D'Essay
Essay-les-Nancy
Nancy, France

Kragsterman B, MD
Department of Surgery
University Hospital
Uppsala, Sweden

Kretschmer G, MD
Department of Surgery, Division of Vascular Surgery
AKH Vienna,
Vienna
Austria

Kuiper JW, MD
Department of Interventional Radiology
Erasmus Medical Center
Rotterdam, The Netherlands

Lakshmi G
Polyclinique D'Essay
Essay-les-Nancy
Nancy, France

Lawrence-Brown MMD, MBBS FRACS
Consultant Vascular Surgeon
Mount Medical Centre
Mount Hospital
Perth, Western Australia

Lee JT, MD
Research Fellow
Division of Vascular Surgery
Harbor-UCLA Medical Center
Torrance, California, USA

Lipsitz EC
Assistant Professor of Surgery
Montefiore Medical Center and
   Albert Einstein College of Medicine
New York, NY, USA

Ljungman C, MD PhD
Department of Surgery
University Hospital
Uppsala, Sweden

Mahmood A, MRCS
Vascular Fellow
Departments of Vascular Surgery
University Hospital Birmingham NHS Trust
Selly Oak Hospital.
Birmingham, UK

Malina M, MD, PhD
Department of Radiology
Malmo University Hospital
Malmo, Sweden

Marro J, BSc
Trial Co-ordinator ACST
St George's Hospital
London, UK

McCollum CN, MBChB MD FRCS
Professor of Surgery
Department of Academic Surgery
South Manchester University Hospitals NHS Trust
Wythenshawe Hospital
Manchester, UK

Mingazzini PM, MD
Associate Professor of Vascular Surgery
Bassini/San Gerardo Teaching Hospital
Cinisello Balsamo (Milan), Italy

Moss JG, MB ChB FRCS FRCR
Consultant Interventional Radiologist
North Glasgow Hospital University NHS Trust
Gartnavel General Hospital
Glasgow, UK

Murphy KPM, MBBCh BAO MRCPI FFR(RCSI) FRCR
Vascular Radiologist
Bristol Royal Infirmary
Bristol, UK

Nevelsteen A MD PhD
Head, Department of Vascular Surgery
University Hospital Gasthuisberg
Leuven, Belgium

Nevin C
Radiology Research Nurse
Freeman Hospital
Newcastle upon Tyne, UK

Nicholson T, MSc FRCR
Department of Vascular Radiology
Hull & East Yorkshire Hospitals NHS Trust
Kingston upon Hull, UK

Ohki T MD
Associate Professor of Surgery
Montefiore Medical Center and
    Albert Einstein College of Medicine
New York, NY, USA

Ouriel K, MD FACS FACC
Chairman, Department of Vascular Surgery
The Cleveland Clinic Foundation
Cleveland, USA

Pfeiffer T, MD
Clinical Assistant in Vascular Surgery
Heinrich-Heine-University
Dusseldorf, Germany

Piquet P, MD
Professor of Vascular Surgery
Hôpital Sainte Marguerite
Marseille, France

Powell JT
University Hospitals Coventry & Warwickshire NHS
    Trust
Coventry, UK

Prager M, MD
Department of Surgery, Division of Vascular Surgery
AKH Vienna,
Vienna, Austria

Raithel D, MD PhD
Head, Department of Surgery
Klinikum Nuernberg Sued
Nuremberg, Germany

Rasoul-Rockenschaub S, MD
Department of Surgery, Division of Vascular Surgery
AKH Vienna,
Vienna, Austria

Rath PC
Polyclinique D'Essay
Essay-les-Nancy
Nancy, France

Ray S, MA MS FRCS
Department of Surgery
Imperial College School of Medicine
Charing Cross Hospital
London, UK

Reekers J, MD
Department of Radiology
Academic Medical Centre
Amsterdam, The Netherlands

Rodway A, MRCS
Clinical Research Fellow
Department of Surgery
Charing Cross Hospital
London, UK

Rollet G, MD
Department of Vascular Surgery
Hôpital Sainte Marguerite
Marseille, France

Rose J, FRCR
Consultant Vascular Radiologist
Freeman Hospital
Newcastle upon Tyne, UK

Ruckley CV MBChM FRCSE FRCPE
Formerly Professor of Vascular Surgery
Royal Infirmary of Edinburgh
Edinburgh, UK

Salas C, MD
Clinical Research Fellow
Department of Vascular Surgery
Leicester Royal Infirmary
Leicester, UK

Sandmann W, MD PhD
Professor of Surgery
Chairman and Director of Department of Vascular
  Surgery and Kidney Transplantation
Heinrich-Heine-University
Dusseldorf, Germany

Schol F, MD
Antwerp Blood-Vessel Centre
Antwerp, Belgium

Semmens JB, PhD
Director, Centre for Health Services Research
School of Population Health
University of Western Australia
Crawley, Western Australia

Shearman CP, BSc MS FRCS
Professor of Vascular Surgery
Department of Vascular Surgery
Southampton General Hospital
Southampton, UK

Shiram R
Polyclinique D'Essay
Essay-les-Nancy
Nancy, France

Simms MH, FRCS
Consultant Vascular Surgeon
Department of Vascular Surgery
University Hospital Birmingham NHS Trust
Selly Oak Hospital
Birmingham, UK

Sonesson B, MD PhD
Department of Radiology
Malmo University Hospital
Malmo, Sweden

Taylor PR, MA MChir FRCS
Consultant Vascular Surgeon
Guy's & St Thomas' Hospital
London, UK

Thelin S, MD PhD
Department of Thoracic Surgery
University Hospital
Uppsala, Sweden

Vanhandenhove I, MD
Antwerp Blood-Vessel Centre
Antwerp, Belgium

van Dijk LC, MD
Department of Interventional Radiology
Erasmus Medical Center
Rotterdam, The Netherlands

van Sambeek MRMH, MD
Department of Vascular Surgery
Erasmus Medical Center
Rotterdam, The Netherlands

van Urk H, MD PhD FRCS (Ed)
Department of Vascular Surgery and Interventional
  Radiology
Erasmus Medical Center
Rotterdam, The Netherlands

Veith FJ, MD
Professor of Surgery
Montefiore Medical Center
New York, NY, USA

Vercaeren P, MD
Antwerp Blood-Vessel Centre
Antwerp, Belgium

Verhoeven ELG, MD
Consultant Vascular Surgeon
Freeman Hospital
Newcastle upon Tyne, UK

Vorwerk D, MD
Professor and Chairman
Department of Radiology
Klinikum Ingolstadt
Ingolstadt, Germany

White GH, FRACS
Endovascular Research Unit, Department of Surgery
University of Sydney
New South Wales, Australia

White RA, MD
Chief, Divison of Vascular Surgery
Harbor-UCLA Medical Center
Torrance, California, USA

Wilson L
Vascular Research Nurse
Freeman Hospital
Newcastle upon Tyne, UK

Wyatt MG, MSc MD FRCS
Consultant Vascular Surgeon
Freeman Hospital
Newcastle upon Tyne, UK

Yadav JS, MD FACC FSCAI
Director of Vascular Intervention
Department of Cardiovascular Medicine
The Cleveland Clinic Foundation
Cleveland, Ohio, USA

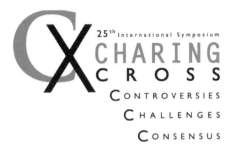

1978-2003

25 YEARS

25th International Symposium
CHARING CROSS
CONTROVERSIES
CHALLENGES
CONSENSUS

Preface

This is our 25th year. We are marking the Silver Jubilee with a Global Endovascular Forum which is concerned with new techniques, new technologies and new horizons. At this forum there will be much use of cine and video and the contents of this forum are best viewed in that medium rather than in book form. The reader will have to attend the event to benefit from that special Jubilee event.

The two days of the traditional Charing Cross meeting are once again convened as a series of debates. The authors have written the chapters long in advance and these have been edited and the book produced so as to be ready for the participants at the time of the meeting. The programme directors have identified key debate topics. These will be performed by the authors on the day and televised.

What is the importance of the book? It is up to date and well referenced and it contains the bullet points made by the speakers in debate form. Each speaker has been asked to review the evidence and put one side of the argument and *not* to give a balanced view. Editorial comments towards consensus follow. It is a feature of the chapters that the authors have not seen the comments of their adversaries and the Editor has read both when he wrote the editorial comments. In 2002, this format was hailed as a new format for top class international meetings and there has been a call for a repeat. In our 25th year we follow the Global Endovascular Forum with two days of controversies and challenges leading to consensus.

R M Greenhalgh

February 2003

Open audit is a waste of time

For the motion
JT Powell

Introduction

Open audit is a waste of time – well almost. What is open audit trying to achieve? (Fig. 1). Audit is a quality improvement and performance management tool, that should seek to improve patient care by systematic audit of consecutive patient cases against predetermined outcome measures. The results of such clinical audit should be discussed in an open forum so that they can spearhead the implementation of change and the improvement of patient care. These improvements should be in turn audited for a process of continuous quality improvement (Fig. 2).

How much does open audit in vascular surgery, alias vascular surgical registries, fulfil this function. It also is important to discuss whether the outcome data from these registries have led to any major scientific or health and social care advance. Perhaps the best known of the vascular registries is Swedvasc. This registry, which is supposed to capture, all vascular surgical procedures in Sweden, has been running since the late 1980s. This important and comprehensive registry, requires the input of considerable manpower to maintain and update. The costs of maintaining the registry have not been documented; these costs are the inputs to the registry. The outputs of the registry include 17 papers published between 1991 and 1999 (Table 1). All have been published in Scandinavian or European surgical journals. What notice have health care workers in Europe or further afield taken of the output of Swedvasc? This is a question that I have tried to address. Swedvasc is a general registry of all surgical procedures. There are also in existence registries of specific surgical or endovascular procedures, particularly relating to endovascular treatment of vascular surgical problems. For example, RETA is a British registry of endovascular repair of abdominal aortic aneurysm.

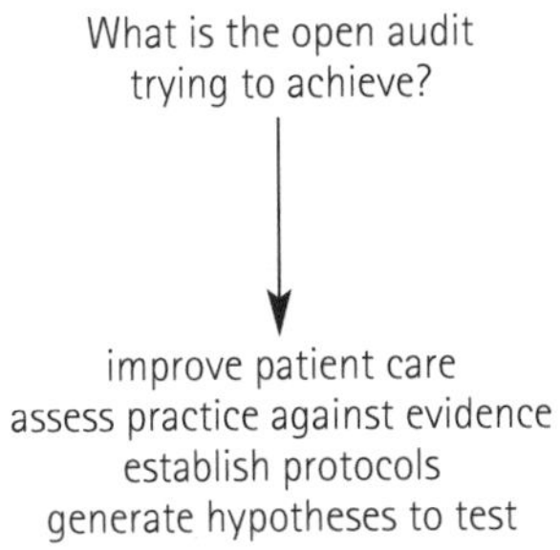

What is the open audit
trying to achieve?

↓

improve patient care
assess practice against evidence
establish protocols
generate hypotheses to test

Figure 1.

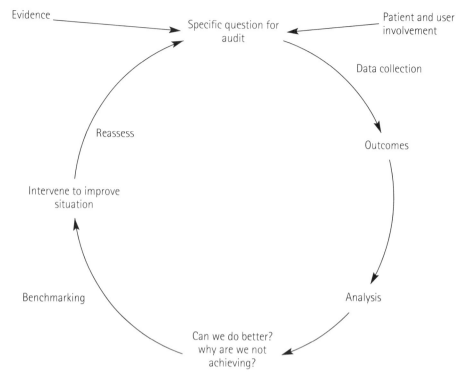

Figure 2.

Methods

I have used two separate mechanisms to assess the impact of the publications from Swedvasc. First, I randomly identified four papers, numbers a, d, g, j from Table 1 above, and then searched for a comparable publication on the same topic in the same year. I then subjected these sets of publications to a citation index scrutiny (Scientific Citation Index on-line). I then identified a further paper from the list in Table 1, paper n, which provides a decision tree approach in the choice of strategy in the treatment of intermittent claudication. Again, I searched for citation index and also searched to identify whether the decision tree approach had been implemented in Sweden or further afield. A similar approach was used to monitor the efficacy of RETA.

Citation indices of Swedvasc papers and comparators

None of the publications from Swedvasc chosen for study (a, d, g, j, Table 1) appear to have been cited in other publications. Two of these papers related to intestinal ischaemia following aortoiliac surgery, the first (paper j) being published in 1996 by Bjorck *et al.*, with a cohort of 2930 patients. The estimated incidence of bowel ischaemia was 2.8%. The conclusions of the paper were that the incidence of bowel ischaemia in this study, was not different from previous reports. In contrast, in the same year, a paper was published by Piotrowski titled 'Colonic ischemia: the Achilles

Table 1. Publications from Swedvasc 1991–2001

	Publication
a	Ahari A, Bergqvist D, Troeng T *et al*. Diabetes mellitus as a risk factor for early outcome after carotid endarterectomy – a population-based study. *Eur J Vasc Endovasc Surg* 1999; **18:** 122–126.
b	Troeng T, Bergqvist D, Norrving B *et al*. Complications after carotid endarterectomy are related to surgical errors than one-fifth of cases. Swedvasc – The Swedish Vascular Registry and The Quality Committee for Carotid Argery Surgery. *Eur J Vasc Endovasc Surg* 1999; **18:** 59–64.
c	[No authors listed] Auditing surgical outcome. 10 years with the Swedish Vascular Registry Swedvasc. *Eur J Surg Suppl* 1998; **581:** 1–48.
d	Bjorck M. Intestinal ischaemia after aortoiliac surgery – a case-control study within Swedvasc Registry. *Eur J Surg Suppl* 1998; **581:** 37–9.
e	Troeng T. Examples of studies performed within Swedvasc. *Eur J Surg Suppl* 1998; **581:** 33–36.
f	Bergqvist D, Troeng T, Elfstrom J *et al*. Auditing surgical outcome: ten years with the Swedish Vascular Registry Swedvasc. The Steering Committee of Swedvasc. *Eur J Surg Suppl* 1998; **581:** 3–8.
g	Zdanowski Z, Troeng T, Norgren L. Outcome and influence of age after infrainguinal revascularisation in critical ischaemia. The Swedish Vascular Registry. *Eur J Vasc Endovasc Surg* 1998; **16:** 137–141.
h	Bergqvist D, Troeng T. Vascular surgery is steadily increasing in Sweden. Lakartidningen 1998; **95:** 2940–2943.
i	[No authors listed] Reoperations, redo surgery and other interventions constitute more than a third of vascular surgery. A study from Swedvasc (the Swedish Vascular Registry). The Swedish Society for Vascular Surgery. *Eur J Vasc Endovasc Surg* 1997; **14:** 244–251.
j	Bjorck M, Bergqvist D, Troeng T. Incidence and clinical presentation of bowel ischaemia after aortoiliac surgery. 2930 operations from a population-based registry in Sweden. *Eur J Vasc Endovasc Surg* 1996; **12:** 129–144.
k	Troeng T, Bergqvist D, Elfstrom J *et al*. Outcome assessment in vascular surgery – the Swedish experience. The Steering Committee of Swedvasc. *J Vasc Surg* 1995; **22:** 810–811.
l	Bergqvist D, Troeng T, Einarsson E *et al*. Vascular surgical audit during a 5-year period. Steering committee of the Swedish Vascular Registry (Swedvasc). *Eur J Vasc Surg* 1994; **8:** 472–477.
m	Troeng T, Bergqvist D, Janson L. Incidence and causes of adverse outcomes of operation for chronic ischaemia of the leg. *Eur J Surg* 1994; **160:** 17–25.
n	Troeng T, Bergqvist D, Janzon L *et al*. The choice of strategy in the treatment of intermittent claudication – a decision tree approach. *Eur J Vasc Surg* 1993; **7:** 438–443.
o	Troeng T, Janzon L, Bergqvist D. Adverse outcome in surgery for chronic leg ischaemia – risk factors and risk prediction when using different statistical methods. *Eur J Vasc Surg* 1992; **6:** 628–635.
p	Troeng T, Bergqvist D, Einarsson E *et al*. Experiences from Swedvasc/VRISS. *Ann Chir Gynaecol* 1992; **8:** 248–252.
q	Troeng T, Bergqvist D, Einarson E *et al*. [A number of problems within vascular surgery should be objects for quality assurance] *Lakartidningen* 1991; **88:** 4436–4438.

heel of ruptured aortic aneurysm repair'.[1] This paper reported the important finding that revascularization of patent inferior mesenteric arteries had little effect on outcome. The incidence of ischaemia did not appear to depend upon the presence of a patent of occluded inferior mesenteric artery. This paper with slightly more meaningful conclusions for clinical practice, has been cited three times.

Table 2 Comparator publications for the RETA registry 1999 results of endovascular abdominal aortic aneurysm repair

	Publication	Citations
a	May J, White GH, Waugh R *et al.* Endovascular treatment of abdominal aortic aneurysms. *Cardiovasc Surg* 1999; **7**: 484–490.	12
b	Ohki T, Veith FJ. Patient selection for endovascular repair of abdominal aortic aneurysms: changing the threshold for intervention. *Semin Vasc Surg* 1999; **12**: 226–234.	6
c	Walker SR, Macierewicz J, MacSweeney *et al.* Mortality rates following endovascular repair of abdominal aortic aneurysm. *J Endovasc Surg* 1999; **6**: 233–238.	4
d	Moore WS, Kashyap VS, Vescera CL *et al.* Abdominal aortic aneurysm: a 6-year comparison of endovascular versus transabdominal repair. *Ann Surg* 1999; **230**: 298–306.	48
e	De Virgilio C, Bui H, Donayre C *et al.* Endovascular vs open abdominal aortic aneurysm repair: a comparison of cardiac morbidity and mortality. *Arch Surg* 1999; **134**: 947–950.	0
	These publications are comparators for ref 5, Thomas *et al. Br J Surg* 1999; **86**: 711.	

The follow-up paper by Bjorck (paper d, Table 1) on intestinal ischaemia published in 1998, was published in a journal supplement and, perhaps for this reason, might not be included on the database that searches for citations, because it is indeed surprising that this later paper did not cite the earlier publication by the same author. This later paper in 1998 on intestinal ischaemia was compared with a paper by El-Sabrout *et al.*[2] The paper by El-Sabrout *et al.* also had no citations. Similarly, the paper by Zdanowski *et al.* on Swedvasc data (paper g, Table 1), like the comparator publication by Jansen *et al.*,[3] had no further citations. In contrast, although the most recent output of Swedvasc concerning diabetes mellitus as a risk factor for outcome after carotid endarterectomy, published in 1999, had no citations, a very similar paper by Ballotta *et al.*[4] already has collected three citations. The conclusions of both these papers, were that carotid endarterectomy can be performed safely with minimal perioperative morbidity and mortality rates in diabetic patients. However, the paper by Ballotta *et al.* was published in a North American journal with a higher impact factor than the European journal chosen for the publication of the data from Swedvasc.

In summary, the publication outputs from Swedvasc appear to have had little impact on the practices, scientific or clinical, of other vascular surgeons as evidenced by citation rate.

Citation index for an endovascular aneurysm repair registry (RETA) and comparative papers

In Britain the registry of endovascular aneurysm repairs has been kept in Sheffield and the results for over 300 endovascular repairs were described in the *British Journal of Surgery* in 1999.[5] Five comparative papers were identified for this paper from the RETA registry, and these are shown in Table 2. Although the paper published from the RETA registry has had no citations, the papers published shown in Table 2 have had 12, 6, 4, 48 and 0 citations respectively. Even when journals of contrasting impact factors, *Cardiovascular Surgery* which has a low impact factor, and *Surgery* which has a high impact factor, are used as the comparators, the citation indices are much higher than the registry paper.

Follow-through towards improving patient care from registry data

A single paper published early on in the history of Swedvasc was selected. This paper concerned the choice of strategy in the treatment of intermittent claudication – a decision tree approach (paper n, Table 1). The authors, Troeng *et al.* 1993, confirm that clinical decision analysis is a method that is used to assist in making risky choices in the clinical arena. The treatment of intermittent claudication continues to be the subject of considerable controversy and clinical trials. Troeng *et al.* also point out that the relevant adverse outcome to avoid is not death or amputation, but rather the lack of improvement after surgery. Therefore, they propose that surgery is the preferred strategy for the management of intermittent claudication when suprainguinal reconstruction is an option. They also point out that clinical data from routine care or the registry can be used for an economic assessment of relevant strategies in the management of intermittent claudication, and point out that these data are awaited. I have seen no evidence that these data have evolved from Swedvasc, although there is abundant evidence in the literature that others have pursued economic assessment and cost-effectiveness in the management of intermittent claudication. Were the Swedish Vascular Registry acting as a formal agent of audit, one might have anticipated that, following the publication by Troeng *et al.* in 1993, an attempt might have been made to implement a protocol where only suprainguinal reconstruction was performed in patients with intermittent claudication. The effectiveness of this protocol should then have been reported. Again, it was not possible to find any evidence that such a protocol had been implemented and evaluated.

The decision analysis and economic assessment data has been advanced most strongly by the Dutch group of Hunink.[6-8] Their analysis showed that for 65-year-old men with either disabling claudication and femoropopliteal stenosis or 65-year-old men with chronic critical limb ischaemic and femoropopliteal stenosis, initial angioplasty increased the quality-adjusted life expectancy by somewhere from between 2 and 13 months, as well as resulting in a decrease in accumulated health costs over their lifetime.[3] Hunink *et al.* also made a comparison of treatment of intermittent claudication by angioplasty and surgery.[3] Results from a sensitivity analysis showed that angioplasty would be the preferred initial treatment, provided the angioplasty 5-year patency rate exceeded 30%. Therefore, in most instances angioplasty would be the preferred initial treatment in patients with disabling claudication. Bypass surgery should be reserved as an initial treatment for those patients with chronic critical limb ischaemia. After 4 years, this paper should be a valuable adjunct to our knowledge base, but nevertheless has only been cited once in the medical literature. The same group have also identified the precise costs associated with revascularization procedures (Hunink *et al.*, 1994[7]; Jansen *et al.*, 1998[3]). They showed that the presence of coronary artery disease, female sex or advanced age increased the cost of the procedure by up to 30%. This group has gone on to investigate the cost-effectiveness of other therapies for intermittent claudication, including exercise therapy.[8] Interestingly, in contradistinction to the British current preference for exercise treatment, this group concluded that, if angioplasty was performed wherever feasible, this would be more effective than exercise alone.

Clearly the investigation of carefully and precisely formulated questions or hypotheses appears to provide more valuable and specific recommendations than the analysis of data from a registry. As such one would have to conclude that open audit from registry data is almost worthless.

From registry data to clinical trial

There is one important use of registry data, though perhaps registries have not been sufficiently used to capitalize on this. The data from open audit or registries can be used to generate hypotheses and provide data for power calculations to enable the design of effective prospective studies. This is an example area of where the RETA registry has been of value. This registry provided ball-park figures for 30-day mortality following endovascular aneurysm repair, for endovascular procedures undertaken during the period of the UK Small Aneurysm Trial.[9] For relatively fit patients, the 30-day operative mortality in RETA improvede from 8.3% in 1996 to 1.1% in 1998, and from the UK Small Aneurysm Trial for elective surgery the 30-day mortality was 5.6%. Therefore, in the design of the endovascular aneurysm repair trials, this allowed power calculations to be performed to evaluate the number of patients that would be needed to randomize to either endovascular or conventional open repair, to determine whether there was a benefit in 30-day operative mortality associated with endovascular repair. This is a valuable use of registry data.

In the next few years we are likely to see increasingly the introduction of new technologies in the management of vascular disease: coated stents, pharmacotherapy, and others. In the United States there is to be a formal re-evaluation of chelation therapy.

Many of these new and advancing technologies are subject to rapid development and change. There are those that argue that such processes should be audited rather than subjected to clinical trials; others would argue that it is never too early to start a clinical trial.[10] However, national registries of those using novel technologies can be valuable in identifying potential participants in formal clinical trials of evaluation, and determining how many procedures might have to be conducted as part of an operator learning curve. These are the data from registries which are invaluable. Otherwise, registries appear to be largely a waste of time.

Registries: where next?

I have put forward a hard, scientific, polarized view. I have omitted to comment on the value of registries in providing governments and national bodies with the total number of vascular surgical procedures performed each year. This benefit has been explored previously.[11] Bergqvist *et al.*[11] also comment on some of the other weaknesses of Swedvasc. These include missed procedures, poor accuracy and reproducibility in completing some data fields and use of 'soft' or imprecise variables.

The patient has rightly become the central point of health-care and patient preference is important. Patient consent is not required for local audit in Britain, since this is expected to improve local patient care (Fig. 2). However, patient consent is now required for research conducted from registries. This is a tight-wire along which future registry managers must tread, if they do not formally seek patient consent for inclusion of patient details in registries.

I have chosen Swedvasc and RETA as examples of registries. There are many others that could have been used as examples. The success of both clinical audit and scientific advance depends on the framing of carefully formulated questions. For example, a local clinical audit might seek to evaluate whether patients with poor cardiac prognosis are prescribed ß-blockers for the period around vascular surgery.[12] A scientific investigation as to whether an occluded inferior mesenteric artery leads to complications of bowel ischaemia after aortoiliac surgery is meritorious, since clinical knowledge will be gained.[1]

The best evidence often comes from prospectively answering important questions in a randomized clinical trial. Two or more trials can be better than one, particularly where the conclusion is the same. A good example is provided by the UK and American small aneurysm trials, both of which tested the hypothesis that early elective surgery for small abdominal aortic aneurysm (4.0–5.5 cm in diameter) would provide a long-term survival benefit. Both trials showed that early surgery did not provide long-term survival benefit.[13,14]

So general vascular surgery registries fail because they do not ask specific questions prospectively and their findings are not implemented into new protocols and evaluated to benefit patient care. Therefore, the use of registries should be confined to the evaluation of new technologies and procedures.

Summary

- Data from vascular surgery registries have had minimal impact in improving patient care.

- The use of vascular surgery registries should be confined to evaluation of new technologies and procedures.

References

1. Piotrowski JJ, Ripepi AJ, Yuhas JP *et al.* Colonic ischemia: the Achilles heel of ruptured aortic aneurysm repair. *Am Surg* 1996; 62: 557–560.
2. El-Sabrout RA, Reul GJ. Suprarenal or supraceliac aortic clamping during repair of infrarenal abdominal aortic aneurysms. *Tex Heart Inst J* 2001; 28: 254–264.
3. Jansen RM, de Vries SO, Cullen KA *et al.* Cost-identification analysis of revascularization procedures on patients with peripheral arterial occlusive disease. *J Vasc Surg* 1998; 28: 617–623.
4. Ballotta E, Da Giau G, Renon L. Is diabetes mellitus a risk factor for carotid endarterectomy prospective study. *Surgery* 2001; 129: 146–152.
5. Thomas SM, Gaines PA, Beard JD. Vascular surgical society of Great Britain and Ireland: RETA registry of endovascular treatment of abdominal aortic aneurysm. *Br J Surg* 1999; 86: 711.
6. Hunink MG, Wong JB, Donaldson MC *et al.* Revascularization for femoropopliteal disease. A decision and cost-effective analysis. *J Am Med Assoc* 1995; 274: 165–171.
7. Hunink MG, Cullen KA, Donaldson MC. Hospital costs of revascularization procedures for femoropopliteal arterial disease. *J Vasc Surg* 1994; 19: 632–641.
8. De Vries SO, Visser K, de Vries JA *et al.* Intermittent claudication: cost-effectiveness of revascularization versus exercise therapy. *Radiology* 2002; 222: 25–36.

9. UK Small Aneurysm Trial Participants. Mortality results for randomised controlled trial of early elective surgery ultrasonographic surveillance for small abdominal aneurysms. *Lancet* 1998; **352**: 1649–1655.

10. Lilford RJ, Braunholtz DA, Greenhalgh R, Edwards SJ. Trials and fast changing technologies: the case for tracker studies. *Br Med J* 2000; **320**: 43–46.

11. Bergqvist D, Einarsson E, Nargren L, Troeng T. A comprehensive regional vascular registry: How is the population served? In: *The Maintenance of Arterial Reconstruction.* Greenhalgh RM, Hollier LH (eds). London: Saunders, 1991: 441–454.

12. Poldermans D, Boersma E, Bax JJ *et al.* The effect of bisoprolol on perioperative mortality and myocardial infarction in high-risk patients undergoing vascular surgery. Dutch Echocardiographic Cardiac Risk Evaluation Applying Stress Echocardiography Study Group. *N Engl J Med* 1999; **341**: 1789–1794.

13. Lederle FA, Wilson SE, Johnson GR *et al.* Immediate repair compared with surveillance of small abdominal aortic aneurysms. *N Engl J Med* 2002; **346**: 1437–1444.

14. UK Small Aneurysm Trial Participants. Long-term outcomes of immediate repair with surveillance of abdominal aortic aneurysms. *N Engl J Med* 2002; **346**: 1445–52.

Open audit is a waste of time

Against the motion
Peter Harris

Introduction

For centuries open audit has been the foundation of quality assurance in professional practice, including that of medicine, and it is a device that has stood the test of time. Allied to thoughtful clinical judgement, based upon learning and experience, and skilful administration of treatment, audit is central to good clinical practice.

Randomized controlled trials (RCT), are a recent invention. Harris *et al.* published one of the first in vascular surgery in 1987.[1] They compared the patency of reversed and *in situ* saphenous vein grafts for femoropopliteal bypass and found no difference. Today, conventional wisdom dictates that no treatment, either medical or surgical, can be considered to have merit unless and until it has been subjected to an RCT. This has become a modern obsession of doctors and therefore of peer-reviewed journals. The Cochrane Review, which collects and analyses data from RCTs while rejecting all other sources of evidence, is symptomatic of this obsession.

Moreover, sponsors of health care, whether insurance companies or government agencies, have also started to show a keen interest in RCTs. In the UK the National Institute for Clinical Excellence (NICE) formulates treatment protocols based mainly upon the results of RCTs, and the recommendations of NICE are 'backed up' by a regulatory body for Clinical Governance with statutory powers – the Council for Health Care Improvement (CHI). No doubt these government agencies have been created with the interests of patients in mind but, there may be some misguided individuals who are tempted to conclude that if treatments can be decided by RCTs and implemented through easy-to-follow protocols, it follows that expensive clinical judgement, i.e. doctors, can be largely dispensed with. This Orwellian concept, if acted upon, would have disastrous consequences for patients.

In opposing the proposition, this chapter aims to demonstrate that, far from being a waste of time, open audit continues to have immense value in everyday vascular surgical practice. It does not claim that RCTs are all bad – they do have a place, alongside open audit, in informing clinical judgement and surgical decision-making.

Levels of scientific evidence

Table 1 is a scale showing different levels of scientific evidence.

The point to be made here is that the highest levels of evidence are required to establish only the most obscure facts. The blindingly obvious, for example the fact that insulin injections lower blood sugar levels in diabetic patients, does not require

Table 1. Levels of scientific evidence

1a	Meta-analysis of randomized controlled trials
1b	At least one randomized controlled trial (phase 2 – efficiency studies)
2a	Controlled study without randomization
2b	Quasi-experimental study (phase 1 – feasibility studies, open registries, performance studies)
3	Descriptive study (comparative case reports etc.)
4	Expert committee reports, opinions, clinical experience, anecdotes

a meta-analysis of aggregated RCTs involving tens of thousands of patients to be accepted by most rational clinicians. A very simple open, observational study is sufficient. Higher, more sophisticated – and expensive – levels of evidence do not make the obvious any more obvious. Indeed it is wasteful extravagance to undertake RCTs when simple, open observational or audit studies will suffice.

When is it appropriate to undertake an RCT? When two or more treatment alternatives exist, of broadly similar efficacy, in order to determine whether, on a balance of scientific probabilities, the efficacy of one is superior to the others. The efficacy of the treatment options under consideration should be sufficiently close that the responsible physician is himself genuinely unsure which is superior. If he/she believes one treatment to be better he/she cannot ethically deny it to some of his/her patients by subjecting them to an RCT. Thus, it follows that an RCT is necessary to establish the presence or absence of marginal differences in treatment outcomes only. It can also be argued, quite reasonably, that marginal differences matter considerably less than wider ones. If the annual rupture rate of an 8cm abdominal aortic aneurysm is 20% and carries a mortality risk of 90%, while surgical repair carries a once only mortality risk of 5%, it does not take an RCT to determine that surgery will, on a balance of probabilities, prolong the patient's life. However, if open and endovascular alternatives for surgical repair of the aneurysm carry similar mortality risks, an RCT is required to determine, on a balance of probabilities, whether the chances of survival are better with one than with the other.

It follows that a pre-requisite for an RCT is that closeness of the efficacy of the treatment options under consideration should have been established already. This demands that open audit studies must be carried out first. Even those with an obsession for RCTs must acknowledge, for this reason alone, that open audit is not a waste of time.

When is it not appropriate to undertake an RCT?

1. When lower levels of evidence are adequate to establish proof of efficacy.
2. In order to convince others, i.e. those with financial responsibility for the health service, of something of which you are already convinced. This is a spurious justification for an RCT, which amounts to an abuse of money and patients.

A valuable characteristic of open audit is that the information yielded is dynamic in that it demonstrates changes over time. In contrast an RCT provides only a 'snapshot' of information at one time point. It is of dubious validity to extrapolate the results of a RCT to other times and circumstances.

Evidence

Examples of open audit studies that are not a waste of time

Personal or unit audit

Good professional practice demands that clinicians should maintain records in order to monitor the results of the treatment they administer to their patients. Sadly, in the UK and elsewhere this has now become a statutory requirement rather than a professional obligation and it is overseen by chief executives of hospital Trusts rather than by representative bodies of the profession such as the Surgical Royal Colleges.

At a personal or unit level comparison of treatment outcomes from different time periods or with an aggregated national 'norm' followed by 'closure of the audit loop' in response to any anomalies identified is an essential aid for improving the standard of care provided. Government-inspired publication of league tables relating to hospitals or individual clinicians is as yet of undetermined effect, but it has potential to be detrimental and beneficial in equal measure.

National audit

Examples of well established national vascular surgical audit projects are to be found particularly in Scandinavia with the Swedevasc and Finvasc registries.

In the UK and Ireland plans are at an advanced stage for the establishment of a National Vascular Database organized by the Vascular Surgical Society (VSS).[2] The main objective of the Scandinavian and British and Irish National Registries is to determine a 'norm' or acceptable range of outcomes for standard vascular surgical procedures against which individuals can compare their own performance. In its pilot studies the VSS has evaluated POSSUM[3] and Bayesian analyses to permit comparison of results from different centres with different populations and case-mix. Sadly, one of the prime incentives for national audit projects of this type is defensive: to provide a 'Shield For Our Profession'[2] in an increasingly litigious society. However, large-scale open audit also provides reliable data to inform clinical decision-making and patient management in everyday vascular surgical practice and, in contrast to RCTs, it demonstrates the impact of changing clinical practice over time.

New treatments and technologies: endovascular aortic aneurysm repair

It is agreed universally that the introduction of any new treatment must be controlled, carefully, in the interests of all stakeholders. In the case of endovascular aneurysm repair the principal stakeholders are the patients, the clinicians, health care administrators and the commercial companies responsible for the manufacture and marketing of the devices. The process of defining the role of this new technology in standard vascular surgical practice involves three basic steps. The first, and most important, step is to establish safety, the second to evaluate its clinical efficacy and the third to compare its performance against that of the established standard treatment – assuming that step two shows its performance to be similar to that of open repair. In the UK a National Registry of Endovascular Treatment of Aortic Aneurysms

(RETA) was established in 1996 – in the same year the European EUROSTAR Registry was established. These two open audit projects have provided a wealth of data, both good and bad, about the safety and efficacy of endovascular aneurysm repair (see below). In addition data from the RETA Registry has been used for power calculations for the UK EVAR trials that are now in progress to compare the efficacy of the endovascular and open operations.

Originally established under the auspices of the Vascular Surgical Society and the British Society for Interventional Radiology (BSIR) the RETA project has now been extended with the involvement of British Cardiologists to collect and analyse data on endovascular techniques for repair of thoracic aortic aneurysms and dissections. NICE has indicated that it will support this initiative subject to data collection being comprehensive i.e. registration of all patients treated by this method in the UK. Thus it can be appreciated that the UK Registry Project – an open audit – is a source of valuable data with major impact upon clinical vascular surgical practice (see below).

EUROSTAR

In Europe there are two large international open audit studies relating to vascular surgery – EUROSTAR, (European Collaborators on Stent-graft Techniques for Aortic Aneurysm Repair), and EUROCAST, (European registry of Carotid Artery Stenting Techniques). Of these EUROSTAR is the largest and best established. With over 4500 patients registered and the involvement of vascular surgeons and radiologists throughout all the countries of Europe, it represents an outstanding example of open audit.

Key achievements of EUROSTAR include:

1. It has established that the early results of endovascular aneurysm repair are characterized by a high initial success rate (97%) and low 30-day mortality rate (2.5%).
2. It has demonstrated that late results associated with first- and second-generation endovascular devices are marred by a high rate of secondary intervention (approx 10% per year) including conversion to open repair (Fig. 1) (cumulative rate rising to 25% at 6 years) and an increasing rate of rupture (cumulative rate rising to 12.7% at 6 years) (Fig. 2).
3. Following from these findings, it has illustrated the need for long-term post-operative surveillance after endovascular aneurysm repair – and indicated the optimum schedules and procedures for follow-up.
4. It has made possible the identification of risk factors for (causes of) late failure of endovascular aneurysm repair (Table 2). These data have informed the processes of a) further technological evolution of endovascular devices and b) clinical application of the new technologies, especially patient selection.
5. It has confirmed that steps to close the audit loop, in this way, have been accompanied by significantly improved clinical results with the newer generations of endovascular devices i.e. it has shown evidence of beneficial change in clinical outcomes over time (Figs 3,4).

Data from EUROSTAR cannot tell us whether endovascular repair is, on a balance of probabilities, a better option that open repair for patients with abdominal aortic aneurysms, but it does tell us that a randomized trial is justified to answer this question, and like RETA it provides valuable information needed to construct the RCT to provide a reliable answer.

Table 2. Independent risk factors for abdominal aortic aneurysm rupture after EVAR (multivariate analysis)

	Risk ratio	p
Last diameter of abdominal aortic aneurysm	1.057	0.0028
Stent migration	5.335	0.0156
Type 3 endoleak (structural failure of endograft)	7.474	0.0024

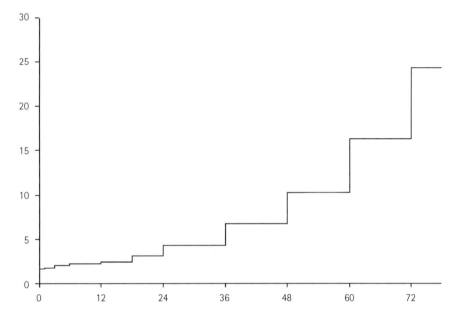

Figure 1. EUROSTAR data. Life table analysis: cumulative rate of late conversion (% x axis) plotted against time after EVAR (months).

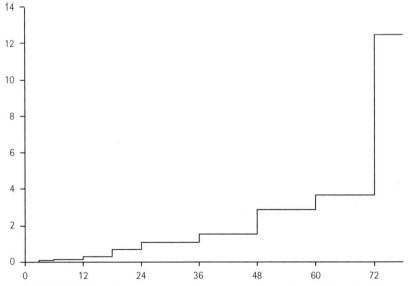

Figure 2. EUROSTAR. Life table analysis: cumulative rate of rupture (% x axis) plotted against time after EVAR (months).

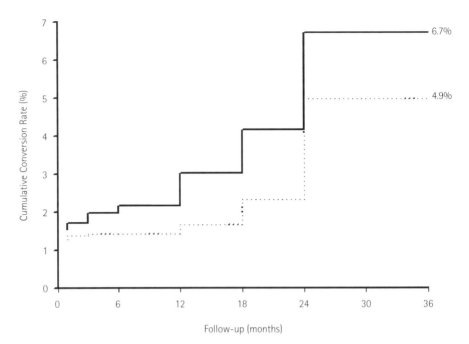

Figure 3. EUROSTAR data. Life table analysis of cumulative rate of conversion after EVAR: comparison of first-generation (solid line) and second-generation (dotted line) endografts (p=0.03, log rank test).

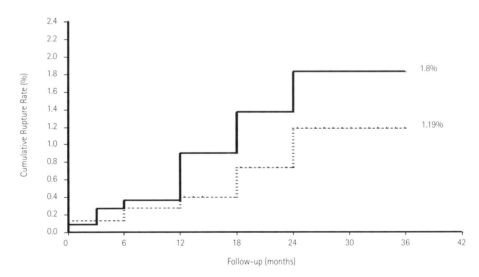

Figure 4. EUROSTAR data. Life table analysis of cumulative rate of rupture after EVAR: comparison of first-generation (solid line) and second generation (dotted line) endografts (p=0.14, log rank test).

Summary

- The function of RCTs is to determine whether, on a balance of scientific probability, there is a difference in outcome of treatments with broadly similar outcomes, i.e. to identify marginal differences in outcomes.

- Marginal differences in outcome matter less than wider differences that can be determined by open audit.

- Open audit is an essential pre-requisite to RCTs in order to establish that the treatments under study do have similar outcomes.

- RCTs provide a 'snap-shot' comparison of treatments at one time point only. Extrapolation to other circumstances and times may not be valid.

- Open audit is 'dynamic' i.e. it can track changes in the outcome of a treatment over time.

- Personal audit is an essential component of 'good practice' in medicine and surgery.

- National outcomes audit is an essential 'shield for our profession' in an increasingly litigious society.

- EUROSTAR is an example of open audit with major influence upon the evolution of a new therapeutic technology and its clinical application.

- Open audit is NOT a waste of time.

References

1. Harris PL, Jones DR, How TV. A prospectively randomised clinical trial to compare reversed and *in situ* vein grafts for femoro-popliteal bypass. *Br J Surg* 1987; **74**: 252–255.
2. Earnshaw JJ. Clinical outcomes audit in vascular surgery: a shield for our profession. *Ann Roy Coll Surg Eng* (in press).
3. Whitely MS, Prytherch DR, Higgins B *et al.* A P-POSSUM type risk model that includes non-operative patients. *Br J Surg* 2001; **88**: A752.

Open audit is a waste of time

Charing Cross Editorial Comments towards Consensus

Professor Janet Powell commences in typical robust style. 'Open audit is a waste of time – well almost'. She asks the question 'what is open audit trying to achieve?'. You would hope that it would improve patient care, assess practice against evidence, establish protocols and generate hypotheses to test. Janet has moved from the leadership of a prolific vascular biology group to be a medical director. She is now in a world where audit is demanded as the 'order of the day'.

Peter Harris, opposing the motion, has no such constraints in the position he holds but finds audit helpful. He writes 'for centuries open audit has been the foundation of quality assurance in professional practice....' '....it is a device that has stood the test of time'. The essence of the opposition argument is that open audit is of immense value and in no sense do they need to show that random controlled trials are all bad. The opposition will not pose the question 'audit or random controlled trial?', but will say that audit, when performed, is useful. We are in for a lively debate.

Roger M Greenhalgh
Editor

Heterografts and homografts have their place

For the motion

Thomas Hölzenbein, Manfred Prager, Christoph Domenig, Susanne Rasoul-Rockenschaub, Georg Kretschmer

Introduction

Autologous saphenous vein is regarded as the graft of choice for limb-threatening ischaemia. It has been proven to be effective for proximal bypass procedures to the above- and below-knee popliteal artery as well as for distal reconstructions to tibial arteries[1] and the arteries of the foot.[2] Although there are reports advocating prosthetic graft material as first choice for above-knee femorodistal bypass reconstructions, saphenous vein is unrivaled with regard to versatility, infection resistance and long-term performance.

There are circumstances, when no saphenous vein is available, either because of inferior quality of the vein or previous removal for varicose vein disease or vein harvest for a bypass procedure at the legs or for coronary artery bypass. Alternate sources of vein will provide reasonable results for femorodistal bypass surgery. This has been proven for lesser saphenous vein,[3] as well as arm veins[4,5] or even the deep femoral vein.[6] There are opposing opinions regarding in which sequence these alternate veins should be harvested for a distal bypass procedure.[1,4] This issue is mostly influenced by local policies for revascularization.[4] Thus currently there are no prospective comparisons available. Although technically feasible, the results of bypass procedures with alternate vein sources do not match results obtained with ipsilateral greater saphenous vein.[7] The reason for this may be the fact that most of these bypass procedures are performed as secondary or tertiary procedures, for failed or failing previous graft.[4] Distal target arteries are located at more distal sites, usually at the tibial level, and the graft material is often barely sufficient to reach the distal anastomosis, even with distal origin bypass grafts.[1]

When no autologous vein is available, only a few options are possible. The surgeon may choose a prosthetic graft material, such as Dacron or expanded polytetrafluoroethylene (ePTFE) for bypass construction. Yet the long-term results of prosthetic bypass to tibial or pedal arteries are not promising.[8] This has led to the development of adjunctive procedures, with the goal of improving the compliance mismatch at the anastomotic site. There have been reports on distal patches, such as the Linton or Taylor patch, both presenting improved patency rates.[9,10] Another solution was the addition of vein cuffs at the anastomotic sites such as the Miller cuff[11] or the St Mary's boot,[12] or complex distal anastomoses with the construction of a distal arteriovenous (AV)-fistula.[13] Although these adjuncts may improve the primary patency of artificial grafts in experienced hands, overall results remain disappointing. Therefore a durable, but easy to use alternative is needed for vascular surgery in patients, who require distal bypass in the absence of suitable autologous graft material. Therefore, heterografts and homografts may be a helpful adjunct in the armamentarium of the vascular surgeon .

Table 1. Vascular grafts currently in clinical use for femorodistal bypass surgery

Autologous vein	Homografts	Heterografts	Prosthetic graft	Tissue engineered graft
Greater saphenous vein	Cryopreserved saphenous vein	Sheep collagen graft	ePTFE	seeded ePTFE
Lesser saphenous vein	Cryopreserved femoral artery	Bovine internal mammary artery	Dacron	
Cephalic vein	Lyophilized saphenous vein	Bovine ureter		
Basilic vein	Non-preserved saphenous vein			
Deep femoral vein	Human umbilical vein			

Human umbilical vein

The glutaraldehyde tanned human umbilical vein graft (HUV) was introduced by Herbert Dardik in 1976.[14] The graft is prepared from segments of human umbilical cords. The umbilical arteries are separated and the remainder of the cord with the vein in the centre is surrounded by a Dacron mesh. The graft is stored in the tanning solution containing glutaraldehyde for preservation. The graft is mounted on a rod, ready for use. Before implantation the graft needs to be rinsed several times with heparinized saline solution to remove excess preservation fluid. Routine vascular surgery techniques are applied during implantation. Yet, great care must be employed when performing the anastomoses, to include the mesh into the suture line thereby preventing anastomotic suture line aneurysms.

Since its introduction, HUV has become one of the most popular biological graft materials available, and has been used widely as an arterial substitute when no saphenous vein is available. There are three studies available comparing ePTFE and HUV in the femoropopliteal segment. All trials presented randomized multicentre evidence that HUV bypass grafts perform better than ePTFE grafts.[15-17]

For above-knee bypass 1-year patencies of 53% at 5 years can be expected. For tibial bypass 6-year patencies of 26% without adjuncts and 47% with distal AV-fistula have been achieved.[18] A 28-year experience summarizing the experience in 1275 patients has been published recently by Dardik,[18] demonstrating a considerable improvement in the preparation of the graft over time, leading to a significant reduction in biodegradation, such as aneurysm formation and dissection.

Heterografts

There are several heterografts under evaluation for peripheral vascular reconstruction. Yet, most reports are short and long-term follow-up is incomplete. The only extensive experience has been reported for the use of sheep collagen grafts. The graft was introduced in the late 1980s[19] and is produced by implantation of a mandrel into the subcutaneous tissue of sheep. The mandrel is then explanted with the surrounding tissue and a graft is formed. The resulting collagen tube is afterwards tanned with glutaraldehyde and reinforced with a polymer mesh.

The graft has been used in the absence of suitable vein for femorodistal bypass surgery. Mid-term results have been promising with up to 62% primary patency for above-knee revascularization at 3 years.[20] For below-knee revascularization primary patency has been reported between 35% and 55%, and for tibial bypass 28% at 2 years.

Another heterograft under evaluation is made from bovine internal mammary artery. The artery is harvested in a typical manner and stabilized with dialdehyde. The resulting graft is about 35 cm in length. Experimental data show that the graft behaves well with regard to wall stability and compliance within the arterial circulation in a canine model.[21] Until now there is only one report of human use available: a small-scale report using the graft for coronary revascularization, but mid-term results have been discouraging.[22]

Another vascular graft is made from glutaraldehyde stabilized ureter, both of human and bovine origin. The bovine graft was introduced in 1989,[23] and has been tested in a canine model. Although the authors conclude that the graft might have an excellent potential no published data are available so far for human use. The human ureteral graft has been evaluated in a rabbit model only so far.[24]

Early days of homograft

Homografts were the first grafts to be used in vascular surgery. Their use dates back to Alexis Carrell, who used homografts to show the feasibility of vascular grafting in the canine and feline circulation.[25] Carrell used fresh homografts stored in a cold saline solution without any pre-treatment up to 4 weeks. The grafts were used as homografts within the same animal species and as xenografts. The problem of an immune response of the recipient was then of minor importance compared with the technical challenge of performing two anastomoses without vascular clamps and suitable suture material. Nevertheless Carrell recognized the importance of late graft failure due to degradation.[26]

Later, in the 1950s, homografts became popular for repair of aneurismal and obliterative aortic lesions. Dubost performed his first abdominal aortic aneurysm repair with a fresh homograft prepared the night before implantation.[27] It soon became evident, that a large number of grafts would be necessary, and storage modalities of human aortic tissue became essential. Grafts were lyophilized or frozen, to make them readily available and independent from sudden donor shortages. Despite improvement in graft procurement and preparation techniques since Carell's time, biodegredation of the grafts was a significant problem.[28] Interest in homografts faded, when synthetic graft material became available, which proved to be easy to handle and more durable.

New era of homografts

New interest in homograft use started in the late 1980s, when technical advances in vascular surgery allowed routine use of alternative vein grafts for femorodistal bypass procedures. Aggressive revascularization policies necessitated use of alternative vein grafts even for primary procedures.[1,4] Depletion of venous resources will occur in multimorbid patients requiring bypass surgeries in the leg and heart. Consequently there is a need for bypass grafts in adverse situations, usually for limb salvage. The prerequisites for such a graft are: sufficient length, infection resistance, and toleration of low graft flow velocities without thrombosis. Artificial grafts are deemed unsuitable in this setting. This has renewed the interest for homografts for distal bypass surgery.[29,30]

Cryopreserved venous homografts

Cryopreserved human saphenous vein grafts are either prepared during multi-organ harvest from brain-dead organ donors[31] or from deceased patients donating human tissue for further use.[32] In any case the veins are carefully removed, and prepared as for femorodistal bypass surgery. The prepared grafts are then rinsed several times with antibiotic solutions and then immersed in a bactericide and fungicide medium containing dimethylsulphoxide (DMSO) and serum before freezing. The freezing process is performed stepwise and under controlled conditions to –80° Celsius. The grafts are then stored at this temperature until use. The grafts are either stored locally or shipped in special containers in liquid nitrogen. At surgery the grafts are rapidly thawed in a water bath and rinsed several times in heparinized saline. The implantation of such grafts is performed with standard vascular surgery techniques.

There are only a few series with cryopreserved homografts where results are published in recent literature. All of them conclude that handling and implantation of a venous homograft is comparable with a distal bypass procedure with autologous saphenous vein. As expected, long-term results are not as good as with autologous vein. The mid-term patency rates are reasonable with reports between 23% and 87% at 1 year and 23.6% after 3 years. Limb salvage could be achieved in 78–88% after 2 years[31,33] and 62% after 3 years.[32] Aneurysm formation and biodegradation is within tolerable limits. Cryopreserved vein is the only homograft currently commercially available.

Cryopreserved arterial homografts

Cryopreserved arterial homografts are harvested similar to venous homografts from brain-dead organ donors.[34–36] There are no reports on arterial homograft harvest in deceased donors. The preservation process is similar to that of cryopreserved vein. The artery is rinsed with heparinized solution and stored in a bactericide and fungicide solution for 48 hours to reduce antigenicity. Then, the preservation medium is changed to a medium containing DMSO and serum. The freezing is performed stepwise until the graft can be stored in liquid nitrogen. After shipping the graft in special containers it is rapidly thawed in a water bath. The graft is rinsed several times before implantation to remove remnants of the storage solution. Implantation is performed using standard vascular principles.

Results of femorodistal bypass procedures with arterial homografts seem to be similar to those achieved with cryopreserved vein: 1-year patency rates can be achieved between 49% and 68%.[34, 36, 37] A long-term observation up to 3 years is available from Albertini, reporting 35% primary patency. Limb salvage at 1 year is reported between 80% and 93%.[34, 36, 37] Cryopreserved arterial homografts are currently used in controlled studies and within study groups and are not commercially available.

The need for immunosuppression in cryopreserved grafts

Although it is generally believed that cryopreserved homografts lose their immunogenicity during the preparation process, there are still signs of cellular rejection or rejection-like mechanisms in mid-term explants.[38] The endothelial lining can be lost in arterial grafts.[36] There seems to be an immune response to the matrix layers of these grafts as well, despite the general belief that cryopreservation may eliminate this problem.[39] Therefore some centres have adopted the concept to subject homograft recipients to a mild immunosuppressive regimen. This has been reported for homologous vein grafts only.[40]

Own experience – arterial transplantation

Our own longstanding experience with kidney and liver transplantation showed that arteries supplying the transplant rarely become aneurysmatic or thrombosed, even during follow-up periods of 20 years or longer. An intact endothelium in a vital matrix seems therefore the prerequisite for long-term patency of homologous arterial grafts. Based on this hypothesis we obtained approval from the local ethics committee (study permit: EK 456/1999) for a clinical observational trial.[41] All patients gave informed consent to the experimental design of the protocol. All data are collected prospectively.

Patients were operated on from May 1999 until August 2002. They underwent at least one revascularization procedure at the diseased extremity. In none of them was sufficient autologous material (contralateral saphenous vein, arm vein, lesser saphenous vein, deep femoral vein) available to construct the needed femorodistal bypass. All the patients were operated on for limb salvage.

The arterial homografts were harvested from brain-dead organ donors, together with multiple organ harvest. All donors were screened for human immunodeficiency virus (HIV), hepatitis B and C, cytomegalovirus (CMV) infection. The graft was harvested by a separate vascular surgical team. The arteries of the left leg were harvested from the aortic bifurcation to the tibioperoneal trunc. The hypogastric artery, the profunda femoris artery and the anterior tibial artery were left long to serve as patch plasty, angiography access or biopsy site. All side branches were tied at a distance of 2–3 mm to the main graft in order to preserve the vasa vasorum.[42] The graft was perfused and stored with a preserving agent (HTK-Solution or UW-Solution). Before use all grafts were subjected to angioscopy to detect segments unsuitable for implantation. Grafts were harvested especially for each patient according to a 'waiting list'. The Department runs a busy transplantation programme finding about 70 organ donors a year. The average waiting time for a suitable graft was 4 weeks.

Implantation of the graft was performed as soon as possible after harvest, thereby minimizing cold ischaemia. The mean cold ischaemia time was 9 hours (3–15 hours). Grafts were implanted with standard vascular surgery techniques, performing the proximal anastomosis first. After reperfusion of the graft the artery was gently stretched before tailoring of the graft and suturing the distal anastomosis. All grafts were placed subcutaneously to facilitate follow-up by clinical means and duplex ultrasound surveillance.

Patients received a mild immunosupressive regimen with prednisolone, cyclososporin A and mofetil mycophenolate. Immunosuppression was discontinued after permanent graft loss.

To date, 14 patients have received 15 grafts. Indication was limb salvage in all patients. There were two grafts to the popliteal artery; all other grafts were to distal tibial or pedal outflow arteries. The mean number of previously failed ipsilateral leg

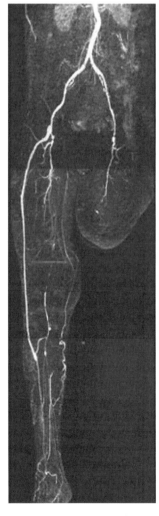

Figure 1. Postoperative magnetic resonance angiogram of Patient 6 after receiving a fresh arterial homograft (common femoral artery to anterior tibial artery). The anastomotic sites of the previous bypass grafts can be clearly appreciated (popliteal artery above- and below-knee). The patient underwent contralateral above-knee amputation 4 years ago.

revascularizations was two[1-6] There was one early graft failure due to anastomotic disruption (30-day patency: 93.3%). Primary 1-year patency was 53.3%; secondary 1-year patency was 66.6%. Two small aneurysms had to be repaired at the site of the common femoral artery of the donor artery. Both were successfully repaired with short lesser saphenous vein interposition grafts. Limb salvage observed at 1 year was 80%.

No patient experienced serious adverse effects from the additional immunosuppressive therapy. Wound healing was similar to that in patients receiving an autologous vein bypass. Results may be not as good as for cryopreserved grafts, but all of these patients presented with end-stage arterial disease and a longstanding vascular history. In all, 50% of the patients had more than three vascular surgeries on the ipsilateral leg before receiving the arterial graft. There are no reports available of patient series with a comparable long-term vascular history.

Future aspects

There are reports on the construction of biocompound grafts with the scaffold made from standard ePTFE seeded with endothelial cells harvested either from autologous veins, usually arm veins. Mid-term studies are available demonstrating primary patency of 70% for infrageniculate grafts.[43] Tissue engineering of vascular grafts using a biodegradable polymer has been undertaken. The scaffold of the grafts is made from polyglycolic acid and polyglactin co-polymers. The inner surface of the graft is then coated with autologous endothelial cells. Although microscopic studies and biomechanical testing demonstrate that these grafts closely resemble native arterial tissue, mid-term patency is usually not achieved.[44,45]

Discussion

With increasing aggressive revascularization policies, depletion of autologous vein sources will occur more frequently. Despite difficult circumstances extension of limb salvage in these patients is possible by the use of heterografts and homografts. HUV has been used with good success and early problems of graft preparation seem to be solved. Published data support the currently renewed interest in bypass procedures with the HUV graft.[18]

Xenografts from different animal sources are tanned with glutaraldehyde, and do not require immunosuppressive therapy. Yet there is only one large series published with most of the procedures being performed to the above-knee popliteal artery.[20] Long grafts to tibial arteries have been performed, but results seem to be disappointing.

Cryopreserved homografts have a long tradition in vascular surgery since its very beginnings. Homografts have been used as a vascular substitute at times when no artificial grafts were available.[27,28] The renewed interest for homografts has been triggered by the need for replacement of infected vascular grafts[35] and the lack of autologous grafts in distal revascularization.[31-41]

Homografts are relatively easy to handle and versatile in their use. They can be implanted in virtually any place in the human circulation accessible to vascular surgery. The decision whether to use self-prepared cryopreserved vein grafts,[31] commercially available cryopreserved vein grafts[32,33] or non-cryopreserved vein grafts grafts[46] or cyropreserved arteries[36,37] largely depends upon the surgeons' preference and local resources. Commercially available grafts tend to be rather expensive, making their widespread use unattractive. The concept of arterial transplantation, using fresh allografts and immunosuppression necessitates close collaboration with an organ transplantation unit, and may not be available in every instance.

Future research is directed towards tissue engineering using either non-biodegradable or biodegradable scaffolds seeded with autologous cells. Although small-scale single-centre studies are available, the general use of such grafts is limited by the availability of a tissue laboratory technically capable of cell seeding.

Summary

- Modern cardiovascular surgery depletes autologous vein sources.

- There is increasing need for biological graft material.

- Human umbilical vein is a good alternative in experienced hands.

- Homograft veins and arteries are easy to handle and provide reasonable graft patency and limb salvage.

- Immunosupression is probably necessary for all homograft procedures.

- Heterografts still play an insignificant role in clinical practice.

References

1. Taylor LM Jr, Edwards JM, Porter JM. Present status of reversed vein bypass grafting: five-year results of a modern series. *J Vasc Surg* 1990; **11**: 193–205.
2. Pomposelli FB Jr, Marcaccio EJ, Gibbons GW *et al.* Dorsalis pedis arterial bypass: durable limb salvage for foot ischemia in patients with diabetes mellitus. *J Vasc Surg* 1995; **21**: 375–384.
3. Chang BB, Paty PS, Shah DM, Leather RP. The lesser saphenous vein: an underappreciated source of autogenous vein. *J Vasc Surg* 1992; **15**: 152–156.
4. Hölzenbein TJ, Pomposelli FB Jr, Miller A *et al.* Results of a policy with arm veins used as the first alternative to an unavailable ipsilateral greater saphenous vein for infrainguinal bypass. *J Vasc Surg* 1996; **23**: 130–140.
5. Hölzenbein TJ, Pomposelli FB Jr, Miller A *et al.* The upper arm basilic-cephalic loop for distal bypass grafting: technical considerations and follow-up. *J Vasc Surg* 1995; **21**: 586–592.
6. Sladen JG, Reid JD, Maxwell TM, Downs, AR. Superficial femoral vein: a useful autogenous harvest site. *J Vasc Surg* 1994; **20**: 947–952.
7. Brochado-Neto FC, Albers M, Pereira CA *et al.* Prospective comparison of arm veins and greater saphenous veins as infrageniculate bypass grafts. *Eur J Vasc Endovasc Surg* 2001; **2**: 146–151.
8. Parsons RE, Suggs WD, Veith FJ *et al.* Polytetrafluoroethylene bypasses to infrapopliteal arteries without cuffs or patches: a better option than amputation in patients without autologous vein. *J Vasc Surg* 1996; **23**: 347–354.
9. Batson RC, Sottiurai VS, Craighead CC. Lintonpatch angioplasty. An adjunct to distal bypass with polytetrafluoroethylene grafts. *Ann Surg* 1984; **199**: 684–693.
10. Taylor RS, Loh A, McFarland RJ *et al.* Improved technique for polytetrafluoroethylene bypass grafting: long-term results using anastomotic patches. *Br J Surg* 1992; **79**: 348–354.
11. Miller J, Foreman R, Ferguson L, Faris I. Interposition vein cuff for anastomosis of prosthesis to small artery. *Aust NZ J Surg* 1984; **54**: 283–285.
12. Tyrell MR, Wolfe JH. New prosthetic venous collar anastomotic technique: combining the best of other procedures. 1991; *Br J Surg* **78**: 1016–1017.
13. Ascer E, Gennaro M, Pollina RM, *et al.* Complementary distal arteriovenous fistula and deep vein interposition: a five-year experience with a new technique to improve infrapopliteal prosthetic bypass patency. *J Vasc Surg* 1996; **24**: 134–143.

14. Dardik HD, Ibrahim IM, Spryregen S, Dardik II. Clinical experience with modified human umbilical cord vein for arterial bypass. *Surgery* 1976; **79**: 618–624.

15. Eickhoff JH, Buchart Hansen HJ, Bromme A *et al.* A randomized clinical trial of PTFE versus human umbilical vein for femoropopliteal bypass surgery. Preliminary results. *Br J Surg* 1983; **70**: 85–88.

16. McCollum C, Kenchington G, Alexander C *et al.* PTFE or HUV for femoropopliteal bypass: a multi-centre trial. *Eur J Vasc Surg* 1991; **5**: 435–443.

17. Johnston WC, Lee KK. A comparative evaluation of polytetrafluoroethylene, umbilical vein, and saphenous vein bypass grafts for femoro-popliteal above-knee revascularization: a prospective randomized Department of Veterans Affairs cooperative study. *J Vasc Surg* 2000; **32**: 268–277.

18. Dardik, H, Wengerter K, Qin F *et al.* Comparative decades of experience with glutaraldehyde-tanned human umbilical cord vein graft for lower limb revascularization: an anlysis of 1275 cases. *J Vasc Surg* 2002; **35**: 64–71.

19. Ramshaw JA, Peters DE, Werkmeister JA, Ketharanathan V. Collagen organization in mandrel-grown vascular grafts. J Biomed Mater Res 1989; **23**: 649–669.

20. Koch G, Gutschi S, Pascher O *et al.* Analysis of 274 Omniflow vascular prostheses implanted over an eight-year period. *Aust NZ J Surg* 1997; **67**: 637–639.

21. Welz A, Triefenbach R, Murrmann G *et al.* Experimental evaluation of the dialdehyde starch pre-served bovine internal mammary artery as a small diameter arterial substitute. *J Card Surg* 1992; **7**: 163–169.

22. Craig SR, Walker WS. The use of bovine internal mammary artery (Bioflow) grafts in coronary artery surgery. *Eur J Cardiothorac Surg* 1994; **8**: 43–45.

23. Burns, O. Eswards GA, Roberts GR *et al.* Performance of a new vascular xeno prosthesis. *ASAIO Trans* 1989; **35**: 214–218.

24. Uematsu M, Masyoshi O. A modified human ureter graft tanned by a new crosslinking agent poly-epoxy compound for small diameter arterial substitutions: an experimental preliminary study. *Artific Organs* 1998; **22**: 909–913.

25. Carrell A. Heterotransplantation of blood vessels preserved in cold storage. *J Exp Med* 1912; **15**: 226–228.

26. Carrell A. Ultimate results of aortic transplantation. *J Exp Med* 1912; **15**: 389–393.

27. Dubost C. First successful resection of an abdominal aorta with restoration of the continuity by a human arterial graft. *World J Surg* 1982; **6**: 256–257.

28. Szilagyi DE, Rodriguez FJ, Smith RF, Elliott JP. Late fate of arterial allografts. Observations 6 to 15 years after implantation. *Arch Surg* 1970; **101**: 721–733.

29. Moneta GL, Porter JM. Arterial substitutes in peripheral vascular surgery: a review. *J Long Term Eff Med Implant* 1995; **5**: 57–67.

30. Callow AD. Arterial homografts. *Eur J Vasc Endovasc Surg* 1996; **12**: 272–281.

31. Lesèche G, Penna C, Bouttier S *et al.* Femorodistal bypass using cryopreserved venous allografts for limb salvage. *Ann Vasc Surg* 1997; **11**: 230–236.

32. Harris L, O'Brien-Irr M, Ricotta JJ. Longterm assessment of cryopreserved vein grafting success. *J Vasc Surg* 2001; **33**: 528–532.

33. Buckley CJ, Abernathy S, Lee SD *et al.* Suggested treatment protocol for improving patency of femoral-infrapopliteal cryopreserved saphenous vein allografts. *J Vasc Surg* 2000; **32**: 731–738.

34. Albertini JN, Barral X, Brancherau A *et al.* Long-term results of arterial allograft below-knee bypass grafts for limb salvage: a retrospective multicenter study. *J Vasc Surg* 2000; **31**: 426–435.

35. Chiesa R, Astore D, Piccolo G *et al.* Fresh and cryopreserved arterial homografts in the treatment of prosthetic graft infections: experience of the Italian Collaborative Vascular Homograft Group. *Ann Vasc Surg* 1998; **12**: 457–462.

36. Alonso M, Segura RJ, Prada C *et al.* Cryopreserved arterial homografts. Preliminary results in infra-geniculate arterial reconstructions. *Ann Vasc Surg* 2001; **13**: 261–267.

37. Castier Y, Lesèche G, Palombi T *et al.* Early experience with cryopreserved arterial allografts in below-knee revascularization for limb salvage. *Am J Surg* 1999; **177**: 197–202.

38. Couvelard A, Lesèche G. Scoazec JY, Groussrad O. Human allograft vein failure: immunohisto-chemical arguments supporting the involvement of an immune-mediated mechanism. *Hum Pathol* 1995; **26**: 1313–1320.

39. Carpenter JP, Tomaszewski JE. Human saphenous vein allograft bypass grafts: immune response. *J Vasc Surg* 1998; **27**: 492–499.

40. Posner MP, Makhoul RG, Altman M *et al.* Early results of infrageniculate arterial reconstruction using cryopreserved homograft saphenous conduit (CADVEIN) andcombination of low-dose sys-temic immunosuppression. *J Am Coll Surg* 1996; **183**: 208–216.

41. Prager M, Hölzenbein Th, Aslim E. Fresh arterial homograft transplantation: a novel concept for critical limb ischemia. *Eur J Vasc Endovasc Surg* 2002; **24**: 314–321.

42. Da GamaAD, Sarmento C, VieiraT, Do Carmo GX. The use of arterial allografts for vascular reconstruction in patients receiving immunosupression for organ transplantation. *J Vasc Surg* 1994; **20**: 271–278.

43. Meinhart JG, Deutsch M, Fischlein T *et al.* Clinical autologous *in vitro* endothelialization of 153 infrainguinal ePTFE grafts. *Ann Thorac Surg* 2001; **7**: S327–S331.

44. Teebken OE, Haverich A. Tissue engineering of small diameter vascular grafts. *Eur J Vasc Endovasc Surg* 2002; **23**: 475–485.

45. Shum-Tim D, Stock U, Hrkach J *et al.* Tissue engineering of autologous aorta using a new biodegradable polymer. *Ann Thorac Surg* 1999; **68**: 2298–2305.

46. Rebane E, Tikko H, Tunder E *et al.* Venous allografts for infrainguinal vascular bypass. *Eur J Vasc Endovasc Surg* 1997; **5**: 21–25.

Heterografts and homografts have their place

Against the motion
Jonathan Beard, Peter Lee Chong

Introduction and definitions

As yet the ideal vascular graft has not been found. Autografts are the best conduits currently in use with regard to long-term patency and resistance to infection, but are not always available or of adequate quality.[1]

Autografts (autogenous or autologous) are harvested from the same individual and may be either arterial or venous. The long saphenous vein is the most commonly used autograft. Biological grafts can also be obtained from another human source (homografts or allografts) or from other species (heterografts or xenografts).

Homografts are usually obtained from the arteries of brain-dead donors or from human umbilical veins (HUV). Homografts were first used in the 1940s and 1950s as arterial substitutes. Fresh homografts rapidly underwent rejection. Homografts preserved by glutaraldehyde, irradiation or freeze-drying fare better in the short term but still suffer from subsequent atheromatous degeneration and aneurysm formation (Fig. 1).[2] The increasing incidence of revision surgery and graft infection have led to a renewed interest in homografts and heterografts.

Evidence for the use of homografts and heterografts

Homograft replacement following removal of an infected prosthetic graft seems an attractive alternative to extra-anatomic reconstruction and proponents for this technique suggest that it permits *in-situ* reconstruction with better resistance to infection than prosthetics.[3] While this may be true, there is no level I evidence to support this claim. The same applies when the questions of long-term patency and degeneration are raised.

The short-term results for homografts and heterografts vary widely and few studies with long-term outcomes are available. One confounder when analysing outcomes is the different methods of preservation. Other confounding issues are the varying indications and sites of implantation as well as the use of different pharmacological adjuncts such as immunosuppressive agents or Warfarin.[4]

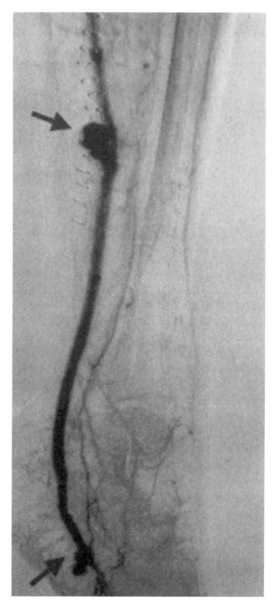

Figure 1. Arteriogram showing two acute pseudoaneurysms in a femorodistal cryopreserved venous homograft. Reproduced from *J Am Coll Surg* 1996; **183**: 208–216.

Risks of homografts and heterografts

Fresh homografts rapidly undergo rejection and thrombosis due to a strong anti-human leucocyte antigen (HLA) response.[5] Cryopreservation with liquid nitrogen and 15% dimethyl sulphoxide, an oxygen radical scavenger, may decrease the host immunological response and the risk of viral transmission[6] but there is no evidence that this preservation technique confers any advantage in terms of patency or freedom from late degeneration. Recent studies suggest that cryopreservation has no significant influence on antigenic suppression of homografts or heterografts[7] and may cause sensitization of future renal transplant candidates.[8] Cryopreserved venous homografts and glutaraldehyde-tanned bovine carotid arteries have been used for angio access but high rates of graft infection and rupture have been reported[9] as well as the usual problems of late degeneration.[10]

Immunosuppression may reduce the risk of rejection[11] and seems essential for fresh homograft transplantation.[12] Immunosuppression impairs wound healing and increases the possibility of opportunistic infection in vulnerable patients who often have other predisposing risk factors such as diabetes and impaired renal function.

Homografts and heterografts carry a low but measurable risk for the transmission of viruses including human immunodeficiency virus (HIV), hepatitis B and C, cytomegalovirus (CMV) infection and bovine spongiform encephalopathy (mad cow disease).

Costs and limitations of homografts and heterografts

Arterial and venous homograft procurement will usually take place as part of a multi-organ harvest procedure along with the kidneys, heart, liver etc. Harvesting will require a vascular surgeon and increase the duration and cost of the harvesting procedure.

The principles of tissue and blood matching to reduce rejection also apply to homografts. The need for ABO and HLA cross-matching, preservation agents, tissue banks and immunosuppressive agents significantly increase the costs.

The limited availability of donors is a problem inherent in this concept just as it is for organ transplantation. Revascularization will be subject to the same 'waiting list' problems, limiting widespread use of this technique.

Infrainguinal reconstruction
Arterial and venous autografts

The commonest small-calibre autologous conduit in clinical use is the long saphenous vein. It is freely available, easily harvested, available in adequate length and adapts well to placement in the arterial circulation. In a minority of cases long saphaenous vein is not available, either due to previous harvesting, inadequate vein calibre or length, previous phlebitis or structural defects within the vein. Alternate vein sources include the short saphenous vein[13] and arm veins.[14] Michaels performed a meta-analysis of approximately 40 studies of femoropopliteal grafts and concluded that autogenous vein was superior to prosthetic grafts with a mean 5-year patency rate of 62% vs 43% respectively for above-knee grafts and 68% vs 27% respectively for below-knee grafts.[15] However, a recent Cochrane review suggested that only one of these trials was of adequate design and size, and that the advantages claimed in favour of vein grafts might be overestimated.[16]

Arterial autografts have many appealing features that make them ideal as arterial substitutes. They retain their viability due to an intact intrinsic blood supply, demonstrate proportional arterial growth when used in children, do not degenerate with time, heal in an infected field and exhibit normal flexibility at joints. The more widespread use of arterial autografts is limited by lack of availability and short length.

Small calibre arterial autografts may be obtained from arteries that are dispensable, such as the internal mammary[17] gastroepiploic[18] and radial arteries.[19] These grafts can be harvested without the need for replacement. Others such as the superficial femoral artery may also be harvested but require replacement by a prosthetic graft. However, if chronically occluded, the superficial femoral artery may be used after endarterectomy without the need for replacement. Arterial autografts have patency rates superior to that of saphenous vein grafts and have good resistance to infection.

Cryopreserved venous and arterial homografts

In the rare case when autografts are unavailable, prosthetic bypass grafts have been shown to produce patency rates which cannot be bettered by the use of cryopreserved vein grafts.[20] Much research has focussed on ways of improving the patency of prosthetic grafts including the use of arteriovenous (AV) fistulas and venous cuffs.[21] A randomized study of 261 femoropopliteal expanded polytetrafluoroethylene (ePTFE) grafts performed by the Joint Vascular Research Group[22] showed a significant patency rate advantage for below-knee anastomoses when a vein cuff was used (80% vs 65%).

Pre-cuffed ePTFE grafts have recently become commercially available, on the premise that the benefit comes from the shape of the cuff, not the vein. Carbon coating of ePTFE grafts (Impra-Carboflo) have shown reduced platelet deposition.[23] Fluoropolymer coating of Dacron grafts (Vascutek-Fluoropassiv) has also been shown to cause less thrombogenicity and tissue reaction.[24] Heparin-bonded, small calibre, collagen-sealed Dacron (HBD) grafts have also been developed (Intervascular-Intergard).

A randomized trial of 209 patients undergoing femoropopliteal bypass[25] has shown a significantly better patency rate for HBD than ePTFE (70% and 55% at 1 and 3 years compared with 56% and 42% respectively).

Endothelial seeding remains an unfulfilled promise. Although several authors have reported encouraging results with improved endothelial coverage and patency rates the technique seems too technically demanding to warrant widespread use (Thompson *et al.* 1994).[26] However, future advances in cell culture and recombinant DNA technology may allow endothelial cells to be used as the vehicle for specifically targeted gene therapy aimed at reducing graft thrombogenicity and myointimal hyperplasia in both prosthetic and autologous vein grafts.[27]

In a large, well followed-up study of 115 cryopreserved vein homografts implanted in 87 limbs, Martin *et al.*[28] demonstrated no added benefits compared with less costly prosthetic grafts for below-knee arterial reconstruction. The patency rates at 24 months are uniformly poor for both types of conduits. A retrospective multicentre study of 165 cryopreserved arterial homografts for below-knee bypass reconstruction showed poor patency rates of 83% at 30 days, and 49%, 35% and 16% at 1, 3 and 5 years respectively (Fig. 2).[29] It is difficult to compare directly cryopreserved venous or arterial homografts with prosthetic grafts because there are no randomized trials comparing the two conduits. In the absence of such trials there seems little justification for using more expensive and risky homografts.

Human umbilical vein grafts

The glutaraldehyde-tanned HUV graft (Biograft-Biovascular Inc.) was introduced in 1975. The HUVs are placed on mandrils and tanned for extended periods in 1% glutaraldehyde solution. Cross-linking of the amino groups of the polypeptide collagen

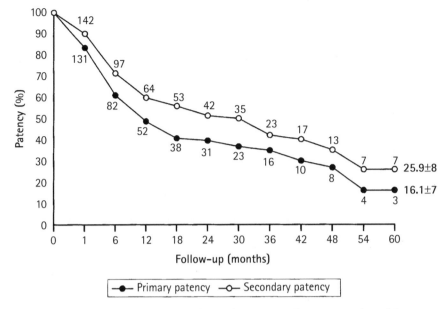

Figure 2. Life table analysis for primary and secondary patency of cryopreserved arterial homografts. Reproduced from *J Vasc Surg* 2000; **31**: 426–435.

chains produces a non-antigenic conduit. The frequent occurrence of aneurysm formation in HUV grafts (as high as 65% after 5 years in some studies) led to improvements in tanning and shaping of the tissue.[30] Despite these manufacturing changes, aneurysms still occur in up to 17% of cases and increase in frequency with time.[31]

In the largest study on the use of HUV, Jarrett *et al.*[32] analysed 171 patients undergoing 211 consecutive femoropopliteal bypass grafts since 1977. These patients were followed up at regular intervals for as long as 10 years. The cumulative patency rates as calculated by the life table method was 70% at 1 year, 45% at 5 years and 26% at 10 years. Infection and aneurysm rates were 3%. The results of the study suggest that HUV grafting produces no better results than the use of any prosthetic graft. A similar report by Dardik *et al.*[33] using HUV produced patency results similar to prosthetic grafting but considerably less than that obtained with autologous vein.

There are no large randomized trials comparing any combination of PTFE, Dacron or HUV in femorodistal bypass. Therefore, as before, there seems little justification for using HUV rather that ePTFE or Dacron if autologous vein or artery is unavaible.

Suprainguinal reconstruction

Autologous long saphenous vein is of insufficient calibre for most suprainguinal reconstructions, but prosthetic grafts have excellent patency rates in this position due to higher flow rates. The reported 5-year patency rates are over 90% for Dacron aortobifemoral bypass grafts,[34] 60–90% for femorofemoral crossovers[35] and 30–80% for axillobifemoral bypass grafts.[36] Therefore homografts and heterografts offer no advantage in terms of patency over prosthetics in the suprainguinal position.

The main use of homografts and heterografts in the suprainguinal position might be to reduce the risk of graft infection or to replace infected prosthetic grafts, because of claims that they possess an increased resistance to infection.[37] Prosthetic vascular graft infection has become a serious problem, particularly if an aortic graft is involved. Most graft infections are due to implantation of bacteria at the time of operation. Despite optimum prophylactic antibiotic schedules, 1–3% of prosthetic grafts become infected.

Patients with an infective source such as distal skin necrosis, or having re-operative surgery, particularly for a graft infection, are at extra risk. Unfortunately, there is no evidence that *in-situ* replacement of an infected graft with a cryopreserved homograft or heterograft is any better than excision of the infected graft and remote bypass grafting through a clean field.[38] Koskas *et al.*[39] have reported one of the largest series of 83 *in-situ* cryopreserved arterial homografts for infected aortoiliac protheses. The mortality was 18%; four patients developed early complications due to disruption of the grafts and 15 developed late occlusive lesions. The same group has also shown that fresh and cryopreserved homografts, like prosthetic grafts, are highly susceptible to infection.[40]

Antibiotic bonding may help to reduce the risk of prosthetic graft infection.[41] There have been two randomized controlled trials of rifampicin-bonded Dacron grafts with adequate follow-up. The first study from Italy involved 600 patients receiving aortofemoral grafts[42] and the second from the UK involved 250 patients having extra-anatomical bypasses.[43] Early wound infection rates were significantly reduced but at 2-year follow-up the reduction in graft infection rate was not significant. This may be because the low infection rate meant the power of the trials was inadequate. Other antibiotic/antibacterial combinations such as the silver graft[44] and the Triclosan-bonded graft[45] are now commercially available.

Gibbons *et al.*[46] and Nevelsteen *et al.*[47] have demonstrated the effective use of autologous femoropopliteal deep veins as a vascular conduit, even in the presence of sepsis when combined with debridement and appropriate antibiotic therapy (Fig. 3). Superficial femoral and popliteal vein is preferable to long saphenous vein in the suprainguinal position because of its greater calibre and possibly because its thicker wall may be more resistant to infection. Original fears that lower limb oedema after

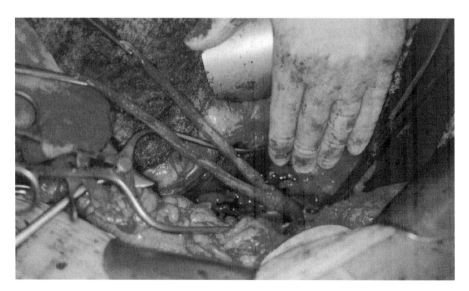

Figure 3. Aortic bifurcation graft fashioned from two superficial femoral veins, used for *in-situ* replacement of an infected aortic prosthetic graft. Reproduced with thanks to Mr C Gibbons.

deep vein harvesting would be prohibitive have not been realised in practice. Good long-term patency rates using superficial femoral and popliteal vein for primary fem-pop bypass have also been reported.[48] Therefore it seems that superficial femoral and popliteal vein is probably the conduit of first choice for the replacement of an infected suprainguinal prosthetic graft.

Renal artery revascularization in children is best achieved by an internal iliac artery autograft as saphenous vein in this context results in a high incidence of aneurysmal dilatation.[49] Arterial autografts may also be used to replace short arterial segments in contaminated or infected fields and for the repair of visceral artery aneurysms.

Summary

- Arterial and venous autografts should be used whenever possible because of their excellent patency rates and resistance to infection.

- Homografts and heterografts suffer from problems of early rejection and late degeneration.

- There is no Level I evidence of any benefit in terms of better patency or resistance to infection of homografts and heterografts compared with prosthetic grafts.

- The costs associated with homografts and heterografts raises serious questions about their cost-effectiveness.

- The safety of homografts and heterografts is questionable because of the increase in the prevalence of viruses such as HIV and a greater awareness of the risks of viral transmission between humans and animals.

- Proponents of homografts and heterografts must demonstrate their safety, efficacy and cost-effectiveness in prospective randomized trials, with long-term follow-up.

References

1. Mills JL, Fujitani RM, Taylor SM. The characteristics and anatomic distribution of lesions that cause reversed vein graft failure: a five-year prospective study. *J Vasc Surg* 1993; **17**: 195–206.
2. Callow AD. Arterial homographs. *EurJ Vasc Endovasc Surg* 1996; **12**: 272–281.
3. Sarac TP, Huber TS, Back MR. Warfarin improves the outcome of infrainguinal vein bypass grafting at high risk of failure. *J Vasc Surg* 1998; **28**: 446–457.
4. Kieffer E, Bahnini A, Koskas F *et al. In situ* allograft replacement of infected infrarenal aortic prosthetic grafts: results in forty-three patients. *J Vasc Surg* 1993; **17**: 349–356.
5. Mirelli M, Stella A, Fagguioli GL *et al.* Immune response following fresh arterial homograft replacement for aortoiliac graft infection. *EurJ Vasc Endovasc Surg* 1999; **18**: 424–429.
6. Borne CH, Roon AJ, Moore WS. Maintenance of viable arterial allografts by cryopreservation. *Surgery* 1977; **83**: 382–391.
7. Moriyama S, Utoh J, Tagami H *et al.*Antigenicity of cryopreserved arterial allografts comparison with fresh and glutaraldehyde treated grafts. *ASAIO J* 2001; **47**: 202–205.
8. Lopez-Cepero M, Sanders CE, Buggs J, Bowers V. Sensitization of renal transplant candidates by cryopreserved cadaveric venous or arterial allografts. *Transplantation* 2002; **73**: 817–819.
9. Bolton WD, Cull DL, Taylor SM *et al.* The use of cryopreserved femoral vein grafts for haemodialysis access in patients at high risk for infection: a word of caution. *J Vasc Surg* 2002; **36**: 464–468.
10. Brems J, Castaneda M, Garvin PJ. A five-year experience with the bovine heterograft for vascular access. *Arch Surg* 1986; **121**: 941–949.

11. de Gama AD, Sarmento C, Vieira T, do Carmo GX. The use of arterial allografts for vascular reconstruction in patients receiving immuno-suppression for organ transplantation. *J Vasc Surg* 1994; **20**: 217–218.

12. Prager M, Holzenbein T, Aslim E *et al.* Fresh arterial homograft transplantation: a novel concept for critical limb ischaemia. *EurJ Vasc Endovasc Surg* 2002; **24**: 314–321.

13. Weaver FA, Barlow CR, Edwards WH *et al.* The lesser saphenous vein: Autogenous tissue for lower extremity revascularisation. *J Vasc Surg* 1987; **5**: 687.

14. Andros G, Harris RW, Salles-Cunha SX *et al.* Arm veins for arterial revascularization of the leg: Arteriographic and clinical observations. *J Vasc Surg* 1986; **4**: 416.

15. Michaels JA. Choice of material for above-knee femoro-popliteal bypass graft. *Br J Surg* 1989; **76**: 7–14.

16. Mamode N, Scott RN. Graft type for femoro-popliteal bypass surgery (Cochrane Review). In: *The Cochrane Library*; Issue 4, Oxford: Update Software, 1999.

17. Boylan MJ, Lytle BW, Loop FD *et al.* Surgical treatment of isolated left anterior descending coronary stenosis. Comparison of left internal mammary artery and venous autograft at 18 to 20 years of follow-up. *J Thorac Cardiovasc Surg* 1994; **107**: 657–662.

18. Dietl CA, Benoit CH, Gilbert CL *et al.* Which is the graft of choice for the coronary and posterior descending arteries? Comparison of the right internal mammary artery and the right gastroepiploic artery. *Circulation* 1995; 92: (Suppl): 1192–1197.

19. Galajda Z, Jagamoss E, Maros T, Peterffy A. Radial artery grafts: surgical anatomy and harvesting techniques. *Cardiovasc Surg* 2002; **10** (S): 476–480.

20. Robinson BI, Fletcher JP, Tomlinson P *et al.* A prospective randomised multicentre comparison of expanded polytetrafluoroethylene and gelatin-sealed knitted dacron grafts for femoropopliteal bypass. *Cardiovasc Surg* 1999; **7**: 214–218.

21. Harris PL, da Silva AF, How TV. Interposition vein cuffs. *EurJ Vasc Endovasc Surg* 1996; **11**: 257–259.

22. Stonebridge PA, Prescott RJ, Ruckley CV. Randomised trial comparing infrainguinal polytetrafluoroethylene bypass grafting with and without interposition cuff at the distal anastomosis. *J Vasc Surg* 1997; **26**: 543–550.

23. Tsuchida H, Cameron BL, Marcus CS, Wilson SE. Modified polytetrafluoroethylene: Indium 111-labelled platelet deposition on carbon-lined and high porosity polytetrafluoroethylene grafts. *J Vasc Surg* 1992; **4**: 643–649.

24. Khee RY, Gloviezki P, Camria RA, Miller VM. Experimental evaluation of bleeding complications, thrombogenicity and neointimal characteristics of prosthetic patch materials used for carotid angioplasty. *Cardiovasc Surg* 1996; **4**: 746–752.

25. Devine C, McCollum CN. Prosthetic femoro-popliteal bypass: PTFE or heparin bonded dacron? *Br J Surg* 2000; **87**: 491.

26. Thompson MM, Budd JS, Bell PRF. Endothelial seeding of prosthetic vascular grafts. *Vasc Med Rev* 1994; **5**: 225–239.

27. Wilson JM, Birinyi LK, Salomon RN *et al.* Implantation of vascular grafts lined with genetically modified endothelial cells. *Science* 1989; **244**: 1344–1346.

28. Martin RS, Edwards WH, Mulherin JL *et al.* Cryopreserved saphenous vein allografts for below-knee lower extremity revascularisation. *Ann Surg* 1994; **219**: 664–672.

29. Albertini JN, Barral X, Branchereau A *et al.* Long-term results of arterial allograft below-knee bypass grafts for limb salvage: a retrospective multicetre study. *J Vasc Surg* 2000; **31**: 426–435.

30. Nevelsteen A, Smet G, Wilms G *et al. Intravenous* digital subtraction angiography and duplex scanning in the detection of late human umbilical vein degeneration. *Br J Surg* 1988; **75**: 668–670.

31. Strobel R, Boontje AH, Van Den Dungen JJAM. Aneurysm formation in modified human umbilical vein grafts. *EurJ Vasc Endovasc Surg* 1996; **11**: 417–420.

32. Jarrett F, Mahmood BA. Long-term results of femoro-popliteal bypass with stabilised human umbilical vein. *Am J Surg* 1994; **168**: 111–114.

33. Dardik H, Miller N, Darchk A. A decade of experience with the glutaraldehyde-tanned human umbilical vein graft for revascularization of the lower limb. *J Vasc Surg* 1988; **7**: 336–346.

34. Nevelsteen A, Wouters L, Suy R. Aortofemoral Dacron reconstruction for aorto-iliac occlusive disease: a 25 year survey. *Eur J Vasc Surg* 1991; **5**: 179–186.

35. Berce M, Sayers RD, Miller JH. Femorofemoral crossover grafts for claudication: a safe and reliable procedure. *EurJ Vasc Endovasc Surg* 1996; **12**: 437–441.

36. Wittens CHA, Van Houtte HJKP, Van Urk H. European prospective multicentre axillo-bifemoral trial. *Eur J Vasc Surg* 1992; **6**: 115.

37. Knosalla C, Goeau-Brissonniere O, Leflon V *et al.* Treatment of vascular graft infection by *in-situ* replacement with cryopreserved aortic allografts: an experimental study. *J Vasc Surg* Apr 1998; **27**: 689–698.

38. Yaeger RA, Taylor LM, Moneta GL *et al*. Improved results in conventional management of infrarenal aortic infection. *J Vasc Surg* 1999; **30**: 76–83.

39. Koskas F, Plissonnier D, Bahnini A, Ruotolo C, Kieffe E. *In-situ* arterial allografting for aorto-iliac graft infection: a 6-year experience. *Cardiovasc Surg* 1996; **4**: 495–499.

40. Camiade C, Goldschmidt P, Koskas F *et al*. *Opimization* of the resistance of arterial allografts to infection: comparative study with synthetic prostheses. *Ann Vasc Surg* 2001: **15**: 186–196.

41. Strachan CJL, Newsom SWB, Ashton TR. The clinical use of an antibiotic bonded graft. Eur *J Vasc Surg* 1991; **5**: 627–632.

42. D'Addato M, Curti T, Freyvic A. Prophylaxis of graft infection with rifampicin bonded Gelseal graft: 2-year follow-up of a prospective clinical trial. Italian Investigators Group. *Cardiovasc Surg* 1996; **4**: 200–204.

43. Earnshaw JJ, Whitman B, Heather BP on behalf of the Joint Vascular Research Group. Two-year results of a randomised trial of rifampicin-bonded extra-anatomic dacron grafts. *Br J Surg* 2000; **87**: 758–759.

44. Illingworth B, Tweden K, Schroeder RF *et al*. *In vivo* efficacy of silver coated (Silzore) infection resistant polyester fabric against biofilm producing bacteria, *Staphylococcus epidermidis*. *J Hrt Valve Dis* 1998; **7**: 524–530.

45. Hernandez-Richter T, Schardey HM, Lohlein F *et al*. The prevention and treatment of vascular graft infection with a triclosan (Irgasan™) bonded dacron graft: an experimental study in the pig. *Br J Surg* (in press).

46. Gibbons CP, Ferguson CJ, Edwards K *et al*. Use of superficial femoropopliteal vein for suprainguinal arterial reconstruction in the presence of infection. *Br J Surg* 2000; **87**: 771–776.

47. Nevelsteen A, Lacroix H, Suy R. Autogenous reconstruction with the lower extremity deep veins: an alternative treatment of prosthetic infection after reconstructive surgery for aortoiliac disease. *J Vasc Surg* 1995; **22**: 129–134.

48. Schulman ML, Badhey MR, Yatco R, Pillari IG. An 11-year experience with deep leg veins as femoropopliteal bypass grafts. *Arch Surg* 1986; **121**: 1010–1015.

49. Novick AC, Stewart BK, Straffon RA. Autogenous arterial grafts in the treatment of renal artery stenosis. *J Urol* 1977; **118**: 919.

Heterografts and homografts have their place

Charing Cross Editorial Comments towards
Consensus

The Vienna experience is quite persuasive. The argument begins that the renal arteries at renal transplantation rarely become aneurysmal or thrombosed over periods of up to 20 years. The authors have harvested arteries from brain-dead organ donors. The patients were immunosuppressed with prednisolone, cyclosporin A and mofetil mycophenolate. The primary patency rate of 53% is quoted in a short follow-up. Our proposers argue for the use of arterial homografts when a vein is not available, although this group are against heterografts. They say that all homografts require immunosuppression. One wonders about human umbilical vein when immunosuppression was not recommended. Should it have been?

The opposition stress the rejection and thrombosis risk. They say that these homografts and heterografts are no better resistors to infection than prosthetic grafts and that results are inferior to venous and arterial autografts. They believe that the proponents of homografts and heterografts must demonstrate their safety, efficacy and cost-effectiveness.

Roger M Greenhalgh
Editor

Endovascular abdominal aortic aneurysm repair should be carried out as a day-case procedure

For the motion

Jacques Bleyn, François Schol,
Inga Vanhandenhove, Peter Vercaeren

Introduction

We started endovascular repair of abdominal aortic aneurysms (AAA) in 1995 in our department and switched to bilateral percutaneous access in 1998 with a suture mediated closure system (Perclose®). In November 1999 we did our first ambulatory repair of an AAA.

This evolution was directed by the four principles that were outlined for the Antwerp Blood-vessel Centre (ABC) at its conception:

1. Endovascular treatment whenever possible.
2. Percutaneous access.
3. Local anaesthesia.
4. Outpatient treatment.

These treatment options were followed to reduce the cost of endovascular treatment and to enhance the patient's comfort, safety and acceptance.

Technique

1. Indication and preoperative work-up for AAA endovascular repair are done with echography and magnetic resonance arteriography in our outpatient clinic.
2. The patient undergoes a 2-day bowel preparation preoperatively, at home, comparable with a rectoscopy bowel preparation.
3. On the day of surgery he or she can take a liquid breakfast and is admitted at 9 a.m. A mild anxiolytic drug (Lysanxia® 10mg) is administered orally. Both groins are shaved and two peripheral venous lines are installed; no arterial line, no central venous line.
4. At 10 a.m. the patient is transferred to the endovascular suite and hooked up to non-invasive monitoring: blood pressure every minute, oxygen tension, and electrocardiogram (ECG). A urinary catheter is placed in position.

5. After preparation and drape, 10 cc of Xylocaine 2% with adrenaline is injected in both groins at the femoral artery level. With a retrograde puncture a 10 Fr introducer is inserted on the main access side, a 6 Fr controlateral.

6. A graduated pigtail catheter is than inserted through the controlateral introducer over a 0.035 Terumo® guidewire and positioned at the renal artery level.

7. Digital substraction arteriography (DSA) in apnoea locates the renal artery origins and checks the measurements for the planned endograft.

8. Deployment of the sutures of the 10Fr Perclose® is done at this stage whenever the final introducer size is bigger then 12 Fr – a technique called 'Preclose'. This is necessary because as the maximum Perclose® size is 10 Fr, it is mandatory to deploy the sutures in the arterial wall before dilating the puncture site to the size of the final introducer (18-23 Fr). These sutures are held by a mosquito clamp during the procedure and tied at removal of the introducer at the end of the procedure.

9. The big bore introducer for main body insertion is guided over a Lunderquist guidewire to the level of the renals and pressurized with heparinized saline solution (2500 IU/litre).

10. It is important to note that **no general heparinization** is used.

11. Deployment of the main body of the graft is performed after a magnified DSA of the juxtarenal aorta is performed through the pigtail catheter that is still in place from the controlateral 6 Fr introducer, to position the proximal part of the graft as close as possible to the renal arteries. After changing the controlateral introducer to its final size, the controlateral limb is deployed.

12. A 'go-home arteriogram' confirms the technical perfection of the repair.

13. The Perclose® system of both access sites and steristrips is put in place. The urinary catheter is removed.

14. Around noon the patient is observed for 2 hours in the recovery room with full monitoring. He or she is given a cup of coffee and may telephone home.

15. At 2 p.m. the patient is transferred to his/her room inside the ABC and eats lunch.

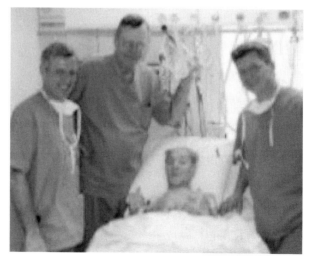

Figure 1. Patient in recovery room in Antwerp immediately after end of operation.

16. In the late afternoon a haematocrit and renal function test is done to detect concealed bleeding or renal problems.
17. Postoperative instructions are given with the family present and the patient is allowed to **walk** home: the use of a wheel chair is not allowed!
18. After 2 weeks an ambulant computerized tomography (CT)-scan and a plain two-plane abdominal X-ray and physical examination are used to control the correct positioning of the endoprosthesis and detect the presence of endoleaks.

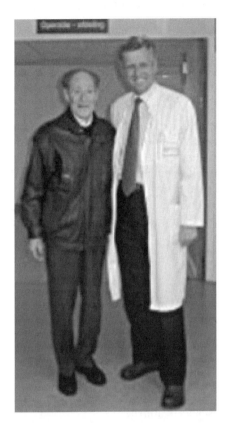

Figure 2. Patient walks home in the afternoon in Antwerp.

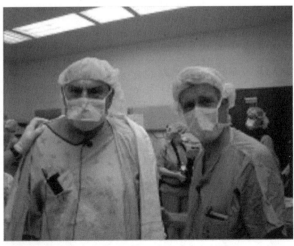

Figure 3. Patient in Chicago walks away from the operation table at the end of the case and is "ready for steak and eggs".

Material

From November 1999 to January 2002, 23 patients with 21 AAA and two iliac aneurysms were treated out of a total of 32 endovascular AAA patients treated in that same period.

Indications for ambulatory treatment were essentially social and insurance-linked. The hospitalized patients were treated in the same way. Mean age was 72 (66–83) in this all male cohort and mean aneurysm diameter (including the two iliac aneurysms) was 55 mm.

Results

Mean operative time was 100 min. There were no conversions, no mortality and no postoperative bleeding. One patient planned as ambulatory had to stay overnight because of a closure device problem.

There were three endoleaks at follow-up (one type I and two type II) but this is no different from results in hospitalized patients.

One patient had a slight fever (38°C) on day 2. Not a single patient had to be read-mitted urgently for postoperative complications that could not be handled by the general practitioner.

Contraindications

Obvious contraindications for our technique are:

1. Unstable patients.
2. Ruptured AAA.
3. Social isolation.
4. AAA not suitable for endovascular treatment.

Discussion and conclusion

As hospital and medical financial resources become a major issue for the century, our new endovascular treatment options offer a short period of time in hospital and local anaesthesia as a way of fighting cost and invasiveness. Ambulatory treatment saves 50% of hospital beds that would be used for a one-night stay. It can be performed safely with adapted surgical and anaesthesia techniques and a dedicated organization of care.

In this elderly population of patients that is more and more informed about the risks of a hospital stay and of general anaesthesia, our treatment options as described above are not only very well accepted but also very popular.

This is definitely the way for the future and at the same time a great marketing tool to promote the excellence of a unit to the general public and to referring physicians.

Summary

- Ambulatory endovascular repair can be performed safely under local anaesthetic.

- We had experience of 23 procedures using a percutaneous approach.

- No mortality, no urgent readmittance.

- A very cost-effective way to treat AAA.

Further reading

1. Henretta JP, Hodgson KJ, Mattos MA *et al.* Feasibility of endovascular repair of abdominal aortic aneurysms with local anesthesia with intravenous sedation. *J Vasc Surg* 1999; 29: 793–798.
2. Leotta L, Merlo M, Bitossi G *et al.* Mid-term results of endovascular repair for abdominal aortic aneurysm, with loco-regional anesthesia, in high-risk patients. *Minerva Cardioangiol* 2001; 49: 23–29.

Endovascular abdominal aortic aneurysm repair should be carried out as a day-case procedure

Against the motion
RJ Hinchliffe, BR Hopkinson

Introduction

To perform endovascular aneurysm repair (EVAR) and discharge the patient from hospital on the same postoperative day is unquestionably feasible but not sensible. Proponents of the day-case approach would suggest that it is economically attractive and safe. This premise is based on observations that EVAR is quick, percutaneous, easy to perform and without complication.

Quick

It is generally perceived as possible to perform EVAR more rapidly than open repair. In a recent 6-year experience EVAR was found to take on average over $3\frac{1}{2}$ hours.[1] Therefore to describe it as a 'quick' procedure is clearly nonsense. Furthermore, complex cases and any intraoperative complications will increase the duration of the procedure.

Easy to perform

Small aneurysms with favourable anatomy do represent a group which is relatively straightforward. However, it is not always possible to predict intraoperative technical difficulties, especially in obese patients where intraoperative imaging may be poor. Complex aneurysms with adverse morphological features are associated with more intraoperative technical complications and may require a range of interventions both open and endovascular to ensure aneurysm exclusion.[2]

Percutaneous

The ability to perform EVAR percutaneously may be cited as a reason to facilitate day-case care. Not all patients are suitable for this technique. In a recent study, using a percutaneous vascular surgical device, 15% of patients required conversion to a conventional groin incision and one patient died from retroperitoneal haemorrhage.[3]

Similar results were found in another study.[4] Both publications underscored the importance of careful patient selection. Obesity, scarred groins and calcification in the former study and large sheath size in the latter predicted procedural failure. It may be argued therefore that larger aneurysms with more difficult morphology and patients with greater co-morbidity – just those who are likely to benefit from percutaneous procedures – are most likely to be those who are unsuitable.

Local anaesthesia would appear an attractive technique to reduce the perioperative morbidity associated with EVAR and shorten hospital stay. The technique usually requires intravenous sedation. Any intraoperative difficulties or complications are likely to result in conversion to general anaesthesia. These include procedures resulting in prolonged lower limb ischaemia, the need for retroperitoneal vascular access, femorofemoral bypass or laparotomy.

Even when successfully performed, the local anaesthesia approach to EVAR carries a significant systemic physiological disturbance, albeit less than that associated with general anaesthesia.[5] Importantly, though a recent investigation comparing local anaesthesia and general anaesthesia. was unable to demonstrate any difference in the number of postoperative cardiac or pulmonary complications.[6] A study of 47 patients using local anaesthesia (in which only one conversion to general anaesthesia was performed and no intra- or postoperative complications were observed) found only 30% of patients were suitable for discharge the day following surgery.[7] In another study 27% of patients undergoing local anaesthesia, EVAR required admission to an intensive care unit with an overall median hospital stay of 3 days.[5]

Procedure severity

EVAR is associated with a period of aortic cross-clamping. This may be prolonged if there are intraoperative technical difficulties. Although the ischaemia-reperfusion injury and cytokine response is attenuated it is not abolished following EVAR.[8] Consequently remote tissue damage including lung injury as a result of the inflammatory response remains a possibility in the perioperative period.

Patients undergoing EVAR are frequently those with cardiovascular, respiratory and renal disease. In a review of 229 patients undergoing EVAR, De Virgilio demonstrated that almost a quarter of patients with two preoperative cardiac risk factors developed a major cardiac event following EVAR.[6]

Safe

In the perioperative period, 24% of patients undergoing EVAR developed a complication – 58% of which were described as major. In addition 6% of patients required re-operation or secondary procedures before hospital discharge.[9]

The complications of aortic surgery are not always manifest within hours of the operation. Local groin haematomas and life-threatening haemorrhage, which may be concealed (retro- or intraperitoneal), are not uncommon following EVAR. In a study of uniiliac endovascular stent-grafts 7% of patients developed groin haematomas.[10] Acute renal dysfunction complicating the administration of radiographic contrast is a real phenomenon. In a study of 400 patients who underwent aortography, there was an 11.3% incidence of acute renal dysfunction.[11] This figure is likely to be higher in those patients with pre-existing renal dysfunction. The chance of developing renal dysfunction increases with higher doses of contrast but this relationship is not always predictable. In addition this complication may not become manifest until 24 hours following the procedure.

Although the incidence of bowel ischaemia following EVAR is low its effects may be devastating. Colonic infarction is not necessarily a predictable event and can occur despite preservation of both internal iliac arteries on completion angiography at the end of the operation.[12] Bowel ischaemia may not be manifest for some hours after the operation and usually requires a period of observation to distinguish a self-limiting ischaemia from fulminant infarction. Early recognition of the condition (which may not happen if the patient is at home) and prompt treatment may avert disaster.

Endovascular aneurysm surgery is currently the remit of larger vascular centres. Patients frequently travel great distances to undergo their surgery. To discharge patients home on the first postoperative day would be logistically difficult. Further, any early complications may be managed in local hospitals where experience of EVAR or expertise in endovascular procedures may be limited.

Summary

- EVAR is frequently performed in patients with multiple medical co-morbidities who have difficulty withstanding any intervention no matter how minimally invasive.

- EVAR is less invasive than open repair but its physiological consequences are not insignificant. Local anaesthesia or percutaneous techniques may appear attractive but have not been shown to improve patient outcome.

- Furthermore, a significant number of patients are not suitable for either local anaesthesia or percutaneous access.

- Intraoperative complications (which may not be anticipated from preoperative investigations) potentially increase the severity of the injury and increase the number of secondary procedures.

- Postoperative complications may be severe, are neither always predictable nor manifest within the first few hours. Early recognition of these problems in-hospital facilitates treatment and potentially improves outcome.

- EVAR must not be performed as a day-case procedure. Just because it can be done does not mean it should be done.

References

1. Moore WS, Kashyap VS, Vescera CL, Quinones-Baldrich WJ. Abdominal aortic aneurysm: a 6-year comparison of endovascular versus transabdominal repair. *Ann Surg* 1999; **230**: 298–306.
2. Kalliafas S, Albertini JN, Macierewicz J *et al*. Incidence and treatment of intraoperative technical problems during endovascular repair of complex abdominal aortic aneurysms. *J Vasc Surg* 2000; **31**: 1185–1192.
3. Teh LG, Sieunarine K, van Schie G *et al*. Use of the percutaneous vascular surgery device for closure of femoral access sites during endovascular aneurysm repair: lessons from our experience. *Eur J Vasc Endovasc Surg* 2001; **22**: 418–423.
4. Rachel ES, Bergamini TM, Kinney EV *et al*. Percutaneous endovascular abdominal aortic aneurysm repair. *Ann Vasc Surg* 2002; **16**: 43–49.

5. Bettex DA, Lachat M, Pfammatter T *et al.* To compare general, epidural and local anaesthesia for endovascular aneurysm repair (EVAR). *Eur J Vasc Endovasc Surg* 2001; **21**: 179–184.
6. De Virgilio C, Romero L, Donayre C *et al.* Endovascular abdominal aortic aneurysm repair with general versus local anesthesia: a comparison of cardiopulmonary morbidity and mortality rates. *J Vasc Surg* 2002; **36**: 988–991.
7. Henretta JP, Hodgson KJ, Karch LA *et al.* Feasibility of endovascular repair of abdominal aortic aneurysms with local anaesthesia with intravenous sedation. *J Vasc Surg* 1999; **29**: 793–798.
8. Swartbol P, Truedsson L, Norgren L. The inflammatory response and its consequence for the clinical outcome following aortic aneurysm repair. *Eur J Vasc Endovasc Surg* 2001; **21**: 393–400.
9. Hill BB, Wolf YG, Lee WA *et al.* Open versus endovascular AAA repair in patients who are morphological candidates for endovascular treatment. *J Endovasc Ther* 2002; **9**: 255–261.
10. Walker SR, Braithwaite BD, Tennant WG *et al.* Early complications of femorofemoral crossover bypass grafts after aorta uni-iliac endovascular repair of abdominal aortic aneurysms. *J Vasc Surg* 1998; **28**: 647–650.
11. Martin-Paredero V, Dixon SM, Baker JD *et al.* Risk of renal failure after major angiography. *Arch Surg* 1983; **118**: 1417–1420.
12. Hinchliffe RJ, Armon MP, Tse CC *et al.* Colonic infarction following endovascular AAA repair: a multifactorial complication. *J Endovasc Ther* 2002; **9**: 554–558.

Endovascular abdominal aortic aneurysm repair should be carried out as a day-case procedure

Charing Cross Editorial Comments towards Consensus

Jacques Bleyn has done it. Jacques Bleyn can do it. Possibly Brian Hopkinson can do it. To be able to do it does not mean to say one should do it. It nevertheless shows what can be achieved to be able to perform an elective aortic aneurysm procedure through a percutaneous system and send the patient home the same day. This is a staggering achievement but one has to say, at least one night in hospital after any aneurysm procedure should not be asking too much!

R M Greenhalgh
Editor

Endovascular procedures belong in a sterile operating suite

For the motion
Edward B Diethrich

Introduction

Treatment of vascular disease has been revolutionized by endovascular surgical techniques. The growth of this new field is characterized by innovations that include percutaneous balloon angioplasty, atherectomy, stenting, and endoluminal grafting. Stent technology has been a major breakthrough in the treatment of coronary and peripheral lesions, and endoluminal grafting – in which stents covered with synthetic graft materials are used to treat aneurysms – has already changed the indications for treatment in many centres. As endovascular technology has advanced, it has become clear that establishing a properly designed endovascular suite is a critical factor in the success and safety of these procedures.

There are few complications a surgeon fears as much as infection and the development of sepsis following a procedure. Although many endovascular interventions are still performed in radiographic facilities, such an environment does not generally provide the strict sterile conditions one has access to in an operating room. My own view, based on nearly 30 years experience at the Arizona Heart Institute, has long been that endovascular 'procedures will be performed with the greatest safety in an endovascular suite under full "operative" sterile conditions ... this can be either a standard operating room equipped for endovascular procedures or an angioplasty suite that has been designed to incorporate the requirements of a sterile environment.'[1]

Evidence

Complications of endovascular procedures most often involve device deployment problems and vascular injury with haemorrhage and subsequent thromboembolism. By contrast, reports of infection and sepsis following endovascular procedures are so rare that some investigators have speculated the true incidence of these complications is 'ill-defined'[2] or 'unknown.'[3] Whether or not the reported incidence of septic complications following endovascular procedures is accurate, one fact remains quite clear: the morbidity and mortality associated with these infections is extremely high.[4–24]

While vascular surgical operations are associated with infection rates ranging from 1 to 6%,[25] there is a relative paucity of data describing complications of endovascular procedures. Still, case reports detailing septic complications of percutaneous angioplasty have been available for nearly two decades.[4-7] Since the introduction of endovascular stents and grafts, infections and sepsis associated with these implantable devices have also been described in the literature.[8-24]

It seems clear that breaches in sterile technique are likely to occur more frequently in the radiographic suite than in the operating room.[3,8,11] Dosluoglu and colleagues[21] published an excellent review of infection following stent placement, highlighting 21 cases reported through 1999. In all but two of these cases, stents were placed in an angiography suite; only one patient received pre-interventional antibiotics. The majority of cases were early, acute infections that presented between 2 and 28 days following intervention. *Staphylococcus aureus* was cultured in the blood or at the time of surgery in 16 cases. Morbidity among the 21 patients was high, with most suffering organ failure of some kind; a total of five patients died.

As illustrated above, bacteria associated with septic complications are likely to originate from the skin, which emphasizes the importance of ensuring proper aseptic technique in device deployment, including adequate sterilization of the arterial puncture site, a clear sterile field, and care with scrubbing, gowning, gloving, masking, and capping.[16] *Staphylococcus aureus* is a common skin flora contaminant and cause of infection; seeding of the endovascular device and the artery at the time of the procedure are likely causes of infections that present within several weeks of the intervention.[3,8,12]

Investigators have speculated that '…any indwelling foreign body may act as a nidus for colonization by circulating organisms…' and that '…the [device] may act as a vector for iatrogenic introduction of bacteria if strict sterile procedure is not followed during manufacture, packaging, and placement…'.[9] Indeed, Therasse and colleagues,[8] who reported an infection and fatal outcome following stent placement in the early 1990s, have advocated that 'aseptic methods used in the angiography suite should be similar to those used in the operating room.'

Factors that appear to increase the risk of stent-related infection are:

1. breaks in sterile technique such as occult glove perforations and inadequate skin preparation;[3]
2. the reuse of an indwelling catheter or sheath that is then left in the groin for more than 24 hours;
3. obtaining repeated vascular access via the femoral artery within 7 days of a previous catheterization;
4. local haematoma formation;
5. increased procedure time.[10]

Angioplasty-induced intimal disruption may predispose to arterial infection and lead to weakening of the vessel wall and formation of an aneurysm that eventually ruptures.[17] Stent infections have been shown to arise where the stent comes in contact with the arterial wall, and bacteria may adhere to the stent surface, particularly when the endoprosthesis apposes a long segment of the arterial wall.[20] The use of long wires and catheters and the deployment of multiple stents also increase the potential for infection.[11] Secondary infection of a chronically implanted stent has been reported following endovascular manipulation months after the initial procedure.[13]

Antibiotic prophylaxis has been suggested as a means of reducing the potential for infection following endovascular procedures.[9,11,19] Unfortunately, its success in preventing infection in this setting is unproven, and there are a number of investigators who are not willing to make definitive recommendations.[3,22] Others suggest that while antibiotics may not be routinely indicated[17] they should be considered when contamination is suspected or in patients who require prolonged indwelling catheterization or reintervention.[21] Without results from a prospective trial emphasizing the value of prophylactic antibiotics in endovascular procedures, cost-containment strategies are likely to preclude their routine use.[12]

While antibiotic prophylaxis is undeniably expensive, there are significant costs associated with strict adherence to sterile technique in endovascular procedures as well. For example, in 1999, Fillinger and Weaver[26] estimated that adding operating-room quality airflow to an endovascular suite cost nearly half a million dollars alone. They maintain that prior to the proliferation of stent and endoluminal graft procedures there was, perhaps, 'no need to meet and maintain operating room sterility standards.' While they concede that there is a low rate of prosthetic graft infection, they rightly point out that it would take 'hundreds or even thousands of patients in a randomized, prospective study' to prove the necessity of operating room sterility standards for endovascular procedures. Indeed, they note the 'human and financial cost of even a single infection is very high,' and emphasize the importance of providing sterile conditions in cases where the surgeon must convert quickly from a percutaneous to open procedure—something that is certainly not entirely uncommon. Maintaining a 'standby' operating room in close proximity to the endovascular suite is an expensive compromise that represents a very questionable use of hospital resources. It is clear that rectifying deficiencies that preclude safe and effective treatment in the endovascular suite is a costly effort that ultimately involves a variety of staff, including administrators, architects, and clinicians. Nevertheless, it is incumbent upon us to offer patients the best possible care – care that prevents infection and its attendant morbidity and mortality.

Conclusion

Unprecedented growth in the field of endovascular surgical technology has introduced a variety of new devices and procedures, including stents and endoluminal grafts. These novel methods of correcting pathologies associated with vascular disease have changed the indications for treatment in many centres. The environment in which these procedures are best performed is somewhat controversial, and a great number of endovascular interventions are still completed in radiographic suites that lack strict adherence to the sterile conditions found in operating rooms. While the infection rate associated with endovascular procedures appears quite low, some investigators have suggested these values may underestimate true incidence. At present, we are unable to document significant differences in infection rates based on the venue of the procedure. Nevertheless, even if current incidence rates are accurate, there is no doubt that infections following any surgical procedure – open or endovascular – are extremely serious. Breaches in sterile technique are more likely to occur in environments designed primarily to facilitate radiographic imaging. While the use of pre-procedural antibiotic coverage, such as that generally used in open vascular procedures, may be a means of limiting infection following endovascular intervention, its efficacy has not been proven. Clearly, there is considerable expense associated with antibiotic prophylaxis and with construction of an endovascular suite that adheres to strict sterile conditions, but we owe it to our patients and the future of this technology to provide an optimal setting that offers the greatest likelihood for successful intervention. It seems certain that infections associated with deployment of endovascular devices will increase as clinicians from a variety of disciplines perform these procedures under less-than-ideal conditions.

Summary

- Unprecedented growth in the field of endovascular surgical technology has introduced a variety of new devices and procedures, including stents and endoluminal grafts.

- As endovascular technology has advanced, it has become clear that establishing a properly designed endovascular suite is a critical factor in the success and safety of these procedures.

- Although many endovascular interventions are still performed in radiographic facilities, such an environment does not generally provide the strict sterile conditions one has access to in an operating room.

- Reports of infection and sepsis following endovascular procedures are rare, and some investigators have speculated the true incidence of these complications is not known.

- Even if the low reported incidence of septic complications following endovascular procedures is accurate, the morbidity and mortality associated with these infections is extremely high.

- Septic complications are likely to originate from the skin, which emphasizes the importance of ensuring proper aseptic technique in device deployment, including adequate sterilization of the arterial puncture site, a clear sterile field, and care with scrubbing, gowning, gloving, masking, and capping.

- Antibiotic prophylaxis has been suggested as a means of reducing the potential for infection following endovascular procedures, but its success in preventing infection in this setting is unproven.

- There are significant costs associated with providing sterile conditions in endovascular suites; however, the cost of infection is extremely high as well, both in terms of human life and monetary expenditure.

- It is incumbent upon us to offer all patients the best possible care – care that prevents infection and its attendant morbidity and mortality.

References

1. Diethrich EB. Endovascular intervention suite design. In: White RA, Fogarty TJ (eds). *Peripheral Endovascular Interventions*. St Louis, Missouri: Mosby, 1996: 129–139.
2. Deitch JS, Hansen KJ, Regan JD *et al*. Infected renal artery pseudoaneurysm and mycotic aortic aneurysm after percutaneous transluminal renal artery angioplasty and stent placement in a patient with a solitary kidney. *J Vasc Surg* 1998; **28**: 340–344.
3. DeMaioribus CA, Anderson CA, Popham SSG *et al*. Mycotic renal artery degeneration and systemic sepsis caused by an infected renal artery stent. *J Vasc Surg* 1998; **28**: 547–550.
4. Krupski WC, Pogany A, Effeney DJ. Septic endarteritis after percutaneous transluminal angioplasty. *Surgery* 1985; **98**: 359–362.
5. Weibull H, Bergqvist D, Jonsson K *et al*. Complications after percutaneous transluminal angioplasty in the iliac, femoral, and popliteal arteries. *J Vasc Surg* 1987; **5**: 681–686.
6. Frazee BW, Flaherty JP. Septic endarteritis of the femoral artery following angioplasty. *Rev Infect Dis* 1991; **13**: 620–623.

7. McCready RA, Sierys H, Pittman JN *et al*. Septic complications after cardiac catheterization and percutaneous transluminal coronary angioplasty. *J Vasc Surg* 1991; **14**: 170–174.

8. Therasse E, Soulez G, Cartier P *et al*. Infection with fatal outcome after endovascular metallic stent placement. *Radiology* 1994; **192**: 363–365.

9. Liu P, Dravid V, Freiman D *et al*. Persistent iliac endarteritis with pseudoaneurysm formation following balloon-expandable stent placement. *Cardiovasc Intervent Radiol* 1995; **18**: 39–42.

10. Gordon GI, Vogelzang RL, Curry RH *et al*. Endovascular infection after renal artery stent placement. *JVIR* 1996; **7**: 669–672.

11. Deiparine MK, Ballard JL, Taylor FC. Chase DR. Endovascular stent infection. *J Vasc Surg* 1996; **23**: 529–533.

12. Weinberg DJ, Cronin DW, Baker AG. Infected iliac pseudoaneurysm after uncomplicated percutaneous balloon angioplasty and (Palmaz) stent insertion: A case report and literature review. *J Vasc Surg* 1996; **23**: 162–166.

13. Bunt TJ, Hill HK, Smith DC, Taylor FC. Infection of a chronically implanted iliac artery stent. *Ann Vasc Surg* 1997; **11**: 529–532.

14. Kolvenbach R, El Basha M. Secondary rupture of a common iliac artery aneurysm after endovascular exclusion and stent-graft infection [letter]. *J Vasc Surg* 1997; **26**: 351–353.

15. Sheeran SR, Gestring ML, Murphy TP, Slaiby JM. Endovascular graft-related iliac artery infection *JVIR* 1999; **10**: 877–882.

16. Latham JA, Irvine A. Infection of endovascular stents: an uncommon but important complication. *Cardiovasc Surg* 1999; **7**: 179–182.

17. Schachtrupp A, Chalabi K, Fischer U, Herse B. Septic endarteritis and fatal iliac wall rupture after endovascular stenting of the common iliac artery. *Cardiovasc Surg* 1999; **7**: 183–186.

18. Heikkinen L, Valtonen M, Lepantalo M *et al*. Infrarenal endoluminal bifurcated stent graft infected with Listeria monocytogenes. *J Vasc Surg* 1999; **29**: 554–556.

19. Malek AM, Higashida RT, Reilly LM *et al*. Subclavian arteritis and pseudoaneurysm formation secondary to stent infection. *Cardiovasc Intervent Radiol* 2000; **23**: 57–60.

20. Brodmann M, Stark G, Pabst E, Lueger A, Tiesenhausen K, Szolar D, Pilger E. Osteomyelitis of the spine and abscess formation in the left thigh after stent-graft implantation in the superficial femoral artery. *J Endovasc Ther* 2000; **7**: 150–154.

21. Dosluoglu HH, Curl R, Doerr RJ *et al*. Stent-related iliac artery and iliac vein infections: two unreported presentations and reviews of the literature. *J Endovasc Ther* 2001; **8**: 202–209.

22. Culver DA, Chua J, Rehn SJ *et al*. Arterial infection and staphylococcus aureus bacteremia after transfemoral cannulation for percutaneous carotid angioplasty and stenting. *J Vasc Surg* 2002; **35**: 576–579.

23. Eliason JL, Guzman RJ, Passman MA, Naslund TC. Infected endovascular graft secondary to coil embolization of endoleak: a demonstration of the importance of operative sterility. *Ann Vasc Surg* Online publication 19 August 2002.

24. Baker M, Uflacker R, Robison JG. Stent graft infection after abdominal aortic aneurysm repair: a case report. *J Vasc Surg* 2002; **36**: 180–183.

25. Lorentzen JE, Nielsen OM, Arendrup H *et al*. Vascular graft infection: an analysis of 62 graft infections in 2,411 consecutively implanted synthetic vascular grafts. *Surgery* 1985; **98**: 81–86.

26. Fillinger MF, Weaver JB. Imaging equipment and techniques for optimal intraoperative imaging during endovascular interventions. *Sem Vasc Surg* 1999; **12**: 315–326.

Endovascular procedures belong in a sterile operating suite

Against the motion
Anna-Maria Belli

Introduction

Endovascular procedures have been successfully performed for more than 30 years and used to treat a wide range of vascular problems. Foreign materials have been introduced permanently into the vascular system to control haemorrhage since 1975.[1] Permanent vascular implants in the form of stents have been used in clinical practice since the early 1980s[2] followed by stent-grafts in the early 1990s.[3]

Percutaneous vascular embolization and revascularization procedures were traditionally peformed by physicians in radiology suites. The development of stent-grafts capable of excluding aneurysms has led to the transfer of some endovascular procedures to the operating suite because a combined percutaneous and open surgical approach was required.[4]

This practice has continued in some institutions despite the fact that these procedures may be performed entirely percutaneously with the aid of arterial closure devices and immediate conversion to open repair is now rare. The risk of infection in non-sterile angiography suites is an argument often used to defend the use of operating suites to perform endovascular procedures.

Evidence

The UK Registry for Endovascular Treatment of Aneurysms (RETA) reports that, in 1996, 22% of procedures were performed in radiology suites but by 1999 this had increased to 43%. This is because the technique is dependent on good image guidance and there is a very small risk of immediate open conversion. A 0.3% immediate conversion rate to open surgery was reported by RETA in 1999 compared with 9.1% in 1996. Wound infection is reported in 2.5% of cases submitted to RETA but stent-graft infection has been reported in only two of 1381 cases and both these had been performed in a sterile operating theatre. Although the numbers are small and the follow-up of short duration, this compares favourably with surgery where there is evidence of graft infection in 1.3% after open surgical repair and a 1.6% incidence of enteric fistulae with an average time to development of infection of 6 months after surgery.[5]

Infection of endovascular metallic stents and stent-grafts is limited to case reports. The literature contains at least 12 case reports of iliac stent infection[6-14] and further case reports of stent infection at other sites. There are at least six case reports of eight aortic stent-graft infections[15–20] although four of these were complex cases requiring several endovascular or surgical interventions and it is not clear which procedures may have introduced infection. There are undoubtedly other incidences of infected stents or stent-grafts that have not yet been reported and so the true incidence is difficult to ascertain but the numbers are small when the total number of these procedures is taken into consideration. Some of the case reports do not state whether the procedures were performed in an angiography suite or operating theatre but even assuming that they all occurred after placement in a non-sterile environment, the rate of infection is comparable with that of open surgical repair. In fact, some recent reports suggest that endovascular therapy may be a suitable alternative to open surgery in infected fields.[21]

Stent-graft placement is an image-guided intervention. The only open surgical aspect of stent-graft insertion is the common femoral arteriotomy unless this is inadequate for access because of common femoral or iliac occlusive disease. In this situation an open surgical approach on to the iliac artery or abdominal aorta may be required.

Even open arteriotomy is unnecessary as demonstrated by reports that stent-graft placement can be safely performed with percutaneous femoral arterial closure devices.[22] One series reported a reduced wound complication rate using such devices (0.9%) compared with open arteriotomy (3.6%).[23] In these situations there is no open surgery whatsoever, the stent-grafts remain within their packages until the last minute and many remain within a closed delivery sheath until they are ready for deployment within the body.

There is supportive evidence from other interventions that have been safely transferred from sterile operating theatre conditions to non-sterile radiology suites. For example, Hickman central venous catheters are often placed in patients who are immunocompromised and early studies confirmed that the placement of these could be safely transferred to radiology where they could be placed more accurately under image-guidance with no increase in the risk of infective complications.[24] It is now routine practice that these catheters are placed under image-guidance outside sterile operating suites.

The cost implications should also be considered. Digital subtraction angiographic equipment is expensive. Top of the range angiographic equipment costs approximately £800 000, or £240 000 per annum to lease with £20 000 annual services charges. Image-guided endovascular procedures are wide ranging and an interventional radiology service will treat a wide variety of conditions which fall outside the vascular surgical remit. For a hospital to invest in such expensive equipment in the operating theatre, it would have to be used on a daily basis to make it cost-effective. Such equipment would be used more effectively in radiology. If sterile conditions are absolutely essential, it would be much more efficient to make the radiology suite sterile!

Summary

- Endovascular procedures rarely require immediate open conversion.
- Excellent imaging facilities with a range of catheters, guidewires and radiation protection measures are required to encompass all endovascular procedures.
- Endovascular aortic aneurysm repair is still a new and developing technology but reported infection rates are low, despite half the stent-graft procedures being performed in radiology suites.

- Expensive equipment is used more frequently and in a wider variety of endovascular procedures if based in radiology.

- Endovascular procedures belong in an imaging suite, and if necessary it is more cost-effective to make this sterile.

References

1. Gianturco C, Anderson JH, Wallace S. Mechanical devices for arterial occlusion. *Am J Roentgenol Rad Ther Nucl Med* 1975; **124**: 428–435.
2. Sigwart U, Puel J, Mirkovitch V *et al*. Intravascular stents to prevent occlusion and restenosis after transluminal angioplasty. *N Engl J Med* 1987; **316**: 701–706.
3. Parodi JC, Palmaz JC, Barone HD *et al*. Transfemoral intraluminal graft implantation for abdominal aortic aneurysm *Annl Vasc Surg* 1991; 5: 491–499.
4. Schneider PA. Balloon angioplasty and stent placement during operative vascular reconstruction for lower extremity ischaemia. *Annl Vasc Surg* 1996; **10**: 589–598.
5. Hallett JW Jr, Marshall DM, Petterson TM *et al*. Graft-related complications after abdominal aortic aneurysm repair: reassurance from a 36-year population-based experience. *J Vasc Surg* 1997; **25**: 277–284.
6. Chalmers N, Eadington DW, Gandanhamo D *et al*. Case report: infected false aneurysm at the site of an iliac stent. *Br J Radiol* 1993; **66**: 946–948.
7. Therasse E, Soulez G, Cartier P *et al*. Infection with fatal outcome after endovascular metallic stent placement. *Radiology* 1994; **192**: 363–365.
8. Deiparine MK, Ballard JL, Taylor FC, Chase DR. Endovascular stent infection. *J Vasc Surg* 1996; **23**: 529–533.
9. Weinberg DJ, Cronin DW, Baker AG Jr. Infected iliac pseudoaneurysm after uncomplicated percutaneous balloon angioplasty and (Palmaz) stent insertion: a case report and literature review. *J Vasc Surg* 1996; **23**: 162–166.
10. Bunt TJ, Gill HK, Smith DC, Taylor FC. Infection of a chronically implanted iliac artery stent. *Annls Vasc Surg* 1997; **11**, 529–532.
11. Hoffman AI, Murphy TP. Septic arteritis causing iliac artery rupture and aneurysmal transformation of the distal abdominal aorta after iliac artery stent stent placement. *J Vasc Intervent Radiol* 1997; **8**: 215–219.
12. Schachtrupp A, Chalabi K, Fischer U, Herse B. Septic endarteritis and fatal iliac wall rupture after endovascular stenting of the common iliac artery *Cardiovasc Surg* 1999; **17**: 183–186.
13. Latham JA, Irvine A. Infection of endovascular stents: an uncommon but important complication. Cardiovasc Surg 1999; **7**: 179–182.
14. Baker M, Uflacker R, Robison JG. Stent-graft infection after abdominal aortic aneurysm repair: A case report. *J Vasc Surg* 2002; **36**: 180–183.
15. Kolvenbach R, Basha ME. Secondary rupture of a common iliac artery aneurysm after endovascular exclusion and stent graft infection. *J Vasc Surg* 1997; **26**: 351–353.
16. Sheeran SR, Gestring ML, Murphy TP, Slaiby JM. Endovascular graft-related Iliac artery infection. *J Vasc Intervent Radiol* 1999; **10**: 877–882.
17. Heikkinen L, Valtonen M, Lepantalo M, Saimanen E, Jaminen A. Infrarenal endoluminal bifurcated stent graft infected with *Listeria monocytogenes*. *J Vasc Surg* 1999; **29**: 554–556.
18. Matsumara JS, Katzen BT, Hollier LH, Dake MD Update on the bifuracted EXCLUDER endoprosthesis: phase 1 results. *J Vasc Surg* 2001; **33**: S150–153.
19. Eliason JL, Guzman RJ, Passman MA, Naslund TC. Infected endovascular graft secondary to coil embolization of endoleak: A demonstration of the importance of operative sterility. *Annls Vasc Surg* 2002; **16**: 562–565.
20. Dattilo JB, Brewster DC, Fan CM *et al*. Clinical failures of endovascular abdominal aortic aneurysm repair: incidence, causes and management. *J Vasc Surg* 2002; **35**: 1137–1144.
21. Krämer S, Pamler R, Seifarth H *et al*. Endovascular grafting of traumatic aortic aneurysms in contaminated fields. *J Endovasc Ther* 2001; **8**: 262–267.
22. Torsello G, Tessarek J, Kasprzak B, Klenk E. Treatment of aortic aneurysm with a complete percutaneous technique. *Deutsche Med Wochens* 2002; **127**: 1453–1457.

23. Rachel ES, Bergamini TM, Kinney EV *et al.* Percutaneous endovascular abdominal aortic aneurysm repair. *Annl Vasc Surg* 2002; **16**: 43–49.
24. Page AC, Evans RA, Kaczmarski R *et al.* The insertion of chronic indwelling central venous catheters (Hickman lines) in Interventional Radiology suites. *Clin Radiol* 1990; **42**: 105–109.

Endovascular procedures belong in a sterile operating suite

Charing Cross Editorial Comments towards Consensus

Ted Diethrich writes as an endovascular surgeon whose specialty has undergone unprecedented growth. His main argument is that a radiological department does not provide the strict sterile facilities that are required. He refers to reports of infection and sepsis and accepts that the incidence is low.

Anna Maria Belli points to the increase of procedural use in the X-ray departments in the United Kingdom over recent years and acknowledges that the facilities are not sterile but says this does not matter. Her main argument is that the prime requirement is excellent imaging facilities. Normally these are available only in the X-ray department but in an environment such as at the Arizona Heart Hospital, excellent imaging facilities in a sterile environment are available.

Both would accept that excellent imaging facilities in a sterile environment would be ideal but there is often a tussle between either having sterility or excellent imaging facilities. There is also a turf tussle between vascular surgery and vascular radiology but perhaps the greatest tussle ahead lies with the cardiologists.

Roger M Greenhalgh
Editor

The majority of carotid interventions before coronary artery bypass grafting are unnecessary

For the motion
David Bergqvist, Martin Björck,
Björn Kragsterman, Christer Ljungman,
Stefan Thelin

Introduction

There has been a debate with oscillating focus over the last 25 years or so concerning the relationship between carotid endarterectomy (CEA) and coronary artery bypass grafting (CABG). Which one has priority? Has the problem no clinical relevance? The issues have been controversial but increasingly raised. One reason for this may be the increasing age of the CABG population, another the positive results for CEA in randomized studies.[1-4] CABG patients are also more frequently screened preoperatively, whereby sometimes tight carotid artery stenoses are detected, albeit asymptomatic.

There are several principal ways to deal with the combination CEA and CABG: staged CEA before CABG, staged CABG before CEA, simultaneous procedure during the same anaesthesia or just performing CABG without considering CEA. The option to perform the CABG first and CEA on a later occasion but within 10 days should in fact be considered contraindicated, the complication rate in a randomized study versus simultaneous operation being unacceptably high (stroke rate 14.4 versus 2.8%;s (p=0.042).[5] The clinical rationale for performing a CEA before CABG would be to prevent post-CABG embolic neurological complications, originating from the carotid bifurcation.

The purpose of this analysis is to scrutinize the literature for evidence on whether or not performing staged CEA before CABG is of any benefit for the outcome after CABG. Let it be made clear that there are no prospective randomized studies on which to base firm conclusions and clinical guidelines.

The use of carotid angioplasty/stenting will not be discussed as it is still under development, and future studies need to prove its efficacy in the treatment of carotid artery disease.

Neurological complications after CABG

The cause of stroke after CABG is multifactorial and complex, and there are more possible mechanisms for stroke development after CABG than after CEA.

Embolization from atherosclerotic lesions in the aortic arch and/or ascending aorta at cross-clamping is probably the most frequent cause.[6,7] Other causes are embolization related to the extracorporeal circulation, cardiogenic embolization, cerebral ischaemia due to hypoperfusion distal to stenosis within the carotid distribution when a low cardiac output is at hand, intracranial bleeding, cerebral oedema due to hyperperfusion and finally embolization from a lesion in the carotid bifurcation.

The incidence of stroke within 30 days of CABG varies widely between 0.6 and 15.8% or even higher.[6,8-14] In addition to potentially true differences in incidence, there could be several other reasons for this remarkable variation such as study design, patient selection, whether some patients have undergone CEA, heterogenous definitions, speciality of assessor, time for follow-up, many small series with large confidence intervals as well as site specific factors. Furthermore there is also a wide variation between studies on how large a proportion of post-CABG strokes are of carotid embolization origin (6-50%).[7,8,13]

Stroke after CABG increases mortality, morbidity, hospital stay and the need for rehabilitation.[8,13] In the review by Naylor *et al.*[13] the case fatality rate after post-CABG stroke was as high as 23%.

A large number of risk factors for the occurrence of adverse neurological outcome after CABG have been reported, again pointing to the complex aetiology of post-CABG stroke.[6,13,15] The factors are summarized in Table I. It is quite obvious that many of these risk factors cannot be overcome by performing CEA. Probably the most important risk factor is atherosclerosis of the ascending and/or aortic arch.[8,16-19] This view is also supported by autopsy data.[20]

Table 1. Risk factors for the development of post-CABG stroke

Age
Female gender
Diabetes mellitus
Hypertension
Pulmonary disease
Peripheral vascular disease
History of neurological disease (prior stroke/TIA)
Carotid artery disease (stenosis > 50%)
History of CEA
Presence of carotid bruit
Carotid occlusion
Smoking
Use of diuretics
History of excessive alcohol consumption
History of unstable angina
History of CABG
Dysrythmia
Recent myocardial infarction
Cardiac failure
Valve disease
Proximal aortic atherosclerotic lesions
Use of intra-aortic balloon pump
Mural thrombus
Prolonged cardiopulmonary bypass
Prolonged cross-clamping time
Cardioplegia
Difficulty in terminating CABG
Large operative drop in haemoglobin
Use of α-adrenergic drugs

Carotid and coronary artery atherosclerotic disease

As atherosclerosis is a generalized disease it is of no surprise that there may be simultaneous lesions in the carotid and coronary territories. It is known that the long-term survival after CEA is significantly better in the absence of coronary artery disease, myocardial infarction being the leading cause of death during follow-up.[21]

The methodological difficulties when establishing the frequency of carotid artery stenosis in CABG patients have been discussed in a recent review by Naylor et al.[13]

Duplex ultrasonography in patients scheduled for CABG reveals a high prevalence of internal carotid artery stenosis. Up to around 25% of the patients have a >50% stenosis and about half of that proportion (ca 12%) a >80% stenosis.[10,11,22–24] The prevalence of severe stenosis increases with age.[25] The incidence of post-CABG stroke is significantly increased in patients with a carotid artery stenosis.[8,18,26,27] There also seems to be an increasing risk of stroke with increasing degree of carotid artery stenotic disease, the highest risk actually being found in patients with occlusion.[13] In these cases hypoperfusion would seem more important than embolism.

The majority of ultrasonographically detected stenoses is asymptomatic, but stenoses that have caused ipsilateral symptomatology seem to increase the risk for post-CABG stroke.[18,25] Asymptomatic carotid artery disease correlates poorly with stroke after cardiovascular surgery but identifies patients at risk dying postoperatively in myocardial infarction.[28]

The results of carotid interventions before CABG

As stated in the introduction, the optimal timing of CEA before or simultaneously with CABG has not been analysed in any prospective randomized study. Nor has it been analysed whether CEA has any beneficial effect at all in CABG patients. Intuitively, there seems to be a reasonable motivation to perform CEA in patients with a symptomatic high-grade stenosis if their coronary circulation is stable. It must, however, be stated that this attitude has not been shown to decrease the stroke rate after CABG, probably because the properly designed studies have not yet been performed.

In the absence of randomized trials, systematic reviews and/or meta-analyses may help in clinical decision making (Table 2). Borger et al.[29] identified 16 studies with a total of 844 patients undergoing combined surgery and 920 undergoing staged procedures. They concluded that combined CABG and CEA may be associated with a higher risk of stroke and death than staged procedures. However, a significantly higher proportion of patients undergoing combined operation had unstable angina. Moore et al.[30] made a similar meta-analysis of 56 reports and came to the conclusion that the staged strategy is useful in a small number of patients with stable and mild coronary disease to allow for 'unprotected' carotid surgery. However, the frequency of myocardial infarction and death was significantly higher when CEA preceded CABG. In their overview, Das et al.[15] reported that the staged procedures reduced the stroke rate to the price of a non-significant higher mortality. However, in their analysis Das et al. included all series, not only those where the authors themselves had compared the two alternatives.

Table 2. Results of CEA performed before or simultaneously with CABG: meta-analyses and reviews (frequencies are given in percent)

	Staged CEA and CABG			Combined CEA and CABG		
	Death	MI	Stroke	Death	MI	Stroke
Moore et al.[30]	9.4	11.5	5.3	5.6	4.7	6.2
Borger et al.[29]	2.9	5.2	3.2	4.7	4.9	6.0
Das et al.[15]	5.9		1.5	3.8		3.9

MI: myocardial infarction.

It is important to remember that meta-analysis is a scientific methodology with its own values and drawbacks. The best yield is obtained when randomized studies are used in the analysis, when each study is too small to draw firm conclusions. When non-randomized studies are added several problems ensue which have to be considered:

1. small sample size
2. groups from different time periods
3. various selection criteria, clinical or other, that may differ between the groups to be compared
4. different or lack of criteria for myocardial infarction, stroke, site of stroke etc.
5. different definitions of important variables
6. lack of risk factor definition
7. dominance of retrospective data.

Concluding remarks

Thus, when analysing the present day knowledge available in the scientific literature neither treatment strategy has been proven to be superior. This means that every single case has to be treated on its own merits in the actual clinical situation. It seems appropriate to use the grades of evidence suggested, to be included when discussing practical guidelines in vascular and endovascular surgery:[31]

1. Beyond any reasonable doubt.
2. On the balance of probabilities.
3. Not proven.

On the basis of evidence thus obtained there are three grades of recommendations. A strong recommendation must be followed and acting otherwise must be compellingly motivated. A recommendation can be made on the basis of evidence but there may be factors which influence the choice of treatment strategy such as health economy, local audit, patient preferences etc. A recommendation may also be suggested, where there is no scientific evidence supporting it, but other reasons are in favour of the recommendation. So far no solid scientific arguments support staged CEA before CABG, but on the other hand there may be individual patients where this treatment option seems reasonable.

The management of patients who are to undergo CABG and who also have carotid artery stenosis is therefore still controversial and debated. Various potential therapeutic options exist. In the absence of randomized studies comparing staged CEA before CABG with either simultaneous surgery or only CABG, the collected data from the literature do not lend support to performing CEA before CABG. There does not seem to be a beneficial effect on either neurological morbidity or mortality. This is said in full awareness of the difficulties comparing the existing data where various selection mechanisms have been involved with risk of bias and false conclusions. To overcome this lack of knowledge a randomized study would be of help. Ideally a randomized trial should be performed on an intention-to-treat basis with independent outcome assessors. If we first presume that half of the post-CABG neurological complications are of carotid artery origin, second that staged CEA before CABG would reduce these complications by 50%, and third if we use the stroke rate of 6.0% in the combined CEA and CABG group as indicated in the meta-analysis of Borger et al.,[29] the randomized study would need a population of around 4000 patients (reduction of carotid stroke rate from 3.0 to 1.5%; α 0.05, β 90%) or of around 9000 patients (reduction of the total stroke rate from 6.0 to 4.5%). If the initial stroke rate is lower than 6%, all other assumptions being equal, the study population has to be even larger. This is true also if the proportion of emboli of carotid bifurcation origin is substantially lower than 50% as suggested by Borger et al.[7] and Naylor et al.[13] – a formidable undertaking not without logistic problems!

Evidence

The scientific evidence today is not strong enough to recommend CEA before CABG on a routine basis, either in all symptomatic or in asymptomatic patients. To summarize, the pro for a staged procedure is reduction of post-CABG stroke risk, and the cons are the necessity of two anaesthesias in a rather short time span, longer total hospital stay with higher cost, the high number needed to treat to prevent one stroke (especially in patients with asymptomatic carotid artery stenosis), risk for coronary complications between the first and the second operation, and most important – the lack of scientific evidence in favour of the staged procedure. At least theoretically, the first operation (CEA) may induce a coagulation activation, which increases the risk of thromboembolic complications at the second operation. Awaiting further evidence, every centre dealing with this problem has to audit their results carefully. In patients with an indication for CABG and symptoms from a carotid artery stenosis, we have chosen the simultaneous approach, which is convenient for the patient and economically beneficial in saving hospital beds.

Summary

- Stroke after CABG is multifactorial, embolization from carotid artery bifurcation being one cause.
- CEA before CABG versus simultaneous operation is controversial.
- There are no randomized studies helping to resolve this controversy.
- Meta-analyses and reviews are partly contradictory.
- Randomized controlled trials are necessary but logistically difficult to perform and need a large sample size.
- So far individual decision making is necessary.

References

1. ACAS. Clinical advisory: carotid endarterectomy for patients with asymptomatic internal carotid artery stenosis. *Stroke* 1994; 25: 2523–2524.

2. ECST. Randomised trial of endarterectomy for recently symptomatic carotid stenosis: final results of the MRC European Carotid Surgery Trial (ECST). *Lancet* 1998; 35: 1379–1387.

3. Barnett H, Taylor D, Eliasziw M *et al.* Benefit of carotid endarterectomy in patients with symptomatic moderate or severe stenosis. North American Symptomatic Carotid Endarterectomy Trial Collaborators. *N Eng J Med* 1998; 339: 1415–1425.

4. Ferguson G, Eliasziw M, Barr H *et al.* The North American Symptomatic Carotid Endarterectomy Trial: surgical results in 1415 patients. *Stroke* 1999; 30: 1751–1758.

5. Hertzer N, Loop F, Beven E *et al.* Surgical staging for simultaneous coronary and carotid disease: a study including prospective randomization. *J Vasc Surg* 1989; 9: 455–463.

6. Roach G, Manchuger M, Mangano M *et al.* Adverse cerebral outcomes after coronary bypass surgery. *N Engl J Med* 1996; 335: 1857–1863.

7. Borger M, Ivanov J, Weisel R *et al.* Stroke during coronary bypass surgery; principal role of cerebral macroemboli. *Eur J Cardiothorac Surg* 2001; 19: 627–632.

8. Borger M, Fremes S. Management of patients with concomitant coronary and carotid vascular disease. *Sem Thoracic Cardiovasc* 2001; 13: 192–198.

9. Cambria R, Ivarsson B, Akins C *et al.* Simultaneous carotid and coronary disease: safety of the combined approach. *J Vasc Surg* 1989; 9: 56–64.

10. Gerraty R, Gates P, Doyle J. Carotid stenosis and perioperative stroke risk in symptomatic and asymptomatic patients undergoing vascular or coronary surgery. *Stroke* 1993; 24: 1115–1118.

11. Brener B, Herman H, Eisenbud D *et al.* The management of patients requiring coronary bypass and carotid endarterectomy. In: *Surgery For Cerebrovascular Disease.* Wesley Moore (ed). London: Saunders, 1996.

12. Roddy S, Darling R, Abrishamchian A *et al.* Combined coronary artery bypass with carotid endarterectomy: Do women have worse outcome? *J Vasc Surg* 2002; 36: 555–558.

13. Naylor A, Mehta Z, Rothwell P, Bell P. Carotid artery disease and stroke during coronary artery bypass; a critical review of the literature. *Eur J Vasc Endovasc Surg* 2002; 23: 283–294.

14. Ivey T. Combined carotid and coronary disease – a conservative strategy. *J Vasc Surg* 1986; 3: 687–689.

15. Das S, Brow T, Pepper J. Continuing controversy in the management of concomitant coronary and carotid disease: an overview. *Int J Cardiol* 2000; 74: 47–65.

16. Gaudino M, Glieca F, Alessandrini F *et al.* Individualized surgical strategy for the reduction of stroke risk in patients undergoing coronary artery bypass grafting. *Ann Thorac Surg* 1999; 67: 1246–1253.

17. Rizzo R, Whitmore A, Couper G *et al.* Combined carotid and cornary revascularization: the preferred approach to the severe vasculopathy. *Ann Thorac Surg* 1992; 15: 1099.

18. D'Agustino R, Svensson L, Neumann D *et al.* Screening carotid ultrasonography and risk factors for stroke in coronary artery surgery patients. *Ann Thorac Surg* 1996; 62: 1714–1723.

19. Nussmeier N. A review of risk factors for adverse neurologic outcome after cardiac surgery. *JECT* 2002; 34: 4–10.

20. Blauth C, Cosgrove D, Webb B *et al.* Atheroembolism from the ascending aorta. An emerging problem in cardiac surgery. *J Thorac Cardiovasc Surg* 1992; 103: 1104–112.

21. Forssell C, Takolander R, Bergqvist D *et al.* Long-term results after carotid artery surgery. *Eur J Vasc Surg* 1988; 2: 93–98.

22. Ricotta J, Faggioli G, Castilone A, Hassett J. Risk factors for stroke after cardiac surgery: Buffalo Cardiac-Cerebral Study Group. *J Vasc Surg* 1995; 21: 359–364.

23. Schwartz L, Bridgman A, Kieffer R, Wilcox R, McCann R, Tawil M, et al. Asymptomatic carotid artery stenosis and stroke in patients undergoing cardiopulmonary bypass. *J Vasc Surg* 1995; 2: 146–153.

24. Ricotta J. The approach to patients with carotid bifurcation disease in need of coronaty bypass grafting. *Semin Vasc Surg* 1995; 8: 62–69.

25. Berens E, Kouchoukos N, Murphy S, Wareing T. Preoperative carotid artery screening in elderly patients undergoing cardiac surgery. *J Vasc Surg* 1992; 15: 313–323.

26. Bilfinger T, Reda H, Giron F, Seifert F, Ricotta J. Coronary and carotid operations under prospective standardized conditions: Incidence and outcome. *Ann Thorac Surg* 2000; 69: 1792–1798.

27. Faggioli G, Curl G, Ricotta J. The role of carotid screening before coronary artery bypass. *J Vasc Surg* 1990; 12: 724–729.

28. Barnes R, Marszalek P. Asymptomatic carotid disease in the cardiovascular surgical patient: is prophylactic endarterectomy necessary? *Stroke* 1981; **12**: 497–500.
29. Borger M, Fremes S, Weisel R *et al.* Coronary bypass and carotid endarterectomy: Does a combined approach increase risk? A metaanalysis. *Ann Thorac Surg* 1999; **68**: 14–21.
30. Moore W, Barnett H, Beebe H *et al.* Guidelines for carotid endarterectomy. A multidisciplinary consensus statement from the ad hoc committee, American Heart Association. *Circulation* 1995; **91**: 566–579.
31. Beard J, Gaines P. *Vascular and Endovascular Surgery* 2nd edn. London: Saunders, 2001.

The majority of carotid interventions before coronary artery bypass grafting are unnecessary

Against the motion
Rachel E Bell, Peter R Taylor

Introduction

Stroke is a devastating complication of coronary artery bypass surgery and is associated with significant mortality (21%).[1] In the last 20 years improvements in perioperative care have led to an overall reduction in the morbidity and mortality following myocardial revascularization. However, the incidence of postoperative stroke has remained unchanged (2%).[2] With the advent of minimally invasive techniques such as coronary angioplasty and stenting, surgical revascularization is limited to patients with severe coronary artery disease. In addition, there has been a significant increase in patients aged over 65 undergoing coronary artery bypass grafting (CABG).[3] Both of these groups of patients have a higher risk of perioperative stroke following CABG. Gardener *et al.* noted that for patients less than 45 years of age undergoing CABG the incidence of stroke was 0.2% and rose to 8.0% for patients over 75.[4] Tuman *et al.* reported an exponential increase in the stroke risk after the age of 65 (0.9% versus 9.9%).[5]

The causes of perioperative stroke are multifactorial and include: emboli from an atherosclerotic ascending aorta or carotid artery,[6,7] ventricular mural thrombi,[8,9] microembolization of air, fat or platelet aggregates formed during cardiopulmonary bypass,[8] hypoperfusion secondary to cerebrovascular disease or perioperative hypotension and more rarely, intracranial haemorrhage.

Studies have shown that the majority of neurological events that occur after CABG are embolic in origin and not related to low flow rates.[10] It is well recognized that cerebral autoregulation is disordered during cardiac bypass so that cerebral blood flow is directly proportional to perfusion pressure. This failure of autoregulation is particularly severe in patients who have suffered previous cerebral infarction.[11] Pump flow rates can be altered to maintain a perfusion pressure of >70 mmHg to avoid cerebral hypoperfusion.

Carotid artery disease can cause perioperative stroke in three ways; emboli arising from carotid plaque, thrombotic occlusion or by contributing to cerebral hypoperfusion.

What do we know?

1. No randomized trial exists.

2. Only a small proportion of patients undergoing CABG have significant carotid artery disease (3.2–8.7%).[9,12]

What is unclear?

1. Do patients with asymptomatic carotid disease have an increased risk of perioperative stroke following CABG?
2. Is there any benefit in performing prophylactic carotid endarterectomy (CEA) either in the perioperative period or the long term?
3. When should this operation be performed?

These questions can be answered by the evidence given below.

Prevalence of carotid disease in population undergoing CABG

The advent of non-invasive carotid duplex imaging has provided information regarding the prevalence of carotid disease in patients requiring cardiac surgery. The reported incidence of significant carotid disease (>75% stenosis) varies from 3.2 to 8.7% (Table 1),[9,12–15] of which the majority (70%) are asymptomatic.[16] The prevalence of significant carotid disease increases with age: 3.8 % in patients aged <60 years, rising to 11.3% for those aged >60.[9] A policy of screening all patients prior to CABG is controversial in view of the low prevalence of carotid disease. Certain groups have advocated screening for all patients and others have limited it to those thought to be at highest risk. Multivariate analysis has shown that lower limb arterial disease, female sex, age, left main stem disease, previous transient ischaemic attack or stroke are all predictors of significant carotid disease (>80%).[14]

Table 1. Prevalence of significant carotid disease in patients undergoing CABG

Series	Unilateral stenosis	Bilateral stenosis	Unilateral stenosis and occlusion	Total
Saladis et al.[13]	3.6%	0.5%	0.5%	4.6%
Berens et al.[14]	3.2%	1%	0.6%	4.8%
Safa et al.[15]	6.4%	1.5%	0.5%	8.4%
Brener et al.[17]	2.1%	0.6%	0.3%	3.0%

Relationship between carotid artery disease and perioperative stroke

Many studies have shown increased postoperative stroke rates in patients with carotid artery disease.[9,14,17] Logistic regression analysis has shown that significant carotid stenosis is the most powerful predictor of perioperative stroke in patients undergoing CABG.[18] Brener et al. reported a 9.2% overall stroke rate in patients undergoing CABG with >50% carotid stenosis and a 20% stroke rate in patients with a carotid stenosis >50% and a contralateral occlusion.[17] Dashe et al. performed preoperative duplex in 224 patients with previous neurological symptoms or a carotid bruit. Half of the patients with 70–99% carotid stenosis had a perioperative stroke and all strokes were ipsilateral to the carotid disease.[19]

Faggioli *et al.* reported that the postoperative risk of stroke was highest in patients with carotid stenoses of >75% compared with rates for people with normal carotid arteries, stenoses of <75% or patients who had simultaneous CEA.[9] The patients who had the highest risk of perioperative stroke were those with; symptomatic carotid disease, asymptomatic bilateral carotid stenosis >80%, asymptomatic carotid stenosis >80% with a contralateral occlusion. Hertzer *et al.* observed a stroke rate of 7.35% in patients with severe bilateral carotid disease compared with 0.94% in patients with unilateral disease.[20] These associations have led to recommendations for staged or combined CEA for patients with significant carotid disease undergoing CABG. In addition, several studies have demonstrated a higher mortality rate (9–13%) for patients with significant carotid disease when compared with patients with no carotid disease (1–4%).[17,21]

Evidence for surgery for symptomatic carotid disease/CABG

It has been well established that patients with symptomatic carotid disease should be treated surgically. Two randomized controlled trials have shown a statistically significant advantage for surgical endarterectomy compared with medical treatment.[22,23] This benefit is seen in terms of freedom from any stroke, any ipsilateral stroke and any stroke or death in patients with symptomatic carotid stenosis >50% by NASCET criteria, the benefit increasing with the degree of stenosis. Carotid surgery should therefore be offered to patients who require coronary revascularization and have symptomatic carotid disease. Rizzo *et al.* reported a stroke rate of 8.2% for patients with symptomatic carotid disease compared with 4.1% for patients with asymptomatic carotid stenosis.[24]

Evidence for surgery for asymptomatic carotid disease/CABG

The risk of stroke in patients with asymptomatic carotid stenosis >60% is about 2% per year (Asymptomatic Carotid Atherosclerosis Study, ACAS).[25] This trial reported that the aggregate risk of ipsilateral stroke and any stroke and death at 5 years was 5.1% for surgical patients and 11.0% for the medical patients. This represented a relative risk reduction of 53% and an absolute risk reduction of 5.9%. In 1993 the Veterans Affairs Cooperative study group reported a significant reduction in the overall incidence of ipsilateral neurological events after CEA in asymptomatic patients with a >50% carotid stenosis.[26] A further meta-analysis of data from all available randomized trials has confirmed a definite benefit of CEA in preventing ipsilateral ischaemic stroke and stroke in any location.[27] Results showing an increased risk of stroke with significant asymptomatic carotid disease are the rationale for performing CEA either prior to or as a combined procedure with CABG. The American guidelines support the practice of CEA for asymptomatic stenoses >60% prior to CABG.[28] The multicentre, randomized Asymptomatic Carotid Surgery Trial (ACST) is still recruiting and the results may well help to clarify this issue.

Timing of CEA

The evidence clearly shows that carotid stenosis increases the risk of stroke during coronary artery bypass surgery. Although logically carotid intervention should be performed before myocardial revascularization, the options are staged (before CABG), combined (or synchronous) CABG and reverse staged CEA (after CABG).

Combined CEA and CABG

Simultaneous carotid/coronary surgery is recommended for patients with unstable angina, left main stem disease or diffuse multi-vessel coronary artery disease with significant carotid disease. The benefits of the combined approach are: decreased anaesthetic time, shorter hospital stay and significant cost saving.[29] The published stroke and mortality rates for combined procedures are summarized in Table 2.[30-44] Schwartz *et al.* reported 37% incidence of left main stem disease in patients having combined CEA and CABG.[45] Clearly, for the CEA to be effective, this needs to be performed before the institution of cardiac bypass.

CEA prior to CABG (staged)

In patients with stable cardiac disease performing the CEA prior to CABG is an option. Improvements in perioperative care have led to a reduction in the number of cardiac events in patients undergoing carotid surgery. The Texas Heart Institute reported a 2% stroke rate and a 3% mortality rate from staged CEA/CABG in patients with stable cardiac disease. These figures are comparable with combined carotid and cardiac surgery.

Table 2. Stroke and death rates for combined carotid and coronary surgery

Series	Year	Number	Death rate	Stroke rate
Jones *et al.*[8]	1984	132	3	1.6
Babu *et al.*[30]	1985	62	4.8	1.6
Reul *et al.*[31]	1986	143	4.2	2.8
Dunn *et al.*[32]	1986	130	4.6	10
Hertzer *et al.*[20]	1989	170	5.3	7.1
Minami *et al.*[12]	1989	116	1.7	4.3
Cambria *et al.*[33]	1989	71	2	2
Rizzo *et al.*[24]	1992	127	5.5	5.6
Vermeulen *et al.*[34]	1992	230	3.5	5.6
Kaul *et al.*[35]	1994	175	3.4	4
Chang *et al.*[36]	1994	189	2	1
Halpin *et al.*[37]	1994	133	0.8	2.3
Akins *et al.*[38]	1995	200	3.5	3
Mackey *et al.*[39]	1996	100	8.0	9.0
Daily *et al.*[29]	1996	100	4	0
Trachiotis *et al.*[40]	1997	88	3.4	4.5
Darling *et al.*[16]	1998	470	2.4	1
Donatelli *et al.*[41]	1998	70	10	0
Terramani *et al.*[42]	1998	30	3.3	0
Bilfinger *et al.*[43]	2000	84	5.9	4.7
Bornardelli *et al.*[44]	2002	64	6.2	0

CEA after CABG (reverse-staged)

Delayed CEA has gone out of favour as several studies have shown that the overall stroke risk is higher (up to 14%) as there is a risk of stroke during the CABG and from the delayed CEA.[20] This is a powerful argument for performing carotid intervention before myocardial revascularization.

Late results

Several studies have confirmed that CEA at the time of CABG measurably reduces the incidence of late stroke in patients with carotid artery disease (91% stroke-free survival at 5years).[20,24,38] In addition Barnes et al. showed that patients with asymptomatic carotid stenosis who have CABG alone have a 33% incidence of a neurological event in the first 3 years after surgery.[21]

Future

'Off-pump' coronary revascularization

CABG without cardiac bypass has been shown to have very favourable results particularly in the elderly. In addition the perioperative stroke rate for 'off-pump' surgery has been significantly lower than that for conventional bypass surgery (0% versus 9.3%).[47]

Carotid angioplasty and stenting

Carotid angioplasty has yet to gain widespread acceptance due to concerns about procedural embolization. However, recent results of carotid stenting using cerebral protection devices have demonstrated that it is possible to perform this procedure safely without the risk of embolic stroke (stroke rate = 4% but all were due to haemorrhagic events).[48] Carotid angioplasty with cerebral protection is currently being compared with CEA in randomized controlled trials. If angioplasty is shown to be of equivalent efficacy, then the arguments for carotid intervention before coronary revascularization become stronger as, theoretically, angioplasty should be associated with fewer myocardial complications than surgical endarterectomy.

Conclusions

Following the Bristol enquiry into perioperative deaths in paediatric cardiac surgery, all cardiothoracic surgeons in the UK have been audited and the results of their surgery published. The audited index operation is first time coronary artery bypass surgery and patients who die from stroke will contribute to adverse statistics. All cardiothoracic surgeons would be well advised to investigate the carotid arteries as described above, and to intervene before revascularizing the coronary circulation. The evidence clearly suggests that carotid intervention should be performed before CABG, and many recent reports of 0-1% stroke rate confirm that this procedure can be performed safely.[16,41,42,44]

Summary

- The prevalence of carotid disease in patients undergoing CABG varies between 3.2 and 8.7%, but increases with age and the severity of coronary disease.

- The most powerful predictor of perioperative stroke during coronary artery bypass surgery is ipsilateral carotid artery stenosis.

- The risk of stroke is highest in patients with symptomatic disease, and asymptomatic patients also have an increased risk.

- The following patients benefit from carotid intervention prior to myocardial revascularization:

  – Symptomatic carotid stenosis >50%

  – Asymptomatic carotid stenosis >70% + a contralateral occlusion

  – Asymptomatic bilateral carotid stenoses > 80%

  – Asymptomatic unilateral carotid stenosis >60%.

- Combined carotid and cardiac surgery can be performed safely.

- If carotid angioplasty with cerebral protection is shown to be of equivalent efficacy to CEA with regard to stroke and death, then it may become the treatment of choice in patients requiring myocardial revascularization.

References

1. Roach GW, Kanchuger M, Mangano CM *et al.* Adverse cerebral outcomes after coronary bypass surgery. *N Eng J Med* 1996; **335**: 1857–1864.
2. Naylor AR, Mehta Z, Rothwell PM, Bell PRF. Carotid artery disease and stroke during coronary artery bypass: a critical review of the literature. *Eur J Vasc Endovasc Surg* 2002; **23**: 283–294.
3. Disch DL, O'Connor GT, Birkmeyer JD *et al.* Changes in patients undergoing coronary artery bypass grafting: 1987–1990. Northern New England Cardiovascular Disease Study Group. *Ann Thorac Surg* 1994; **57**: 416–423.
4. Gardner TJ, Horneffer PJ, Manolio TA *et al.* Major stroke after coronary artery bypass surgery: Changing magnitude of the problem. *J Vasc Surg* 1986; **3**: 684–687.
5. Tuman KJ, McCarthy RJ, Nafaji H, Ivankovitch AD. Differential effects of advanced age on neurologic and cardiac risks of coronary artery operations. *J Thorac Cardiovasc Surg* 1992; **104**: 1510–1517.
6. Bar-El Y, Goor GA. Clamping of the atherosclerotic ascending aorta during coronary artery bypass operations: its cost in stroke. *J Thorac Cardiovasc Surg* 1992; **104**: 469–474.
7. Breslau PJ, Fell G, Ivey TD *et al.* Carotid arterial disease in patients undergoing coronary artery bypass operations. *J Thorac Cardiovasc Surg* 1981; **82**: 765–767.
8. Jones EL, Michalik RA, Murphy DA *et al.* Combined carotid and coronary operations: when are they necessary? *J Thorac Cardiovasc Surg* 1984; **87**: 7–16.
9. Faggioli GL, Curl GR, Ricotta. The role of carotid screening before coronary artery bypass. *J Vasc Surg* 1990; **12**: 724–731.
10. Furlau AJ, Brener AC. Central nervous system complications of open heart surgery. *Stroke* 1984; **15**: 912–915.
11. Lundar T, Lindegaard K, Frysaker T *et al.* Disassociation between cerebral autoregulation and carbon dioxide reactivity during non-pulsatile cardiopulmonary bypass. *Ann Thorac Surg* 1985; **40**: 582–587.
12. Minami K, Sagoo S, Breymann T *et al.* Operative strategy in combined coronary and carotid disease. *J Thorac Cardiovasc Surg* 1988; **95**: 303–309.

13. Salasidis GC, Latter DA, Steinmetz OK et al. Carotid artery duplex scanning in preoperative assessment for coronary artery revascularisation: The association between peripheral vascular disease, carotid artery stenosis, and stroke. J Vasc Surg 1995; 21: 154–162.

14. Berens ES, Kouchoukos NT, Murphy SF, Wareing TH. Preoperative carotid artery screening in elderly patients undergoing cardiac surgery. J Vasc Surg 1992; 15: 313–323.

15. Safa TK, Friedman S, Mehta M et al. Management of co-existing coronary artery disease and asymptomatic carotid artery disease: report on a series of patients treated with coronary artery bypass alone. Eur J Vasc Endovasc Surg 1999; 17: 249–252.

16. Darling RC III, Dylewski M, Chang BB et al. Combined carotid endarterectomy and coronary artery bypass grafting does not increase the risk of postoperative stroke. Cardiovasc Surg 1998; 6: 448–452.

17. Brener BJ, Brief DK, Alpert J et al. The risk of stroke in patients with asymptomatic carotid stenosis undergoing cardiac surgery: A follow-up study. J Vasc Surg 1987; 5: 269–279.

18. Ricotta JJ, Faggioli GL, Castilone A, Hassett JM. Risk factors for stroke after cardiac surgery: Buffalo Cardiac-Cerebral Study Group. J Vasc Surg 1995; 21: 359–364.

19. Dashe JF, Pessin MS, Murphy RE, Payne DD. Carotid occlusive disease and stroke risk in coronary artery bypass graft surgery. Neurol 197; 49: 678–686.

20. Hertzer NR, Loop FD, Beven EG et al. Surgical staging for simultaneous coronary and carotid disease; a study including prospective randomisation. J Vasc Surg 1989; 9: 455–463.

21. Barnes RW, Liebman PR, Marszalek PB et al. The natural history of asymptomatic carotid disease in patients undergoing cardiovascular surgery. Surgery 1981; 90: 1075.

22. European Carotid Surgery Trialists'Collaborative Group. Randomised trial of endarterectomy for recently symptomatic carotid stenosis: final results of the MRC European Carotid Surgery Trial. Lancet 1998; 351: 1379–1387.

23. North American Symptomatic Carotid Endarterectomy Trial Collaborators. Beneficial effect of carotid endarterectomy in symptomatic patients with high-grade stenosis. N Eng J Med 1991; 325: 445–453.

24. Rizzo R, Whittemore AD, Couper GS et al. Combined carotid and coronary revascularisation: the preferred approach to the severe vasculopath. Ann Thorac Surg 1992; 54: 1099–1109.

25. Executive Committee for Asymptomatic Carotid Atherosclerosis Study. Endarterectomy for asymptomatic carotid artery stenosis. JAMA 1995; 273: 1421–1428.

26. Hobson RW II, Weiss DG, Fields WS et al. Efficacy of carotid endarterectomy for asymptomatic carotid stenosis. The Veterans Affairs Cooperative Study Group. N Eng J Med 1993; 328: 221–227.

27. Benavente O, Moher D, Pham B. Carotid endarterectomy for asymptomatic carotid stenosis: a meta-analysis. Br Med J 1998; 317: 1477–1480.

28. Biller J, Feinberg WM, Castaldo JE et al. Guidelines for carotid endarterectomy. A statement for healthcare professionals from a special writing group of the stroke council, American Heart Association. Stroke 1998; 29: 554–562.

29. Daily PO, Freeman RK, Dembitsky WP et al. Cost reduction by combined carotid endarterectomy and coronary artery bypass grafting. J Thorac Cardiovasc Surg 1996; 111: 1185–1193.

30. Babu SC, Shah PM, Singh BM et al. Coexisting carotid stenosis in patients undergoing cardiac surgery: indications and guidelines for simultaneous operations. Am J Surg 1985; 150: 207–211.

31. Reul GJ Jr, Cooley DA, Duncan JM et al. The effect of coronary bypass on the outcome of peripheral vascular operations in 1093. J Vasc Surg 1986; 3: 788–798.

32. Dunn EJ. Concomitant cerebral and myocardial revascularisation. Surg Clin North Am 1986; 66: 385–395.

33. Cambria RP, Ivarsson BL, Atkins CW et al. Simultaneous carotid and coronary disease: Safety of the combined approach. J Vasc Surg 1989; 9: 56–64.

34. Vermeulen FE, Hamerlijnck RP, Defauw JJ et al. Synchronous operation for ischaemic cardiac and cerebrovascular disease: early results and long-term follow-up. Am Thorac Surg 1992; 53: 381–390.

35. Kaul TK, Fields BL, Wyatt DA et al. Surgical management in patients with coexistent coronary and cerebrovascular disease. Chest 1994; 106: 1349–1357.

36. Chang BB, Darling C III, Shah DM et al. Carotid endarterectomy can be safely performed with acceptable mortality and morbidity in patients requiring coronary artery bypass grafts. Am J Surg 1994; 168: 94–96.

37. Halpin DP, Riggins S, Carmichael JD et al. Management of coexistent carotid and coronary disease. Southern Med J 1994; 87: 187–189.

38. Akins CW. Combined Carotid Endarterectomy and Coronary Revascularisation Operation. Ann Thorac Surg 1998; 66: 1483–1484.

39. Mackey WC, Khabbaz K, Bojar R *et al.* Simultaneous carotid endarterectomy and coronary bypass: perioperative risk and long-term survival. *J Vasc Surg* 1996; **24**: 58–64.

40. Trachiotis GD, Pfister AJ. Management strategy for simultaneous carotid endarterectomy and coronary revascularisation. *Ann Thorac Surg* 1997; **64**: 1013–1018.

41. Donatelli F, Pelenghi S, Pocar M *et al.* Combined carotid and cardiac procedures: improved results and surgical approach. *Cardiovascular Surgery* 1998; **6**: 506–510.

42. Terramani TT, Rowe VL, Hood DB *et al.* Combined carotid endarterectomy and coronary artery bypass grafting in asymptomatic carotid artery stenosis. *Am Surg* 1998; **64**: 993–997.

43. Bilfinger TV, Reda H, Giron F *et al.* Combined carotid operations under prospective standardized conditions: Incidence and outcome. *Ann Thorac Surg* 2000; **69**: 1792–1728.

44. Bonardelli S Portolani N, Tiberio GA *et al.* Combined surgical approach for carotid and coronary stenosis. Sixty-four patients and review of literature. *J Cardiovasc Surg* 2002; **43**: 385–390.

45. Schwartz LB, Bridgman AH, Kieffer RW *et al.* Asymptomatic carotid artery stenosis and stroke in patients undergoing cardiopulmonary bypass. *J Vasc Surg* 1995; **21**: 146–153.

46. Bernhard VM, Johnson WD, Petersen JJ. Carotid artery stenosis associated with surgery for coronary artery disease. *Arch Surg* 1972; **105**: 837–840.

47. Ricci M, Karamanoukian HL, Abraham R *et al.* Stroke in octogenarians undergoing coronary artery surgery with and without cardiopulmonary bypass. *Ann Thorac Surg* 2000; **69**: 1471–1475.

48. Macdonald S, Venables GS, Cleveland TJ, Gaines PA. Protected carotid stenting: safety and efficacy of the MedNova Neuroshield filter. *J Vasc Surg* 2002; **35**: 966–972.

The majority of carotid interventions before coronary artery bypass grafting are unnecessary

Charing Cross Editorial Comments towards Consensus

The outcome of this debate may be based on numbers. There can be little doubt that carotid endarectomy (CEA) for a symptomatic lesion must be performed before coronary artery bypass grafting (CABG). The possible exception is for patients with unstable angina where the opposers argue that a combined carotid and coronary procedure could have merit. Certainly an anaesthetist would be concerned about operating on a CEA patient who also has unstable angina. The mortality risk of that carotid procedure would be greatly increased. Often the unstable angina can be corrected without CABG so the combined procedure may not be indicated frequently.

The proposers argue for a lack of evidence in terms of random controlled trial and meta-analysis and argue that the decision taken should be a local decision because the evidence is not absolute. This is the mainstay of their argument that many carotid interventions before CABG are unnecessary.

The opposition lean heavily on the ACAS study which failed to give a clear result in terms of stroke without warning. They state honestly that the Asymptomatic Carotid Surgery Trial results are awaited and surely this implies that there is uncertainty whether asymptomatic carotid arterial disease should be operated upon or not.

The logic would seem to be to submit every asymptomatic carotid surgical patient to random allocation trial until a result is known. We are then likely to know whether the majority of carotid interventions before CABG are unnecessary, but that is the future.

What about the present? Many asymptomatic procedures are clearly performed without strong evidence, which is anxiously awaited.

Roger M Greenhalgh
Editor

Carotid stenting should always be performed with cerebral protection

For the motion
PA Gaines

Introduction

The currently available published Level 1 data support the concept that carotid artery stenting is an effective alternative to carotid endarterectomy in patients with symptomatic high-grade carotid stenosis.[1-3] Despite the prophylactic intent of the treatment both techniques have a peri-procedural stroke and death rate. It is likely that the majority of cerebral ischaemic episodes following carotid artery stenting are due to cerebral embolization. In more than 90% of treatment episodes, emboli are detected by transcranial Doppler.[4] Even so, defined cerebral ischaemia shown by magnetic resonance diffusion-weighted imaging occurs in 15–29% of cases on the ipsilateral side.[5 6] These changes are not limited to carotid artery stenting, ipsilateral diffusion-weighted imaging lesions have also been found following carotid endarterectomy in 34% of cases.[7] It would appear then that the embolic burden to the brain is much higher than can be defined by simple clinical outcome. It would seem prudent therefore to restrict all embolization to the brain during carotid artery stenting.

Question 1

Do cerebral protection systems capture emboli?

Using the system of temporary balloon occlusion Henry and colleagues found debris in all 183 patients treated with the Guardwire system.[8] An average of 74 particles per patient were found, measuring 56-2652 microns (μ) in diameter. Using the AngioGuard filter system Angelina and colleagues found debris in 84% of their 38 patients with particles measuring 1-5043 μ in diameter with an average number of 33.7 plus or minus 5.6 particles.[9] Using the Neuroshield system, macroscopic particles were found in 35% of filters.[10]

Question 2

Do cerebral protection systems reduce neuroembolic complication following carotid artery stenting compared with patients treated without cerebral protection?

Transcranial Doppler shows a significant reduction (p=0.002) of microembolic signals to the middle cerebral artery in patients protected compared with those who are not.[11]

Our own article (in press) shows that in 75 patients treated with cerebral protection compared with 75 patients treated without cerebral protection, the all stroke and death rate fell from 10.7% to 4% and the death and major disabling stroke rate fell from 6.7% to 2.7% in the protected group.

The World Registry collected by Wholey (personal communication) shows that in symptomatic patients the procedural stroke and death rate can be reduced from 5.86% to 2.8% using cerebral protection.

In the UK National Registry the rate of death and disabling stroke fell from 3.4% to 2.08% when cerebral protection was used, and the death and all stroke rate fell from 6.8% to 3.47%.

Can we predict those patients who will benefit form cerebral protection?

The data available to predict which patients will release most emboli are contradictory. When debris is collected using temporary balloon occlusion, Henry showed that hypoechoic plaques released the greater number of particles, but hyperechoic plaque produced the larger debris.[8] However, in an *ex-vivo* model Ohki and colleagues demonstrated that echolucent plaque released a higher number of particles than echogenic plaque.[12] Henry could not find an association with the degree of stenosis and yet Ohki could.

Neither is it reasonable to stent asymptomatic patients on the presumption that the plaque is less friable. These patients still release emboli and still have adverse neurological events following stent placement without cerebral protection.

Summary

- Carotid artery stenting is associated with neuroembolic complications.
- Cerebral protection systems are capable of collecting atheromatous debris during the stenting procedure.
- The number of neuroembolic complications is reduced when using a cerebral protection system.
- We cannot define a sub-group of patients who do not require cerebral protection.
- With the current array of devices available to us there are no technical reasons why a cerebral protection system cannot be used in all patients.
- Cerebral protection should be used in all patients being treated with a carotid artery stent until such time as solid contradictory evidence is available.

References

1. CAVATAS Investigators. Endovascular versus surgical treatment in patients with carotid stenosis in the Carotid and Vertebral Artery Transluminal Angioplasty Study (CAVITAS): a randomised trial. *Lancet* 2001; **357**: 1729-1737.

2. Brooks WM, Jones MR, Coleman TC, Breathitt L. Carotid angioplasty and stenting versus carotid endarterectomy: randomized trial in a community hospital. *J Am Coll Cardiol* 2001; **38**: 1589-1595.

3. Naylor AR, Bolia A, Abbott RJ *et al.* Randomized study of carotid angioplasty and stenting versus carotid endarterectomy: a stopped trial. *J Vasc Surg* 1998; **28**: 326-334.

4. Jordan WJV, Doblart DD, Plyuscheva NP *et al.* Microemboli detected by transcranial Doppler monitoring in patients during carotid angioplasty versus carotid endarterectomy. *Cardiovasc Surg* 1999; **7**: 33-38.

5. Jaeger HJ, Mathias KD, Hauth E *et al.* Cerebral ischemia detected with diffusion weighted MR imaging after stent implantation in the carotid artery. *Am J Neuroradiol* 2002; **23**: 200-207.

6. van Heesewijk HP, Vos JA, Louwerse ES *et al.* New brain lesions at MR imaging after carotid angioplasty and stent placement. *Radiology* 2002; **224**: 361-365.

7. Muller M, Reiche W, Langenscheidt P *et al.* Ischemia after carotid endarterectomy: comparison between transcranial Doppler sonography and diffusion-weighted MR imaging. *Am J Neuroradiol* 2000; **21**: 47-54.

8. Henry M, Henry I, Klonaris C *et al.* Benefits of cerebral protection during carotid stenting with the PercuSurge GuardWire system: midterm results. *J Endovasc Ther* 2002; **9**: 1-13.

9. Angelini AR, Barbera MD, Sacca S *et al.* Cerebral protection during carotid artery stenting. collection and histopathologic analysis of embolized debris. *Stroke* 2002; **33**: 456-461.

10. Al-Mubarak N, Colombo A, Gaines PA *et al.* Multicenter evaluation of carotid artery stenting with a filter protection system. *J Am Coll Cardiol* 2002; **39**: 841-846.

11. Al-Mubarak N, Roubin GS, Vitek JJ *et al.* Effect of the distal-balloon protection system on microembolization during carotid stenting. *Circulation* 2001; **104**: 1999-2002.

12. Ohki T, Marin ML, Lyon RT *et al.* *Ex vivo* human carotid artery bifurcation stenting: correlation of lesion characteristics with embolic potential. *J Vasc Surg* 1998; **27**: 463-471.

Carotid stenting should always be performed with cerebral protection

Against the motion
Philippe Amabile, Serge Cohen, Gilles Rollet,
Jean-Michel Bartoli, Philippe Piquet

Introduction

Carotid endarterectomy is the standard treatment for patients with high-grade carotid stenosis. Randomized controlled trials in both symptomatic[1,2] and asymptomatic[3] patients have demonstrated the safety and efficacy of this treatment over medical therapies. The combined rate of stroke and/or death usually observed after carotid endarterectomy is less than 3% for asymptomatic patients, 5% for symptomatic patients with transient ischaemic attacks (TIAs), and 7% for patients with a prior stroke. To achieve these good results, however, selection criteria are crucial. Carotid endarterectomy in patients with severe co-morbidities is associated with an increased risk of stroke and death.[4,5] If specific angiographic characteristics (controlateral occlusion, ipsilateral carotid siphon stenosis) are present or if the surgical access is difficult (radiation-induced stenosis, restenosis after carotid endarterectomy), the combined rate of stroke and/or death can be as high as 14%.[6,7] Thus, because patients were highly selected in randomized trials, the applicability of these studies to the general population is questioned.[8]

Percutaneous transluminal angioplasty (PTA) and stenting plays an important role in the treatment of occlusive atherosclerotic lesions in all localizations. Because PTA and stenting avoids surgical incision and general anesthesia, the technique is thought to be less invasive. Thus there are more and more reports of treatment of carotid artery stenosis with angioplasty and stenting. Clinical results are highly variable depending on the nature of the lesion (i.e. atherosclerosis, restenosis, radiation-induced stenosis), the clinical status of the patient (asymptomatic, TIAs, stroke) and the angioplasty technique.[9-13]

Considering the lack of controlled data about carotid artery stenting, this technique may be hazardous if used in all patients requiring carotid endarterectomy. In selected high-risk patients, however, carotid artery stenting may be an acceptable alternative to carotid endarterectomy.

The purpose of this retrospective study is to analyse our results on carotid artery stenting in this subset of high-risk patients, including those with high-risk anatomy, restenosis after carotid endarterectomy, radiation-induced stenosis, and severe co-morbidities in order to elucidate the role of endovascular intervention in the treatment of carotid stenosis.

Subjects and methods

Patient selection

From November 1996 to September 2002, 615 patients with carotid artery stenosis were referred to our department for treatment. Among them, 78 patients with 83 symptomatic and asymptomatic common carotid artery or internal carotid artery stenoses >60 % were selected for carotid artery stenting. Before selection all patients underwent a neurological examination by a neurologist and were classified using the Modified Rankin Scale (MRS).

Carotid artery stenting was considered in high-surgical-risk patients with severe co-morbidities (coronaropathy, congestive heart failure, renal insufficiency, chronic obstructive pulmonary disease, and age over 80 years), and/or neurological deficit with MRS score >3 and/or difficult surgical access (previous radical neck surgery with or without tracheostomy, previous cervical irradiation, restenosis after carotid endarterectomy) and/or angiographically defined risk factors (occlusion of the opposite internal carotid artery or stenosis of the internal carotid artery in the region of the siphon). Furthermore technical requirements for carotid artery stenting were favourable vascular anatomy (no major tortuosity), no kinking in the stent area deployment and no intraluminal thrombus. The experimental protocol and informed consent were approved by the Institutional Review Board. All patients were informed of the experimental nature of this procedure and signed an informed consent form.

Procedure

Before procedure, to assess lesion morphology, a colour duplex scan of carotid artery was performed, followed by a carotid digital subtraction angiography for symptomatic stenosis or by magnetic resonance angiography for asymptomatic stenosis. A brain computed tomography (CT) scan was obtained to detect pre-existing cerebral infarction and to exclude intracerebral bleeding lesion. During the same procedure, a carotid bifurcation CT scan was done to measure carotid diameter and lesion length, and to allow stent selection.

In 81 cases (97.5%) the procedure was performed in an angiography suite with patients under conscious sedation with standard monitoring techniques including arterial pressure monitoring, continuous electrocardiography, and oxymetry. An oral regimen of aspirin (300 mg per day) and ticlopidin (500 mg per day) or clopidogrel (75 mg per day) was started 5 days before endovascular treatment.

The last five cases were performed with the concomittent use of GPIIb/IIIa inhibitors. Carotid stenoses were approached through a femoral access with a 7 Fr sheath under local anaesthesia. An intravenous loading dose of heparin (30 U per kilogram of body weight) was given at the beginning of the procedure, after the acquisition of the appropriate diagnosis images.

Then a vertebral catheter was advanced at the level of the aortic arch and pushed into the common carotid artery. A 0.035 soft hydrophilic guidewire was placed into the external carotid artery and then replaced by a 0.035 stiff guidewire (Amplatz Super Stiff; Boston Scientific). In case of carotid tortuosity a 6 Fr guiding catheter (Envoy; Cordis) was advanced over this wire, proximal to the carotid bifurcation; otherwise, a 100 cm, 7Fr sheath (Brite tip; Cordis) was used.

The lesion was crossed with a 0.014 or 0.035 wire depending on the type of stent used. To prevent bradycardia, 0.5 mg of atropin was administered intravenously prior to balloon inflation. In case of very tight stenosis a pre-dilatation was performed with a 3 mm diameter angioplasty balloon (Rapid exchange; AVE-Medtronic). Otherwise, a primary stenting with self-expanding stent (Easy-Wallstent, Magic-Wallstent or Carotid-Wallstent; Boston Scientific) was performed.

Complete stent deployment was achieved with balloon angioplasty inflation within the stenosis (Rapid exchange; AVE-Medtronic or Bypass speedy; Boston Scientific). After stent deployment, intracerebral angiogram including anteroposterior and lateral views was obtained to exclude embolic branch occlusion.

In two cases (2.5%), at the beginning of our experience, common carotid artery lesions were approached through a cervicotomy. Balloon-expandable stent (Palmaz, Cordis) was placed in one case and balloon angioplasty without stent placement was performed in the other.

Postoperative follow-up

Patients were placed on an oral regimen of clopidogrel or ticlopidin plus aspirin for 4 weeks. All patients underwent a carotid duplex scan before discharge and then at 3, 6, and 12 months and yearly thereafter. Follow-up examinations were performed at the same frequency by the neurology team, the vascular surgeons, or the patient's referring physician.

Neurological complications were defined as transient ischaemic attacks with a neurological deficit lasting less than 24 hours. Minor stroke was defined as neurological deficit lasting less than 7 days or persisting with an MRS score <3. Major stroke was defined as disabling neurological deficit (MRS score >3) persisting more than 7 days.

Statistical analysis

Data were expressed as mean ± SD. Nominal variables were analysed with the c^2 test. Statistical significance was assumed at p<0.05. Time to recurrent stenosis >50% was analysed using a Kaplan-Meier analysis. Data were analysed with the SPSS 11.0 software package.

Results

Patient demographics and clinical presentation

The demographic characteristics and co-morbid medical conditions of the patients are listed in Table 1. Inclusion criteria for this study appear in Table 2. Twenty-five patients were selected for severe co-morbidities. Among them, ten patients had one medical risk factor, nine had two medical or angiographic risk factors, and six had three medical or angiographic risk factors. Twenty patients were selected for severe neurological status. Among them 12 patients had an MRS score of 3, and eight had a score of 4. Furthermore, in this neurological group, five patients had one medical or angiographic risk factor and one patient had two of these risk factors. Six patients in the radiation-induced stenosis group and 12 in the restenosis group had one medical or angiographic risk factor. In the restenosis group, two patients had two of these risk factors. One patient selected for a restenosis after carotid endarterectomy, had in his history a neck irradiation for cancer. One patient was selected for the association of

Table 1. Demographic characteristics, medical conditions, risk features and presenting symptoms of the patient population

Factor	n (%)
Age	
Mean	70.4
Range	36–95 years
Age over 80 years	19 (22.9)
Sex	
Male	58 (69.9)
Female	20 (30.1)
Risk factors	
Smoking	50 (60.2)
Hypercholesterolaemia	40 (48.1)
Medical conditions	
Hypertension	54 (65.1)
Neurological symptoms	44 (53)
Qualifying symptoms	30 (36.1)
Amaurosis	1
TIA	3
Stroke	26
Non-qualifying symptoms	14 (16.9)
Amaurosis	2
TIA	4
Stroke	8
Coronary artery disease	30 (36.1)
Lower limbs arteriopathy	17 (20.5)
Diabetes mellitus	15 (18.1)
Controlateral carotid occlusion	11 (13.2)
Congestive heart failure	10 (12)
COPD	5 (6.)
Obesity	4 (4.8)
Hemodialysis	3 (3.6)
Presentation	
Asymptomatic	53 (63.8)
Symptomatic	30 (36.2)
Amaurosis	1
TIA	3
Stroke	26

TIA : transient ischaemic attack.
COPD : chronic obstructive pulmonary disorder.

Table 2. Conditions leading to patients selection for CAS

Indication	n (%)
Severe co-morbidities	25 (30.1)
Severe neurological status	20 (24.1)
Restenosis after carotid endarterectomy	18 (21.7)
Radiation stenosis	17 (20.5)
Radiation stenosis + restenosis	1 (1.2)
Angiographic risk factors	1 (1.2)
Controlateral recurrent laryngeal nerve palsy	1 (1.2)

an occlusion of the controlateral internal carotid artery and a stenosis of the ipsilateral internal carotid artery in the siphon. Finally, one patient was selected because he had a recurrent laryngeal nerve palsy following carotid endarterectomy and a controlateral internal carotid artery stenosis.

Lesion characteristics and technique

Stenoses were located in the internal carotid artery in 65 cases (78.3%), in the common carotid artery close to the bifurcation in 10 (12%) cases, and in the common carotid artery in seven cases (8.5%) and in the internal carotid artery and common carotid artery in one case (1.2%).

Among the stenoses, 47 (56.6%) were atherosclerotic, 17 (20.5%) were radiation-therapy induced, 18 (21.7%) were recurrent after carotid endarterectomy, and one lesion (1.2%) was a restenosis developed after neck radiation-therapy.

The degree of stenosis was defined according to the NASCET angiographic protocol. The mean pre-treatment degree was 75% (60–99%). At the end of the procedure, technical success rate was 98.8 % (one patient had a 40% residual stenosis).

Pre-dilatation occurred in two cases (2.4%). A total of 93 stents were deployed (1.1 per stenosis). All the internal carotid artery and bifurcation stenoses were covered with self-expandable stents (n=73 and n=15 respectively). Common carotid artery stenoses were treated with balloon angioplasty alone in one case, with balloon-expandable stent in one case, and with self-expandable stents in four cases. To achieve an adequate result, two stents were deployed in five cases in the internal carotid artery and in three cases in the carotid bifurcation. In one case, three stents had to be deployed to treat a recurrent stenosis in the internal carotid artery.

One patient underwent combined angioplasty and stenting to treat a stenosis of the intracranial portion of the internal carotid artery.

No acute stent thrombosis occurred in this series. No common carotid artery or internal carotid artery lesion required conversion to conventional surgery.

Procedural complications

No patients died within 30 days of endovascular treatment. Neurological complications ipsilateral to carotid artery stenting arose in nine cases (10.8%) including eight minor strokes (9.6%) and one TIA (1.2%). No thrombosis of intracranial arteries was shown on the angiogram. In four cases these accidents occurred a few hours after carotid artery stenting. All these patients were treated with heparin and anti-platelets and fully recovered within a week. No differences in neurological complications were observed between symptomatic and asymptomatic patients.

Conditions leading to patient selection for carotid artery stenting was not correlated with neurological complications (Table 3a). In the same way, nature of carotid stenosis was not related to poorer neurological outcomes (Table 3b).

Bradycardia occurred in nine cases (10.8%) and resolved with atropin and balloon deflation in all cases. Non-neurological complications occurred in three cases (3.6%). In two cases these complications were related to the femoral access, with one groin haematoma and one acute limb ischaemia caused by an arterial closure device. One patient suffered digestive haemorrhage in relation to a duodenal ulcer. All these complications required surgical intervention and were successfully treated.

Table 3a. Correlation of conditions leading to patients selection for CAS and complications

Indication	Lesion, n	TIA (%)	Minor stroke (%)	Non–neurological complication (%)
Severe co-morbidities	25	1 (4)	2 (8)	0 (0)
Neurological status	20	0 (0)	2 (10)	2 (10)
Restenosis after carotid endarterectomy	18	0 (0)	1 (5.5)	0 (0)
Radiation stenosis	17	0 (0)	3 (17.6)	1 (5.9)
Radiation stenosis + restenosis	1	0 (0)	0 (0)	0 (0)
Angiographic risk factors	1	0 (0)	0 (0)	0 (0)
Controlateral recurrent laryngeal nerve palsy	1	0 (0)	0 (0)	0 (0)
Total	83	1 (1.2)	8 (9.6)	3 (3.6)

TIA : transient ischaemic attack

Table 3b. Correlation of nature of carotid stenosis and neurological complications

Nature of stenosis	Lesion, n	Major stroke (%)	Minor stroke (%)	TIA (%)
Atherosclerosis	47	0 (0)	4 (8.5)	1 (2.1)
Restenosis	18	0 (0)	1 (5.5)	0 (0)
Radiation stenosis	17	0 (0)	3 (17.6)	0 (0)
Re + Ra	1	0 (0)	0 (0)	0 (0)
Total	83	0 (0)	8 (9.6)	1 (1.2)

Re + Ra: restenosis and radiation stenosis; TIA: transient ischaemic attack

Clinical follow-up

Clinical follow-up was maintained in patients. The mean duration of clinical follow-up was 11.6 ± 12.1 months (range 1–47 months). During this period, duplex scan follow-up was obtained in 63 patients out of 78: one patient refused duplex scan follow-up, two patients died before the first duplex scan examination and 12 patients had a period of monitoring between carotid artery stenting and duplex scan examination of less than 3 months. During the follow-up period eight patients died (10.2%). One death was related to a stroke ipsilateral to carotid artery stenting 5 months after the procedure, in a patient with atrial fibrillation. A continuous Doppler examination was performed in the emergency room and showed patent internal carotid artery. Three patients died of cardiac causes (two myocardial infarction and one congestive heart failure), one patient died of septicaemia, another patient died after pneumonectomy, and two deaths were unexplained.

The surviving 71 patients are free of neurological symptoms.

Recurrent stenosis >50% or thrombosis occurred respectively in eight cases and one case after a mean duration of 12 ± 4.9 months (Fig. 1). All these recurrent stenoses and thrombosis were asymptomatic and diagnosed on systematic duplex scan examination. Patients with restenosis after carotid endarterectomy had a higher risk of recurrent stenosis relative to patients with atherosclerotic stenosis or radiation-induced stenosis but this difference was not significant.

Four patients with tight restenosis were treated successfully with further angioplasty.

Discussion

This retrospective study suggests that carotid artery stenting without cerebral protection device in patients with high surgical risk can be performed with mortality and neurological complication rates comparable with those of surgery in the same group of patients. In this series of carotid artery stenting, ten neurological complications occurred after stent deployment, with one TIA and nine minor strokes. These complications are at the same rate of those observed after carotid artery stenting in high surgical risk patients.[14,15] No major stroke occurred within 30 days of carotid artery stenting – and all minor strokes resolved within a week. Non-neurological complications occurred in three cases and were related to puncture site management and anticoagulation therapy. In the 78 patients reported here, there were no procedural deaths or myocardial infarctions.

One of the critical issues of both carotid endarterectomy and carotid artery stenting is the risk of carotid thrombosis and cerebral embolization. In our series, no acute carotid thrombosis was observed immediately after carotid artery stenting, probably because we, like other groups, used anticoagulation, antiplatelet therapy, and primary stenting. No major embolic event was detected in the intracerebral angiograms after carotid artery stenting, thus we can assume that strokes were caused by distal microembolization of atherosclerotic debris.

This well-known phenomenon has been confirmed by previous *in vitro* experimentation and clinical studies that demonstrated debris release during carotid artery stenting, persisting after stent placement.[16-18] Debris release occurs in 80-100% of procedures and during all the steps of carotid artery stenting.[19-21] However, the majority of the particles are released during balloon dilatation and stenting.[16] These embolic particles consist of atherosclerotic debris, organized thrombus and calicified material.[22] The number of particles dislodged from the plaques is highly variable. Echolucent plaques and stenosis over 90% produce a higher number of embolic particles.[22] It is important to note that all the embolic material captured during carotid artery stenting had particles over 300 μm. In 52% of cases, embolic material contained particles over 1000 μm.[20] As a matter of interest, the approximate size of an important cerebral artery may be as small as 100 μm.

Even if distal microembolization of atherosclerotic debris is a usual phenomenon during carotid artery stenting, the rate of neurological symptoms following these embolic events is low. Three large series of carotid artery stenting without cerebral protection report stroke and death rates ranging from 1.6 to 4.3%.[10,23-24] Thus one should question the need for a systematic utilization of cerebral protection device to prevent cerebral infarction. Three types of systems are currently under investigation. One is an occlusion catheter placed proximal to the lesion that allows reversal of flow in the internal carotid artery.[25] Because there is no need to cross the lesion to prevent embolization, occlusion catheters may have an advantage over other devices but no data are available in clinical practice.

The two other systems are occlusion balloons and filters placed downstream from the site of stent implantation. Filters have the theoretical advantage of permitting cerebral perfusion during their deployment but they can also miss small embolic particles. Furthermore a recent study showed that in 3.5% of the cases, the filter could not cross the stenosis. In 6.9 % of the procedures the filter could be advanced through the lesion only after predilatation. In addition, the filter was difficult to retrieve through the stent in 8.4% of the cases requiring endoluminal manoeuvres.[26] Thus safety of these devices is uncertain and needs further investigation.

Occlusion balloon catheters may avoid atherosclerotic debris embolization since they allow total carotid occlusion. Initial results by Théron[12] and Henry[27] were excellent, with stroke rates ranging from 0 to 1.9%. Recent data, however, suggest that despite balloon protection, periprocedural neurological complications occurred in 5.2% of patients who underwent carotid artery stenting; the mean occlusion time of 10.4 ± 4 minutes is a real concern.[19] Embolic complications may occur during the procedure itself or during flush application into the freshly stented bifurcation area through collateral circulation.[28] In addition, Al-Mubarak showed that distal balloon protection significantly reduces Doppler-detected microembolic signals but does not abolish them.[29]

Finally, in our experience half of the strokes did not occur during the procedure but in the hours following carotid artery stenting. Thus, considering that cerebral protection devices increase the complexity of carotid artery stenting without abolishing neurological complications and that these devices are expensive, their systematic utilization is questionable. We favour the selective use of a protection device but we have to first determine high embolization risk patients who will benefit from this technique.

In our study no difference was detected between symptomatic and asymtomatic patients, probably due to the higher risk profile of our population. However, even if not significant considering the small number of patient treated in each group, nature of the stenosis was associated with different outcomes. Among the 18 patients treated for restenosis by carotid artery stenting, one minor stroke occurred in a patient with recurrent CI stenosis 6 years after the initial endarterectomy, resulting probably more from the ongoing atherosclerotic process than from intimal hyperplasia. The other 17 patients did not suffer neurological complications. On the contrary, three patients of 17 treated by carotid artery stenting for radiation-induced stenosis suffered minor strokes. A possible explanation for this difference is the nature of the stenosis itself. Radiation-induced stenoses are related to accelerated atherosclerosis, usually involve long arterial segments, and may reflect a more severe situation than common atherosclerosis.[30] In view of our results we suggest that patients treated for radiation-induced stenosis may benefit from cerebral protection device whereas those with early restenosis following carotid endarterectomy may not. For the remaining patients, further investigation should be performed especially as regards atherosclerotic plaque structure.

Ohki in an experimental study found that echolucent plaques and stenosis over 90% produced a higher number of embolic particles, whereas presence of preoperative symptoms, plaque ulceration or calcification, sex, and diameter of the vessel did not significantly correlate with the number of embolic particles recovered.[22] One large clinical study addressed the outcomes of carotid artery stenting and showed that the only predictors of stroke were age over 80 years and the presence of long or multiple stenosis.[31] Symptomatic or asymptomatic nature of the stenosis was not related to poorer outcomes – a finding similar to our study.

Mechanical cerebral protection is not the only solution to prevent cerebral infarction. Pharmacological protection using GP IIb/IIIa inhibitors should also be addressed since they decrease mortality and morbidity in a number of coronary stent studies.[32,33] Emboli can potentially trigger platelet aggregation and may amplify microvascular obstructions leading to loss of endothelial integrity, release of vasoactive amines from activated platelets, increased vascular tone and subsequent cerebral infarction. GP IIb/IIIa inhibitors have shown cerebral infarction reduction in experimental models of cerebral ischemia and their effect on platelets aggregation last for several days.[34] They also improve outcomes after stroke,[35] and recent clinical findings suggest that abciximab may help to reduce periprocedural adverse events in patients undergoing carotid artery stenting.[23]

In this study, 128 patients received adjuvant therapy with abciximab during carotid artery stenting and for 12 hours following carotid artery stenting. Two patients (1.6%) suffered minor strokes which compares favourably to carotid artery stenting with cerebral protection device. Furthermore, use of GP IIb/IIIa inhibitors during carotid artery stenting appears to be safe with no increase of intracranial bleeding. We have used GP IIb/IIIa inhibitors in our last five cases with no occurrence of stroke but the number of patients treated is too small to draw conclusions.

Microembolization of atherosclerotic debris during carotid artery stenting is usual. Cerebral protection devices can prevent this phenomenon but do not abolish it. Results from non-randomized studies show comparable results between carotid artery stenting with and without emboli protection devices. Thus we do not advocate the routine use of cerebral protection devices during carotid artery stenting. Randomized trials are warranted to define which patients can benefit from these techniques with or without the adjunctive use of GP IIb/IIIa inhibitors. Whatever the technique used, carotid artery stenting is for the moment unwarranted for patients with standard surgical risk.

Summary

- Microembolization of atherosclerotic debris occurs in 80–100 % of carotid artery stenting.

- The majority of the particles are released during balloon dilatation and stenting.

- The number and the size of particles is highly variable.

- Cerebral protection devices can prevent microembolization but do not abolish it.

- Results from non-randomized studies show comparable results between carotid artery stenting with and without emboli protection devices

- Randomized controlled trials are needed

References

1. Randomised trial of endarterectomy for recently symptomatic carotid stenosis: final results of the MRC European Carotid surgery trial (ECST). *Lancet* 1998; 351: 1379–1387.
2. Barnett HJ, Taylor DW, Eliasziw M *et al.* Benefit of carotid endarterectomy in patients with moderate or severe stenosis: North American Symptomatic Carotid Endarterectomy Trial Collaborators. *N Engl J Med* 1998; 339: 1415–1425.
3. Executive Committee for the Asymptomatic Carotid Atherosclerosis Study. Endarterectomy for asymptomatic carotid artery stenosis. *JAMA.* 1995; 273: 1421–1428.
4. Wennberg DE, Lucas FL, Birkmeyer JD *et al.* Variation in carotid endarterectomy mortality in the Medicare population. *JAMA* 1998; 279: 1278–1281.
5. Ouriel K, Hertzer NR, Beven EG *et al.* Preprocedural risk stratification: Identifying an appropriate population for carotid stenting. *J Vasc Surg* 2001; 33: 728–732.
6. Sundt MT, Sandok BA, Whisnanat JP. Carotid endarterectomy: complications and preoperative assessment of risk. *Mayo Clinic Proc* 1975; 50: 301–306.
7. Rothwell PM, Slattery J, Warlow CP. Clinical and angiographic predictors of stroke and death from carotid endarterectomy: systematic review. *Br Med J* 1997; 315: 1571–1577.
8. Barnett HJ, Eliasziw M, Meldrum HE, Taylor DW. Do the facts and figures warrant a 10-fold increase in the performance of carotid endarterectomy on asymptomatic patients? *Neurology* 1996; 46: 603–608.

9. CAVATAS Investigators. Endovascular versus surgical treatment in patients with carotid stenosis in the Carotid and Vertebral Artery Transluminal Angioplasty Study: a randomised trial. *Lancet* 2001; **357**: 1729–1737.

10. Roubin GS, New G, Iyer SS *et al.* Immediate and late clinical outcomes of carotid artery stenting in patients with symptomatic and asymptomatic carotid artery stenosis: a 5-year prospective analysis. *Circulation* 2001; **103**: 532–537.

11. Kirsch EC, Khangure MS, van Schie GP *et al.* Carotid arterial stent placement: results and follow-up in 53 patients. *Radiology* 2001; **220**: 737–744.

12. Théron JG, Payelle GG, Coskun O *et al.* Carotid artery stenosis: treatment with protected balloon angioplasty and stent placement. *Radiology* 1996; **201**: 627–636.

13. d'Audiffret A, Desgranges P, Kobeiter H, Becquemin JP. Technical aspects and current results of carotid stenting. *J Vasc Surg* 2001; **33**: 1001–1007.

14. Gil-Peralta A, Mayol A, Gonzales Marcos JR *et al.* Percutaneous transluminal angioplasty of the symptomatic atherosclerotic carotid arteries: results, complications and follow-up. *Stroke* 1996; **27**: 2271–2273.

15. Shawl F, Kadro W, Domanski MJ *et al.* Safety and efficacy of elective carotid artery stenting in high-risk patients. *J Am Coll Cardiol* 2000; **35**: 1721–1728.

16. Ohki T, Roubin GS, Veith FJ *et al.* Efficacy of a filter device in the prevention of embolic events during carotid angioplasty and stenting: an *ex vivo* analysis. *J Vasc Surg* 1999; **30**: 1034–1044.

17. Martin JB, Pache JC, Treggiari-Venzi M *et al.* Role of the distal balloon protection technique in the prevention of cerebral embolic events during carotid stent placement. *Stroke* 2001; **32**: 479–484.

18. Jordan WD, Voellinger DC, Doblar DD *et al.* Microemboli detected by transcranial doppler monitoring in patients during carotid angioplasty versus carotid endarterectomy. *Cardiovasc Surg* 1999; **7**: 33–38.

19. Tübler T, Schlüter M, Dirsch O *et al.* Balloon-protected carotid artery stenting: relationship of periprocedural neurological complications with the size of particulate debris. *Circulation* 2001; **104**: 2791–2796.

20. Angelini A, Reimers B, Della Barbera M *et al.* Cerebral protection during carotid artery stenting: collection and histolpathologic analysis of embolized debris. *Stroke* 2002; **33**: 456–461.

21. Whitlow PL, Lylyk P, Londero H *et al.* Carotid artery protected with an emboli containment system. *Stroke* 2002; **33**: 1308–1314.

22. Ohki T, Marin ML, Lyon RT *et al. Ex vivo* human carotid artery bifurcation stenting: correlation of lesion characteristics with embolic potential. *J Vasc Surg* 1998; **27**: 463–471.

23. Kapadia SR, Bajzer CT, Ziada KM *et al.* Initial experience of platelet glycoprotein IIb/IIIa inhibition with abciximab during carotid stenting: a safe and effective adjunctive therapy. *Stroke* 2001; **32**: 2328–2332.

24. Criado FJ, Lingelbach JM, Ledesma DF, Lucas PR. Carotid artery stenting in vascular surgery practice. *J Vasc Surg* 2002; **35**: 430–434.

25. Ohki T, Parodi J, Veith FJ, Bates M, Bade M, Chang D *et al.* Efficacy of a proximal occlusion catheter with reversal of flow in the prevention of embolic events during carotid artery stenting: an experimental analysis. *J Vasc Surg* 2001; **33**: 504–509.

26. Reimers B, Corvaja N, Moshiri S *et al.* Cerebral protection with filter devices during carotid artery stenting. *Circulation* 2001; **104**: 12–15.

27. Henry M, Amor M, Henry I *et al.* Carotid stenting with cerebral protection: first clinical experience using the PercuSurge GuardWire system. *J Endovasc Surg* 1999; **6**: 321–331.

28. Théron J, Guimaraens L, Coskun O *et al.* Complications of carotid angioplasty and stenting. *Neurosurg focus* 1998; **5**(6).

29. Al-Mubarak N, Roubin GS, Vitek JJ *et al.* Effect of the distal balloon protection system on microembolization during carotid stenting. *Circulation* 2001; **104**: 1999–2002.

30. Carmody BJ, Arora S, Avena R, Curry KM, Simpkins J, Cosby K *et al.* Accelerated carotid artery disease after high-dose head and neck radiotherapy: is there a role for routine carotid duplex surveillance? *J Vasc Surg* 1999; **30**: 1045–1051.

31. Mathur A, Roubin GS, Iyer SS *et al.* Predictors of stroke complicating carotid artery stenting. *Circulation* 1998; **97**: 1239–1245.

32. Topol EJ, Mark DB, Lincoff AM *et al.* Outcomes at 1 year and economic implications of platelet glycoprotein IIb/IIIa blockade in patients undergoing coronary stenting: results from a multicentre randomized trial: EPISTENT Investigators: evaluation of platelet IIb/IIIa inhibitors for stenting. *Lancet* 1999; **354**: 2019–2024.

33. Lincoff AM, Tcheng JE, Califf RM *et al.* Sustained suppression of ischemic complications of coronary intervention by platelet GP IIb/IIIa blockade with abciximab: one-year outcome in the EPIOLG

trial: evaluation in PTCA to improve long-term outcome with abciximab GP IIb/IIIa blockade. *Circulation* 1999; **99**: 1951–1958.

34. Choudri TF, Hoh BL, Zerwes HG *et al.* Reduced microvascular thrombosis and improved outcome in acute murine stroke by inhibiting GP IIb/ IIIa receptor-mediated platelet aggregation. *J Clin Invest* 1998; **102**: 1301–1310.

35. The abciximab in ischemic stroke investigators. Abciximab in acute ischemic stroke: a randomized, double-blind, placebo-controlled, dose-escalation study. *Stroke* 2000; **31**: 601–609.

Carotid stenting should always be performed with cerebral protection

For the motion

JS Yadav

Introduction

Embolization of the brain has long been considered the Achilles heel of carotid angioplasty and stenting. We were sufficiently concerned with the risk of embolization that in the very first case of carotid angioplasty performed at the University of Alabama we inserted two sheaths and two guiding catheters and placed an occlusion balloon distally to provide emboli protection (Fig. 1).

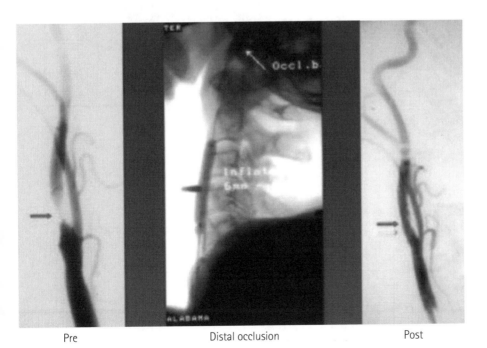

Pre   Distal occlusion   Post

Figure 1. Cerebral protection in 1994.

Evidence

A variety of lines of evidence including *ex-vivo* angioplasty of carotid plaque, transcranial Doppler monitoring, carotid intervention and retrieval of particles with filter type emboli protection devices have conclusively demonstrated that embolization occurs in every carotid intervention procedure (Figs 2-5).[1-3] Fortunately the brain is tolerant of small emboli and only larger emboli appear to cause ischaemic consequences. In a rat model, particles generated after *ex-vivo* carotid plaque angioplasty were fractionated into particles less than 200 microns (μ) in diameter and particles ranging from 200-500μ in diameter and were injected into the rat internal carotid artery. There were two very interesting findings in this study: first, that most of the particles were released during angioplasty and stenting and not during crossing the lesion; second, that only the larger particles in the 200-500 μ range caused neuronal ischaemia at day 3 after injection.[4]

A variety of emboli protection devices have been developed. (Fig. 6) They can be classified into occlusive and non-occlusive devices. (Table 1) Several series have been published, primarily from Europe, demonstrating either reduction in clinical complications or in surrogate endpoints such as the number of emboli measured by transcranial Doppler with a variety of emboli protection devices (Table 2). Several

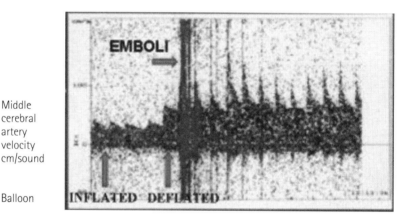

Figure 2. Transcranial Doppler.

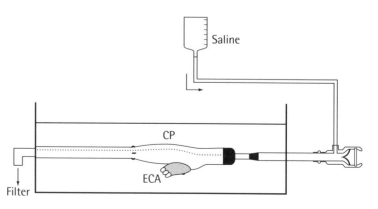

Figure 3. *Ex-vivo* carotid plaque embolization model.[1]

Table 1. Anti-embolization devices

Occlusive
Distal flow arrest
Theron	Balloon occlusion catheter
PercuSurge	Balloon occlusion guidewire

Proximal flow arrest
Arteria	Balloon occlusion guide catheter
MOMA	Balloon occlusion guide catheter

Non-occlusive
Supported filters
AngioGuard	Guidewire filter
MedNova	Guidewire filter
Accunet	Guidewire filter
Trap	Nitinol filter

Unsupported filters
EPI	Guidewire filter
Etrap	Guidewire filter

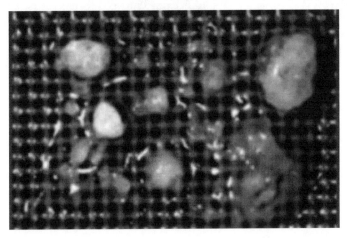

Figure 4. *Ex-vivo* carotid plaque embolization model.[1] Embolic particles were generated from each plaque.

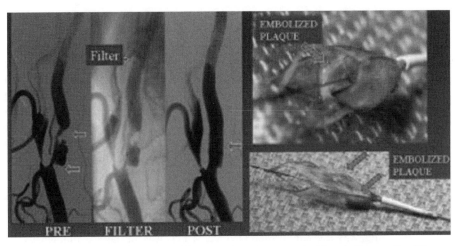

Figure 5. Sx internal carotid arteries with severe ulceration treated with emboli prevention filter.

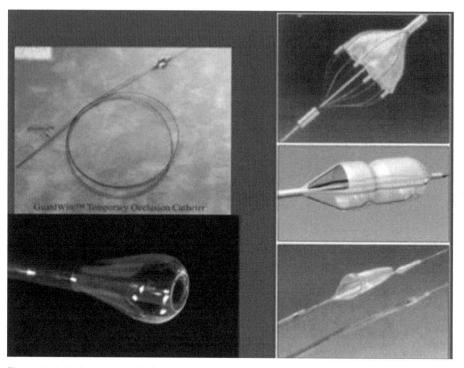

Figure 6. Emboli prevention devices. Left column: balloons; right column: filters.

Table 2. Anti-embolization devices

<u>Randomized controlled trials vs carotid
endarterectomy</u>
AngioGuard (SAPPHIRE)
Accunet (CREST)

<u>Case series</u>
PercuSurge
Mednova

case series have been published with the PercuSurge distal balloon occlusion device. In one series of 43 carotid artery stents there was a 93% technical success rate and one death and no strokes at 30 days post-procedure.[5] In another series 39 carotid stent patients were treated without emboli protection and 37 were treated with the PercuSurge device.[2] This was not a randomized study. Transcranial Doppler monitoring was performed in all patients. There was one stroke in each arm of the study but the number of emboli was 164 ± 108 in the group treated without protection and 68 ± 83 in the group treated with protection ($p < 0.05$). In another study from Germany in which 58 patients were treated with the PercuSurge device there was a correlation between the size of the particles and the risk of a peri-procedural neurological complication, with a particle surface area of >0.8 mm being associated with a 60% risk of a neurological event.[6]

The first filter was the AngioGuard device, which was initially evaluated by Dr Grube in Germany in coronaries and saphenous vein grafts and carotids (Figs 7–11).[3]

- Feasibility Study in Coronaries/SVGs
- Coronaries: 15
  - Acute MI: 2
- SVG: 11
- Vessel diameter: 3.3 ± 0.35 mm(2.8–5.8)
- Stenosis: 89% ± 8.5% (70%–100%)
- Technical success: 96.2%
- Slow flow with filter: 36% SVGs
- MACE: 0

Figure 7. Initial filter experience: AngioGuard.[3] SVG: saphenous vein graft; MI: myocardial infarction; MACE: major adverse cardiovascular events

- University of Minnesota
- Particles recovered from all patients
- Number: 147 ± 111 (20–361)
- Size (area):   0.10 mm² ± 0.5 mm² (0.015–2.0)
- Embolic burden per patient:
  37 mm² ± 36 mm² (0.6 mm²–110 mm²)

Figure 8. Initial filter experience: AngioGuard histopathology.[3]

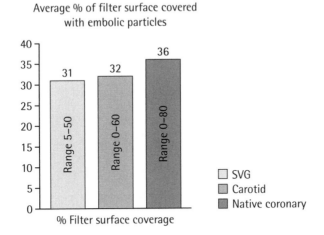

Average % of filter surface covered with embolic particles

Figure 9. Filter surface coverage.

Figure 12 shows AngioGuard filters used in coronary, carotid and saphenous vein graft intervention showing extensive plaque fragments which embolized during the intervention and were captured by the filter. Reimers has published a study evaluating several filter devices: AngioGuard, Mednova and EPI (Fig. 13-14).[7] In a study of the Mednova filter in 162 carotid artery stent cases, there was a high technical success rate of 94%; 8% of the patients did require pre-dilatation and there was a 1% stroke and a 1% death rate.[8] Visible debris was evident in 35% of the filters. In a study

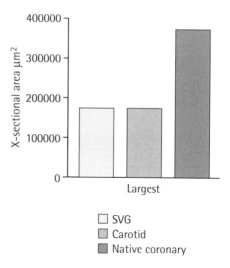

Figure 10. Embolic partical size: maximum partical size recovered.

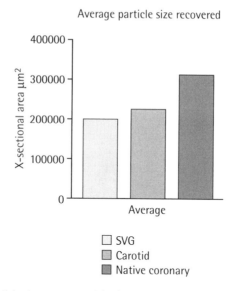

Figure 11. Embolic particle sizeaverage particle size recovered.

from Italy looking at the AngioGuard filter, 83.7% of the filters were found to have debris and 53% of the filter surface was covered by particles.[9]

Two of the emboli protection devices are being evaluated in randomized trails: the AngioGuard device is being evaluated in the SAPPHIRE trial and the Accunet device is being evaluated in the CREST trial. Randomized data from the SAPPHIRE Trial (*Study of angioplasty with protection in patients at high risk for endarterectomy*) comparing carotid stenting with the AngioGuard emboli protection device to carotid endarterectomy should be available before this meeting (Fig. 15).

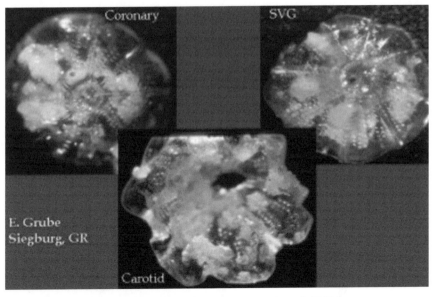

Figure 12. Left: coronary; middle: carotid; right: saphenous vein graft (SVG).[3]

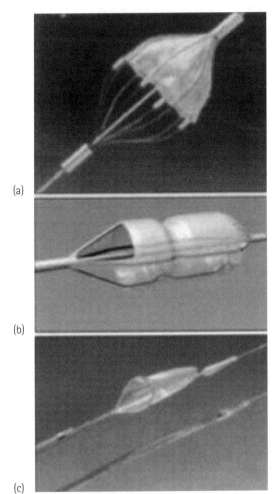

(a)

(b)

(c)

Figure 13. Filters. Ref. 7 [88 CAS; Stenosis: 78.7+ - 10.7%; SX: 35.7%.] (a) Angioguard: 48 (55.8%); (b) Mednova: 30 (34.9%); (c) EPI: 8(9.3%).

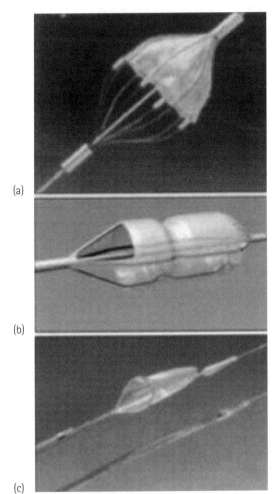

- Technical success: 83/86 (96.5%)
- Stroke: 1 (1.2%)
- Major cardiac: 2 (2.3%)
- Macroscopic debris: 53% of filters

Figure 14. Filters.[7]

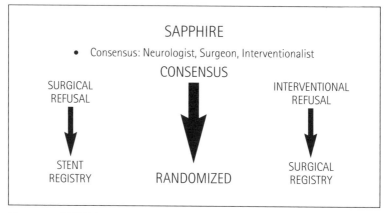

Figure 15. SAPPHIRE.

Conclusions

Multiple lines of evidence indicate the occurrence of embolization during carotid stenting. Several studies have demonstrated retrieval of emboli as well as reduction in stroke during carotid stenting by emboli prevention devices. The pace of technological progress in emboli protection devices has been very rapid and the newer generation devices are much easier to use and lower in profile, and should facilitate the procedure and further reduce the risk of complications.

Summary

- Embolization is very frequent during carotid stenting.
- Neurological events are caused by larger (>200 µ) particles.
- Both occlusive and filter type emboli prevention devices are effective in retrieving particles during carotid stenting.
- Several small studies with emboli prevention devices have demonstrated a reduction in surrogate end points and clinical events.

References

1. Ohki T, Marin ML, Lyon RT *et al*. *Ex vivo* human carotid artery bifurcation stenting: correlation of lesion characteristics with embolic potential. *J Vasc Surg* 1998; **27**: 463–471.
2. Al-Mubarak N, Roubin GS, Vitek JJ *et al*. Effect of the distal-balloon protection system on microembolization during carotid stenting. *Circulation* 2001; **104**: 1999–2002.
3. Grube E, Gerckens U, Yeung AC *et al*. Prevention of distal embolization during coronary angioplasty in saphenous vein grafts and native vessels using porous filter protection. *Circulation* 2001; **104**: 2436–2441.
4. Rapp JH, Pan XM, Sharp FR *et al*. Atheroemboli to the brain: size threshold for causing acute neuronal cell death. *Vasc Surg* 2000; **32**: 68–76.
5. Dietz A, Berkefeld J, Theron JG *et al*. Endovascular treatment of symptomatic carotid stenosis using stent placement: long-term follow-up of patients with a balanced surgical risk/benefit ratio. *Stroke* 2001; **32**: 1855–1859.
6. Tubler T, Schluter M, Dirsch O *et al*. Balloon-protected carotid artery stenting: relationship of periprocedural neurological complications with the size of particulate debris. *Circulation* 2001; **104**: 2791–2796.
7. Reimers B, Corvaja N, Moshiri S *et al*. Cerebral protection with filter devices during carotid artery stenting. *Circulation* 2001; **104**: 12–15.
8. Al-Mubarak N, Colombo A, Gaines PA *et al*. Multicenter evaluation of carotid artery stenting with a filter protection system. *J Am Coll Cardiol* 2002; **39**: 841–846.
9. Angelini A, Reimers B, Della Barbera M *et al*. Cerebral protection during carotid artery stenting: collection and histopathologic analysis of embolized debris. *Stroke* 2002; **33**: 456–461.

Carotid stenting should always be performed with cerebral protection

Against the motion

P Bergeron, V Douillez, P Khanoyan, J Gay

Introduction

For 25 years, carotid angioplasty has been improving[1] with regards to technical evolution and the shifting of daily practice. Routine stenting was the first major technical and clinical step and reduced the rates of immediate complications. Therefore it improved the results of sole balloon angioplasty in cases of recurrent carotid stenoses.[2] Since then, routine carotid stenting has been applied to *de novo* stenosis and has gained enough enthusiastic support to be proposed as an alternative to conventional carotid endarterectomy.

The development of protective devices has been the second major technical step designed to reduce the rate and the seriousness of embolic complications during carotid stenting. A multitude of devices has been developed, based on different concepts and tested with experimental models including animal ones.[3-4] This technology significantly reduced the minor stroke rate as mentioned by Roubin *et al.*[5] Over the 5-year period of interest, the 30-day minor stroke rate decreased from 7.1% during the first year to 3.1% in the fifth.[5]

On the other hand, one must agree that the cerebral protection has increased the complexity of the procedure and the cost of the intervention.

The lack of clinical validation of this latest technology combined with the higher cost, the technical complexity and the competition between the different devices has led us to question the value of the cerebral protection. Reliable data from the current controlled trials may answer this question.

The similarity with routine shunting during carotid endarterectomy is obvious. Most surgeons use selective shunting. Are they to be blamed, in a case of postoperative stroke without shunting?

Technique and illustration

Protective devices started with the occlusive devices. Occlusion of the internal carotid artery (Fig. 1) was proved to be superior to the occlusion of the common carotid artery, due to the maintained flow in the external carotid artery. This has lead to the development of the reverse flow systems (Figs 2, 3).

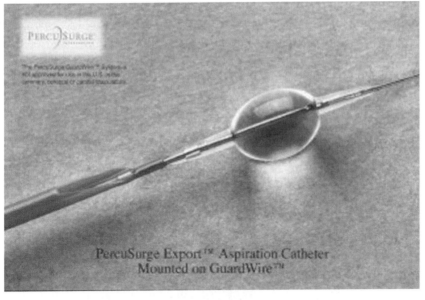

Figure 1. By courtesy of Medtronic AVE, The PercuSurge GuardWire used for distal occlusion of the internal carotid artery.

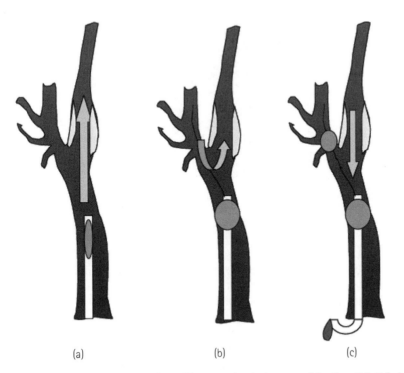

(a)　　　　　　　　(b)　　　　　　　　(c)

Figure 2. By courtesy of ArteriA. This figure illustrates the deployment of the Parodi Anti Emboli System (PAES) protective device. The canulated catheter is deployed in the common carotid artery (a). Then the proximal balloon is inflated and the blood flow only involves the internal and external carotid arteries (b). The external carotid artery is occluded with the help of a second inflated balloon (c) and the blood flow reverses, originating from the brain and being injected through a femoral venous access.

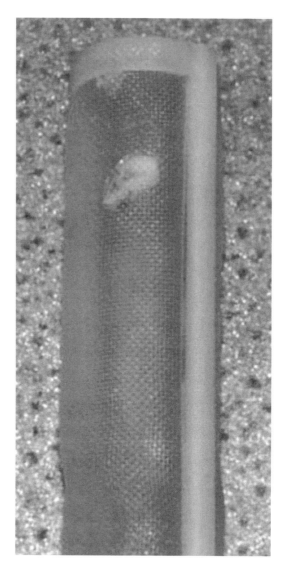

Figure 3. Atheromatous debris collected in the PAES filtering system.

The main drawback of these devices is that the interruption of the cerebral blood flow is not tolerated in up to 10% of the cases[6,7] when the circle of Willis' is not optimal. This may lead to stroke if prolonged.

Filters have been developed in order to make up for these drawbacks, thus allowing a constant blood circulation into the brain (Fig. 4). Many devices are currently in competition. Most filters are now 'monorail' filters, which simplifies the procedure. The drawbacks of these filters mainly consist in the additional manoeuvres, which are time consuming, and the additional cost, what has discouraged most of us. Another drawback of filtering protective devices is that crossing the lesion may lead it to embolize into the brain.[8] Some authors advocate that pharmacological protection, using antiplatelet agents and glycoprotein receptor antagonists can be used to protect the brain. We believe that this is an adjunctive procedure, which might be efficient

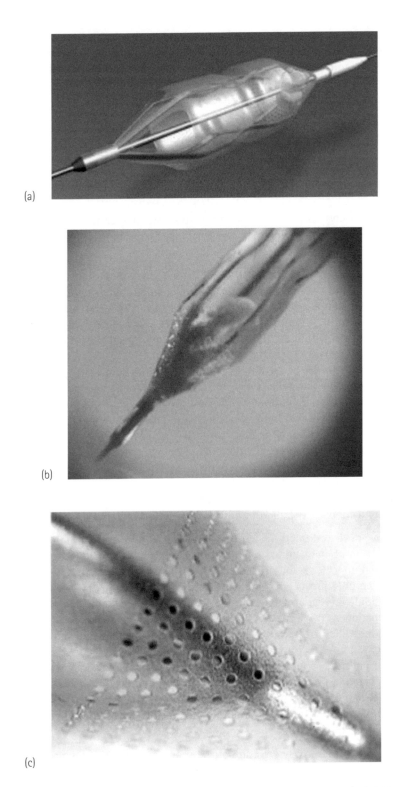

(a)

(b)

(c)

Figure 4. By courtesy of Abbott Vascular Devices. Embolic filters, such as the EmboShield marketed by Abbott Vascular Devices (a), consist of a distally placed basket that prevent embolized debris (b) from entering the cerebral circulation. Figure 4c shows the pores of the filter, allowing blood flow but also being a limiting feature for it allows particles smaller that their diameter to cross the filter.

during the postoperative course, but it cannot avoid mechanical production of debris during carotid stenting. Moreover it could dramatically worsen the evolution of an intracranial haemorrhage, although this also has to be further investigated. This is the reason why, according to Wholey[9] the use of pharmacological protection should only be considered for non-hypertensive patients, with extremely complex types of lesions, and who are free from previous stroke.

Evidence

The evidence is demonstrated in the next 10 points.

1. Most of neurological events happen in the post-stenting course, rather than during the procedure itself. Thus atheroembolism appears to be an ongoing process.

   (a) In our experience,[10] we performed 214 consecutive procedures from 1991 to 2002; half of the new neurological complications happened immediately after the procedure. Out of 37 neurological complications reported, we observed 13 (35%) procedural complications, six transient ischaemic attacks (TIAs) (16%) within the following 24 hours, and seven (19%) added complications from the day 1 to discharge.

   (b) Taking advantage of the data emanating from the Eurocast Registry,[11] one could estimate that almost 45% of the neurological complications reported from the procedure up to 2 years of follow-up happened during the hospital stay. Concerning the usefulness of cerebral protection, the registry showed similar results with and without protective device, and furthermore showed no significant difference between the three types of protective devices.

   (c) Macdonald and Gaines[12] reported procedural or postoperative stroke/death rates of respectively 2% and 4%.

   (d) Qureshi and Hopkins[13] reported in their series 14 cases of neurological complications (13%), of which 10 happened postoperatively.

2. Protective devices do not prevent from all procedural neurological complications. Some authors reported procedural rates up to 10 % for reversible deficit and up to 5.2% for stroke/death rate.[5,14]

3. There is no EBM prospective comparative data comparing carotid stenting with and without cerebral protection. The world survey leaded by Wholey[15] described a 4.2% perioperative stroke/death rate in 1597 patients without cerebral protection, while in 771 consecutive protected patients, the stroke/death rate was only 1.7%.

   In our personal series, the peri-procedural rate of complications was 1.7% without cerebral protection and higher (2.7%) with protective devices, when we considered all types of strokes. However, these two consecutive series are not comparable for the first one only enrolled highly selected lesions, and the second unselected lesions.

4. There is no comparative evaluation of the trapping features of the protective devices. The characteristics and the amount of debris captured during protected procedures are irregular and depend on the plaque structure, but also on the efficacy of the devices. As reported in different experiences using different protective systems[6,16] debris may be found in 40–100% of the cases, depending on the patient selection and the protective device used.

5. There is no ideal system for cerebral protection. In up to 5% of the cases[17] protective devices cannot be used due to either their size or their inability to cross the tortuosities of the internal carotid artery. Sometimes it is the retrieval system that cannot be used. In our experience, combined filters have been necessary when occlusive devices were not tolerated, and it happened that filters could not cross internal carotid artery tortuosities, which were protected with a flow reversal system (Fig. 5).

6. Microembolization with silent cerebral infarction[18] were demonstrated after protected carotid stenting. It can also lead to a possible deficit in cognitive functions and to partial memory loss.

7. We do not know exactly which lesion must be protected and which one is at no risk. Plaque characterization has been strongly investigated[19-21] on the basis of their respective echogenicity, observed during duplex scan examination. A study is currently running to identify which lesion is at risk (ICAROS).[22] The first results based on gray scale (GSM) show that plaques with a GSM>50 are not at risk. Others could benefit from cerebral protection due to their low echogenicity and high risk of potential embolization.

8. Nevertheless, we are awaiting scientific data. Most authors do not use protective devices for some specific lesions such as recurrent stenoses after carotid endarterectomy, radiation-induced stenoses, and lesions at the origin of the supra-aortic vessels.

9. Others[23] do not use any protective device at all, and show similar results with comparable complication rates. These series may be biased by a high selection of the lesions treated. We had also reported a very low rate of complications in a pilot study only enrolling selected lesions of the internal carotid artery.[24]

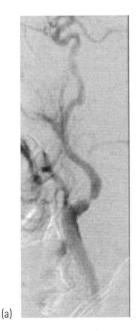
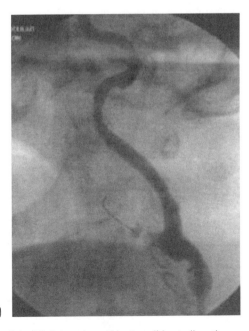

(a)   (b)

Figure 5. In this patient, the tortuosities of the left internal carotid artery did not allow the placement of the filter device (a). The stenting procedure was successfully achieved with the help of the Parodi Anti Embolic System (PAES) protective device (b).

10. Embolic particles may come off the plaques at each step of the carotid stenting procedure, including carotid catheterization from the aortic arch[25] to guide placement through the stenosis.[8] An ideal system for cerebral protection should be effective from the initial step of the procedure until the very last endovascular manoeuvre.

Comments

All these arguments justify further studies comparing protected versus unprotected carotid stenting, assessing the efficacy of the numerous devices, the role of the post-procedural use of drugs, and also evaluating the new generations of stents including covered and coated stents. These studies should include diffusion-weighted magnetic resonance imaging to detect silent infarctions. As we believe that carotid stenting must not have a widespread application, except in high risk patients, protective devices must not always be used. They could be reserved to highly emboligenous plaques associated with thrombus or ulcerations. On the contrary, echolucent regular fibrous plaques could be treated without protection, but this has to be demonstrated.

Symptoms, length of the lesion and age of the patients seem to be valuable predictors of the outcome of carotid stenting. Other factors such as cholesterolaemia and postoperative hypertension must also be considered for the selection of the patients and for the management of the disease.[13,26,27]

Summary

- There is no level I evidence to support the view that protected carotid stenting is superior to unprotected carotid stenting.

- Selected patients can be treated without cerebral protection with comparable results.

- There is no ideal protective device. These are in perpetual technical evolution. A comparative study is also required to assess the efficacy of each.

- Patients at high risk of embolization must be identified.

- Most complications occurring in the postoperative period do not benefit from protective devices, therefore pharmacological protection could be helpful.

- A strict selection is necessary for carotid stenting indications and also for cerebral protection indications.

- There is not yet any clinical evidence to support the view that carotid stenting should always be performed with cerebral protection.

References

1. Mathias K. Overview and history of treatment of carotid artery stenosis. In: Amor M, Bergeron P, Mathias K, Raithel D (eds). *Carotid Artery Angioplasty and Stenting.* Minerva Medica 2002; 1–5.
2. Bergeron P, Chambran P, Benichou H, Alessandri C. Recurrent carotid disease: will stents be an alternative to surgery? *J Endovasc Surg* 1996; 3: 76–79.

3. Ohki T, Roubin GS, Veith F et al. Efficacy of a filter device in the prevention of embolic events during carotid angioplasty and stenting: An ex vivo analysis. J Vasc Surg 1999; 30: 1034–1044.

4. Ohki T, Parodi JC, Veith FJ et al. Efficacy of a proximal occlusion catheter with reversal of flow in preventing embolic events during carotid artery stenting: an experimental analysis. J Vasc Surg 2001; 33: 504–509.

5. Roubin GS, New G, Iyer SS et al. Immediate and late clinical outcomes of carotid artery stenting in patients with symptomatic and asymptomatic carotid artery stenosis: a 5-year prospective analysis. Circulation 2001; 103: 532–537.

6. Henry M, Henry I, Klonaris C et al. Benefits of cerebral protection during carotid stenting with the PercuSurge GuardWire system: midterm results. J Endovasc Ther 2002; 9: 1–13.

7. Adami CA, Scuro A, Spinamano L et al. Use of the Parodi anti-embolism system in carotid stenting: Italian trial results. J Endovasc Ther 2002; 9: 147–154.

8. Coggia M, Goeau-Brissonniere O, Duval JL et al. Embolic risk of the different stages of carotid bifurcation balloon angioplasty: an experimental study. J Vasc Surg 2000; 31: 550–557.

9. Wholey MH, Wholey M, Jarmolowski CR, Eles GR. The growing role of carotid artery stenting. Endovascular Today 2002; 1: 24–28.

10. Bergeron P. Personal communication. Analysis of neurological complications during CAS. International Congress XVI on Endovascular Interventions, Phoenix, AZ; Feb. 2003

11. European Registry on Carotid Angioplasty and Stenting. www.euro-cast.org

12. Macdonald S, Venables GS, Cleveland TJ, Gaines PA. Protected carotid stenting: safety and efficacy of the MedNova NeuroShield filter. J Vasc Surg 2002; 35: 966–972.

13. Qureshi AI, Luft AR, Janardhan et al. Identification of patients at risk for periprocedural neurological deficits associated with carotid angioplasty and stenting. Stroke 2000; 31: 376–382.

14. Tubler T, Schluter M, Dirsch O et al. Balloon-protected carotid artery stenting: relationship of periprocedural neurological complications with the size of particulate debris. Circulation 2001; 104: 2791–2796.

15. Wholey MH, Wholey M, Mathias K et al. Global experience in cervical carotid artery stent placement. Catheter Cardiovasc Interv 2000; 50: 160–167.

16. Cremonesi A, Castriota F. Efficacy of a nitinol filter device in the prevention of embolic events during carotid interventions. J Endovasc Ther 2002; 9: 155–159.

17. Al-Mubarak N, Colombo A, Gaines PA et al. Multicenter evaluation of carotid artery stenting with a filter protection system. J Am Coll Cardiol 2002; 39: 841–846.

18. Jaeger HJ, Mathias KD, Hauth E Christmann A. Cerebral ischemia detected with diffusion-weighted MR imaging after stent implantation in the carotid artery. AJNR Am J Neuroradiol 2002; 23: 200–207.

19. Nicolaïdes AN, Biasi GM, Griffin M et al. Carotid plaque characterization. In: Amor M, Bergeron P, Mathias K, Raithel D (eds). Carotid Artery Angioplasty and Stenting. Minerva Medica 2002: 21–29.

20. Pedro LM, Pedro MM, Goncalves I et al. Computer-assisted carotid plaque analysis: characteristics of plaques associated with cerebrovascular symptoms and cerebral infarction. Eur J Vasc Endovasc Surg 2000; 19: 118–123.

21. Biasi GM, Sampaolo A, Mingazzini P et al. Computer analysis of ultrasonic plaque echolucency in identifying high risk carotid bifurcation lesions. Eur J Vasc Endovasc Surg 1999; 17: 476–479.

22. Biasi GM, Ferrari SA, Nicolaides AN et al. The ICAROS registry of carotid artery stenting. Imaging in carotid angioplasties and risk of stroke. J Endovasc Ther 2001; 8: 46–52.

23. Criado FJ, Lingelbach JM, Ledesma DF, Lucas PR. Carotid artery stenting in a vascular surgery practice. J Vasc Surg 2002; 35: 430–434.

24. Bergeron P, Becquemin JP, Jausseran JM Percutaneous stenting of the internal carotid artery: the European CAST I Study. Carotid Artery Stent Trial. J Endovasc Surg 1999; 6: 155–159.

25. Bergeron P, Massonat J. Angioplasty and stent application for carotid atherosclerosis. In: Leahy AL, Bell PRF, Katzen BT (eds). Minimal Access Therapy for Vascular Disease. London: Martin Dunitz, 2002: 89–102.

26. Dangas G, Laird JR Jr, Satler LF et al. Postprocedural hypotension after carotid artery stent placement: predictors and short- and long-term clinical outcomes. Radiology 2000; 215: 677–683.

27. Mathur A, Roubin GS, Lyer SS. Predictors of stroke complicating carotid artery stenting. Circulation 1998 Apr 7; 97(13): 1239–45.

Carotid stenting should always be performed with cerebral protection

Charing Cross Editorial Comments towards Consensus

Peter Gaines and Jay Yadav argue that carotid stenting should always be performed with cerebral protection. The explanation given by Peter Gaines is that cerebral protection systems are capable of collecting atheromatous debris and that the number of neuroembolic complications is reduced when using a cerebral protection system. Therefore as devices are available he suggests that they should be used in all patients treated with carotid artery stent *until such time as solid contradictory evidence is available*. The normal expectation of introducing a new technique is the new technique needs to be demonstrated to be beneficial to the previous technique. Here the authors argue that the previous technique was poor and this one is better because the device for catching atheroma is available. In short, because it is available, it should be used!

The opposition have reviewed the arguments and draw attention to the lack of high quality evidence to show that protected carotid stenting is superior. They say also that the complications which occur in the postoperative period do not benefit from protective devices used at the same time as the procedure.

R M Greenhalgh
Editor

There is no mandate for intervention for asymptomatic carotid disease

For the motion

Alison W Halliday, Joanna Marro

Introduction

Intervention for asymptomatic carotid disease (ACS) by surgeons and radiologists is unlikely to prevent ipsilateral strokes and death. No evidence exists to support the use of stenting in ACS and the single surgical trial supporting surgery, ACAS (Asymptomatic Carotid Atherosclerosis Study) has been heavily criticized since its publication in 1995.[1]

Evidence

ACAS showed a statistically significant reduction in projected 5-year ipsilateral strokes occurring as a result of surgery for 60–99% ACS, when compared with contemporary medical treatment. It did not show any evidence for reduction in ipsilateral disabling stroke. The small advantage shown (reduction in stroke rate from 2% to 1% per year) depended on patients having their surgery with a <3.0% risk of perioperative stroke or death.[1] In 1999 the Aspirin and Carotid Endarterectomy Trial (ACE) reported a 4.6% risk of stroke and death in patients having surgery for ACS.[2] Other 'real-life' reports have confirmed that morbidity and mortality from surgery often exceeds 4% and operation cannot therefore be justified in these patients.[3-5]

There have been attempts to identify subgroups of patients at higher stroke risk in whom surgery could be justified; women in ACAS had a higher stroke risk and have a lower stroke risk on medical treatment, so do not benefit from operation. Ipsilateral computed tomography (CT) infarction did not indicate high risk in ACAS and other studies have reported similar findings.[6-8] The detection of ipsilateral emboli using transcranial Doppler (TCD) is infrequent and unlikely to prospectively identify patients at increased stroke risk.[9] Increasing duplex stenosis and contralateral occlusion were not risk factors favouring surgery in ACAS. In fact, the 5-year stroke risk in ACAS was lower in patients with contralateral occlusion on medical treatment (3.5%) compared with the surgical group (5.5%); in ACE patients with contralateral occlusion the 30-day perioperative stroke rate was 12%! Operating on left-sided stenoses might be expected to save more dominant hemisphere strokes but, again, the operative risk is higher (6.6% vs 4.2% for the right side in ACE) not supporting this strategy.

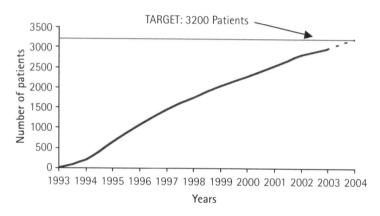

Figure 1. Asymptomatic Carotid Surgery Trial (ACST) recruitment.

The ongoing Asymptomatic Carotid Surgery Trial (ACST) with over 3000 patients is due to report by March 2004 and continues to randomize patients (Fig. 1).[10] This is the last large trial of surgery for ACS. This trial may enable a high-risk group to be identified. The mean follow-up in ACST to date is >3.5 years with some patients now having been followed for 10 years.

In all ACS patients the risk of stroke seems small compared with the risk of death or disability from other vascular causes (mainly cardiac). Nadareishvili and Rothwell reported that non-stroke and myocardial deaths were two to three times commoner than stroke deaths over 10–15 years follow-up in patients with 50–99% stenosis. Although 30% of the stenoses studied progressed between 5 and 15 years after study entry, there was NO association between increasing stenosis and ipsilateral stroke. They concluded that 'prevention strategies should concentrate on coronary risk more than stroke risk'.[11]

Definitive large trials now support the use of medical treatment in stroke prevention. The Prospective Pravastatin Pooling project (PPP) in 2001 analysed three large trials (CARE, LIPID and WOSCOPS) with over 19 000 patients randomized to pravastatin versus placebo. In the secondary prevention trials (CARE and LIPID) the use of pravastatin was associated with a 23% reduction in non-fatal ischaemic strokes (98% CI, 6–37%) (Fig. 2).[12] Supporting this were the results from B-mode ultrasound regression trials documenting the effectiveness of pravastatin in slowing and/or reversing atherosclerosis.[13-15]

The findings from PPP were rapidly followed by the convincing results of the Heart Protection Study (HPS) of 20 536 UK adults with atherosclerosis, hypertension or diabetes who were randomized to simvastatin or placebo.[16] During the 5-year study period all-cause mortality was significantly reduced by 14.7% and there was an 18% reduction in coronary death rate. One quarter reduction in non-fatal or fatal stroke (p<0.0001) was found and the benefits were present irrespective of the subgroup studied (women, peripheral arterial disease, diabetes and lipid levels). Ischaemic strokes were reduced by 30% and the highly significant benefit was seen by year 2 of follow-up and in every subsequent year (Fig. 3).

The number of patients having at least one transient ischaemic attack (TIA) was also significantly reduced (250 to 204, p=0.02). The need for intervention using coronary revascularization (angioplasty or surgery) went down by 30% and the number

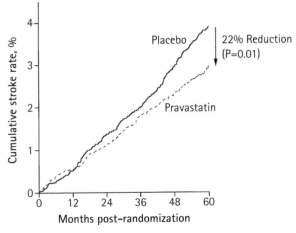

Figure 2. Occurrence of any stroke (fatal or non-fatal) by treatment assignment (CARE and LIPID combined).

Year of follow-up	Simvastatin-allocated	Placebo-allocated	Event rate ratio (95% CI)	
1	481/10269 (4.7%)	527/10267 (5.1%)		
2	377/9745 (3.9%)	538/9683 (5.6%)		
3	359/9288 (3.9%)	509/9055 (5.6%)		
4	331/8818 (3.8%)	436/8463 (5.2%)		
5+	485/8358 (5.8%)	575/7897 (7.3%)		
ALL FOLLOW-UP	2033/10 269 (19.8%)	2585/10 267 (25.2%)		0.76 (0.72–0.81) p<0.0001

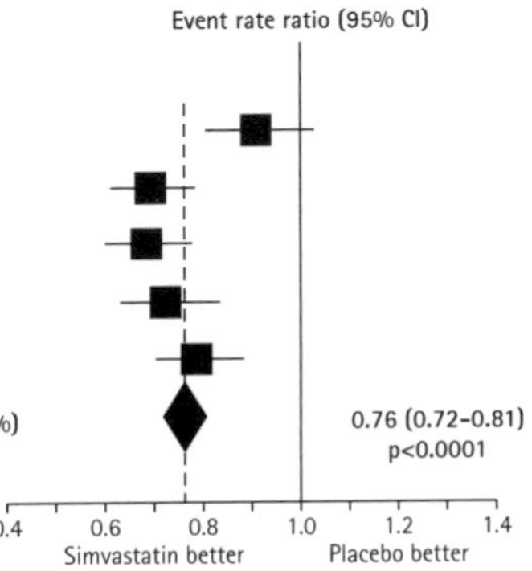

0.4   0.6   0.8   1.0   1.2   1.4
Simvastatin better   Placebo better

Figure 3. Effects of simvastatin allocation on first major vascular event during follow-up: Analyses are of numbers of participants having a first event during each year of follow-up and of those still at risk of a first event at the start of each year.

of carotid endarterectomies and angioplasties was halved in the simvastatin-treated group (42 vs 82, p=0.0003). "Much larger numbers ... suffered a stroke in the HPS than in any previous cholesterol-lowering trial, resolving any remaining uncertainties about the effects of statin therapy on the incidence of stroke". These benefits are **additional** to other treatments such as aspirin and occurred despite non-compliance in up to one-third of patients.

Conclusion

Intervention by surgery or angioplasty for asymptomatic carotid stenosis does not prevent disabling stroke and even in some well-run trials surgery has caused more strokes than it has saved. Lipid lowering therapy effectively prevents at least 50% of ischaemic strokes in patients with ACS and is well-tolerated and safe.

Summary

- No trial has shown that lives or strokes can be saved by stenting asymptomatic carotid artery stenosis.

- In ACAS, operation did not prevent strokes in women or disabling strokes in men or women.

- 'Real life' results of operation are worse than ACAS even in well-run trials such as ACE.

- Unless the Asymptomatic Carotid Surgery Trial (ACST) identifies a 'high-risk group' that might benefit from intervention, none has yet been identified.

- Unjustified increases in stenting and operation cost lives, cause strokes and waste money.

- Medical treatment is more effective than surgery at preventing stroke and death (The Heart Protection Study, Pravastatin Pooling Project).

- There is no place for intervening with surgery or angioplasty in asymptomatic carotid disease.

References

1. Executive Committee for the Asymptomatic Carotid Atherosclerosis Study. Endarterectomy for asymptomatic carotid artery stenosis. *J Am Med Assoc* 1995; **273**: 1421–1428.
2. Taylor DW, Barnett HJ, Haynes RB, Ferguson GG *et al.* Low-dose and high-dose acetylsalicylic acid for patients undergoing carotid endarterectomy: a randomised controlled trial – ASA and Carotid Endarterectomy (ACE) Collaborators. *Lancet* 1999; **353**: 2179–2184.
3. Wennberg DE, Lucas FL, Birkmeyer JD *et al.* Variation in carotid endarterectomy mortality in the Medicare population: trial hospitals, volume, and patient characteristics. *J Am Med Assoc* 1998; **279**: 1278–1281.
4. Smurawska LT, Bowyer B, Rowed D *et al.* Changing practice and costs of carotid endarterectomy in Toronto, Cananda. *Stroke* 1998; **29**: 2014–2017.
5. Goldstein LB, Samsa GP, Matchar DB, Oddone EZ. Multicenter review of preoperative risk factors for endarterectomy for asymptomatic carotid artery stenosis. *Stroke* 1998; **29**: 750–753.
6. Young B, Moore WS, Robertson JT *et al.* An analysis of perioperative surgical mortality and morbidity in the asymptomatic carotid atherosclerosis study: ACAS Investigators. *Stroke* 1996; **27**: 2216–2224.
7. Baker WH, Howard VJ, Howard G, Toole JF. Effect of contralateral occlusion on long-term efficacy of endarterectomy in the asymptomatic carotid atherosclerosis study (ACAS): ACAS Investigators. *Stroke* 2000; **31**: 2330–2334.
8. Kucey DS, Bowyer B, Iron K *et al.* Determinants of outcome after carotid endarterectomy. *J Vasc Surg* 1998; **28**: 1051–1058.
9. Molloy J, Markus HS. Asymptomatic embolism predicts stroke and TIA risk in carotid artery stenosis. *Stroke* 1999; **30**: 1440–1443.
10. Halliday AW, Thomas D, Mansfield A. The asymptomatic carotid surgery trial (ACST). Rationale and design. Steering Committee. *Eur J Vasc Surg* 1994; **8**: 703–710.
11. Nadareishvili ZG, Rothwell PM, Beletsky V *et al.* Long-term risk of stroke and other vascular events in patients with asymptomatic carotid artery stenosis. *Arch Neurol* 2002; **59**: 1162–1166.
12. Byington RP, Davis BR, Plehn JF *et al.* Reduction of stroke events with pravastatin. The Prospective Pravastatin Pooling (PPP) Project. *Circulation* 2001; **103**: 387–392.
13. Crouse JR, Byington RP, Bond MG *et al.* Pravastatin, lipids, and atherosclerosis in the carotid arteries (PLAC-II). *Am J Cardiol* 1995; **75**: 455–459.
14. Salonen R, Nyyssonen K, Porkkala E *et al.* Kuopio atherosclerosis prevention study (KAPS). A population-based primary preventive trial of the effect of LDL lowering on atherosclerotic progression in carotid and femoral arteries. *Circulation* 1995; **92**: 1758–1764.
15. MacMahon S, Sharpe N, Gamble G *et al.* Effects of lowering average of below-average cholesterol

levels on the progression of carotid atherosclerosis: results of the LIPID atherosclerosis substudy. LIPID Trial Research Group. *Circulation* 1998; **97**: 1784–1790.

16. Heart Protection Study Collaborative Group. MRC/BHF Heart Protection Study of cholesterol lowering with simvastatin in 20536 high-risk individuals: a randomized placebo-controlled trial. *Lancet* 2002; **360**: 7–22.

There is no mandate for intervention for asymptomatic carotid disease • **For the motion** • AW Halliday, J Marro

There is no mandate for intervention for asymptomatic carotid disease

Against the motion
Giorgio M Biasi, Paolo M Mingazzini,
Gaetano Deleo, Alberto Froio

Introduction

Stroke is the third leading cause of death and the first among cardiovascular diseases, and a most frequent cause of disability, demanding elevated social costs and needing huge resources to address assistance and rehabilitation.

The prevention of stroke has consequently become of utmost importance in modern health care.

Some 30 years after the introduction on a large scale of carotid endarterectomy (CEA) for the prevention of neurological disturbances from carotid bifurcation plaques, and more than 10 years since the publication of international, prospective randomized studies that seemed to finally allay doubts and uncertainties on the subject,[1-7] transmitting for posterity the message that CEA is the gold standard for the prevention of stroke, some old problems concerning indication and the appropriateness of CEA remain unsolved and some new ones have appeared preponderantly on the international scene.

While there is a substantial consensus that CEA is effective in the prevention of stroke in symptomatic patients with haemodynamic carotid artery stenoses,[8,9] trials have concluded that the evidence of benefit of CEA in asymptomatic patients with a 70% or more carotid stenosis is questionable and in any case minimal, compared with conservative medical treatment.[2,4,5,10]

These data conflict with the diffuse practice worldwide of CEA procedures performed on asymptomatic patients and also with the conclusions of other equally influential and authoritative publications.[7,11,12] The position of these authors, that effective prevention of stroke should also be addressed to asymptomatic carotid stenoses, is justified by data from the literature showing that only a minority of strokes is preceded by transient neurological symptoms/ischaemic attack (TIA).[13]

The facts

Evidence-based data on prevention present some handicaps compared with similar data related to treatment. The most relevant is that the clear benefit of any preventive action, has statistical- rather than clinical-based evidence. The benefit or not of a procedure in preventing a stroke from a carotid bifurcation plaque, depends of course on the study design, the volume of the sample and the duration of the observation. Beyond any doubt, the scarcer and vaguer the risk of neurological disturbances in the natural history of the patient and of the plaque, the lower the operative risk – but this also applies to evidence of benefit of any procedure, and the longer the period of observation and the larger the sample of the patients. Elderly, symptomatic patients presenting with a very tight stenosis of the carotid bifurcation due to a 'complex' plaque, are probably the ideal candidates for a carotid procedure, especially when performed in centres with great experience and a < 3% operative neurological complication rate. In such a group of patients it is very likely that a small sample will be sufficient to obtain statistical evidence in a randomized trial versus best medical treatment. In the case of neurologically asymptomatic, younger individuals, affected by haemodynamic carotid stenoses, a more significant number of parameters and algorithms have to be entered in both arms of a study and a much higher number of procedures over a longer period of observation, have to be performed to provide evidence of the efficacy of the procedure in preventing a stroke.[14,15]

For example, a similar situation was evidenced in the UK Small Aneurysm Trial. In fact, the 9-year follow-up of patients in the trial has provided slightly different results from those that emerged at the conclusion of the study at 5 years.[16] Later on, it may very well be that, for asymptomatic subjects presenting with a ≥ 70% stenosis, with a good life expectancy, in the long run a prophylactic intervention might be beneficial. In any case, late results of study designs in which symptomatic patients and asymptomatic subjects were grouped in the same study, should probably be reconsidered. The impression largely diffused is that data from trials often have to be integrated with epidemiology, extrapolated and finally interpreted. In such circumstances it would be more appropriate to say that we are dealing with a medicine based on 'interpretation of evidence', rather than 'evidence-based medicine'. Furthermore, as subgroups of patients presenting different symptoms can be identified with regard to the risk of stroke, paraphrasing Eric Arthur Blair (who later adopted the pseudonym of George Orwell), *not all asymptomatic subjects are equal,* either.

It has been reported that symptomatic patients may present different behaviour in terms of risk of perioperative stroke and/or death. Ocular symptoms constitute a lesser risk than hemispheric symptoms.[17,18] Subgroups of so-called asymptomatic individuals should similarly be identified. Those presenting with a negative history of neurological symptoms should be regarded as being at a different risk from those who report aspecific symptoms (non-hemispheric or ocular), or do not refer to any recent symptoms (during the previous 180 days) or finally those that have a negative brain CT scan but in which the clinical neurological history might be difficult to collect. In addition, so called 'silent strokes' were observed in from 5% to 12% of asymptomatic carotid stenosis.[19] It has been demonstrated that the longer the time interval from the TIA or non-disabling stroke, the less the likelihood of another neurological event.[20] The reason for this finding is unclear. One can speculate that during the months following the TIA, repair or healing of the plaque can take place. On the other hand, one may then also speculate that other events can occur with eventually more catastrophic and permanent outcomes.

In other words, categorizing patients as candidates for any carotid procedure on the basis of rate of stenosis and presence or absence of neurological symptoms alone, does not identify sufficiently and accurately the real risk presented by the patient.

Several recent randomized trials, have indicated a substantial relative risk reduction in asymptomatic patients with carotid stenosis of 60% or more, when treated surgically, with a 5-year risk of stroke reduced from 11% to 5% in the Asymptomatic Carotid Atherosclerosis Study (ACAS).[7] The expert panel Guidelines of the American Heart Association (AHA) has therefore concluded for a '*grade A recommendation*' of the use of endarterectomy in asymptomatic patients with 60% to 99% stenosis, provided the rate of perioperative stroke and death is less than 3% and life expectancy is at least 5 years.[11, 21]

The National Stroke Association (NSA) has also stated in a consensus panel that, if the risk associated with surgery is assured at less than 3%, endarterectomy can be recommended also in asymptomatic stenoses.[12]

Discussion

Incidence of stroke has increased during recent years and this has been considered as related to an inadequate control of the cerebral risk factors.[22] Asymptomatic carotid artery stenosis has been identified by the National Stroke Association as one of the risk factors for stroke, and CEA has been recommended for prevention of a first stroke in case of asymptomatic carotid stenosis ≥ 60% when surgical morbidity and mortality account for ≤ 3%.[12,21] Literature diffusely reports large series of subjects affected by asymptomatic severe carotid stenosis who have undergone CEA, with very satisfactory results; this has created some concern – for example Barnett's warning of the risk that, on a wave of enthusiasm, too optimistic data would divulge a wrong message leading to an unjustified, dogmatic increase in the indication for CEA procedures.[23] At present there is not sufficient evidence that prophylactic CEA is beneficial in asymptomatic severe carotid stenosis and only the results of ongoing trials might add significative information.[24,25] Nevertheless, it looks as if this message is not clear – and this is confirmed by the fact that between 25% and 60% of CEAs are performed on asymptomatic individuals.[23,26]

Data from well conducted randomized studies, to which we have been referring in this report, are not to be questioned, nevertheless they do not seem to have the final word about the inappropriateness of CEA in asymptomatic severe (>70%) carotid stenosis. Very few topics in medicine have been as deeply, thoroughly and exhaustively analysed and discerned and been given so much attention as CEA in asymptomatic carotid stenosis. The question at this point is why such a relevant number of CEA procedures are still currently performed worldwide on asymptomatic patients[27] if the message is univocal, incontrovertible and incontestable.

Possible reasons to explain this situation are the following:

1. Some surgeons are not aware of the results of these trials.
2. Surgeons do not care for, or confute, the evidence of the trials and continue to treat asymptomatic subjects.
3. Surgeons are aware of the results of the studies but claim better outcomes than those in the natural history of asymptomatic patients.
4. Economical aspects and implications.

Point number 1 does not deserve discussion whereas points 2 and 3 are the key aspects of the matter.

Potential biases of randomized trials, even when impeccably conducted, have been suggested. The criticism is that models adopted in trials usually do not reproduce routine practice.[28] Gender, age, degree of stenosis, neurological symptoms, presence of contralateral lesions or other co-morbidities in the populations selected for trials, selected surgeons, centres and hospitals, different means of assessment of carotid stenoses (ultrasound, magnetic resonance angiography, etc.), time interval of observation, dimension of the population sample, may not be representative of the population as a whole. It is well known that prospective randomized controlled studies are usually conducted in centres of excellence, where a large number of operations are done per year, whereas centres with less experience (where a higher rate of complications should be expected), are generally excluded.[29]

These all represent relevant caveats of randomized trials. In addition, if one considers that parameters and variables, such as the characteristics of the plaque, ulceration, irregularity, grey scale median (GSM), etc. are usually disregarded and not even mentioned in several study designs, skepticism is comprehensible. It has been observed that the characteristics of the plaque, such as surface irregularity or ulcerations, may not relate reliably to symptoms in as much as they are not easily detectable, either by means of ultrasonography or angiography.[30] Nevertheless, these data seem to be surpassed by the present technology.

Considering the prevalent embolic origin of stroke, it is probable that the rate of progression and percentage of stenosis are not so important *per se*, but as related to modifications and remodelling processes inside the atherosclerotic plaque.

Characterization of the plaque is therefore essential for indication – and modern duplex ultrasonography is now superior to angiography in the morphological examination of the plaque, and is recognized as the gold standard in the diagnosis of the carotid plaque.

Different criteria used by the two largest trials, NASCET and ECST, to measure the percentage of stenosis, have generated confusion in comparing data and conclusions from different studies. Now that the gold standard for the diagnosis of carotid bifurcation disease is the duplex scan, we should calculate the percentage of stenosis of diameter reduction of the native artery, with a proportional acceleration in the arterial flow.[31]

Considering plaque morphology, several characteristics are responsible for the increase in the risk of stroke,[32] such as intraplaque haemorrhage,[33,34] ulceration and rupture,[33,35-37] the presence of endoluminal thrombus[35] and the inflammatory reaction with thinning of the fibrous cap of the carotid plaque.[38]

We have found significant correlation between hypoechoic soft plaques with low GSM values and incidence of cerebral events.[38-40]

We have also demonstrated that the rate of neurological complications following carotid stenting in patients with a GSM <25, is statistically higher than that with GSM>25 ($p<0.001$).[41,42,43] The study did not relate to CEA patients, but similar results in these patients may be expected.

If data from trials still leave room for uncertainty among a large group of providers, it becomes reasonable to say that at a certain point other criteria of judgment and discernment need to be introduced.

I realize that statistically it may only be regarded as anecdotal, nevertheless my personal experience is of a retrospective analysis of a series of 504 patients, asymptomatic or presenting with aspecific neurological symptoms, operated on for CEA from May 1996, when the first carotid stenting procedure was performed in my hospital. Of the 504 patients, one had a minor stroke and three had major strokes and there were no deaths, which corresponds to a rate of neurological complications of 0.79%. I think that these results compare favourably with the natural history of asymptomatic severe carotid stenoses.

In our routine practice, potential advantages of the CEA procedure are thoroughly examined and explained to the patients, who are then solicited to express their position and eventually their consent. Data from international trials and statistical analysis, results from clinical, angiographic and especially ultrasound examination with assessment of the GSM of the plaque, are presented and discussed with the patients who must be informed of the potential risk of stroke from an asymptomatic carotid stenosis, detected occasionally at a control. The automatic exclusion from a surgical programme of a patient in this condition, would not be entirely ethical or in his/her clinical interest.

I do not think that point 4, concerning economical aspects and implications, deserve much discussion since the question of the cost-effectiveness of CEA remains substantially unsolved.[44,45]

Conclusions

In conclusion, the automatic exclusion, with lack of critical discernment of neurologically asymptomatic patients, on the basis of raw data represented by rate of stenosis and presence or absence of neurological symptoms, is no longer acceptable.[46] Considering the fact that a remarkable number of asymptomatic patients or patients who have non-specific symptoms are submitted to prophylactic CEA, it is absolutely essential that patients and providers having the most favourable outcome profile be identified.

Subgroups of patients should be defined and characterized on the basis of the features of their plaque.[47] The assumption that plaque heterogeneity should be considered in selecting patients for CEA,[48] has to be seconded and supported.

Our conclusion is that there is a mandate for intervention for asymptomatic carotid artery patients with a good life expectancy, through a selection of candidates for surgery at higher risk of stroke, based on the characteristics of their plaque at duplex sonography.

Summary

- Trials have demonstrated the efficacy of CEA in preventing stroke from carotid bifurcation plaques in high grade, symptomatic stenoses.

- Data tend to demonstrate that CEA is not beneficial in asymptomatic subjects.

- The reliability of only the two classical parameters usually considered in trials: rate of stenosis and neurological symptomatology, on which to base indication to CEA, is debated.

- Not all asymptomatic patients are equal.

- Subgroups of patients should be identified on the basis of the features of the carotid plaque and other co-morbidities in addition to classical parameters and variables, for a correct indication and assessment of efficacy of CEA.

- A less strict and drastic analysis of raw data from trials, would be to the benefit of the patient.

- The automatic exclusion from a surgical programme of an asymptomatic patient presenting with a significative carotid stenosis, would not be entirely ethical or in his/her clinical interest.

References

1. Asymptomatic Carotid Atherosclerosis Study Group: Study design for randomised prospective trial of carotid endarterectomy for asymptomatic atherosclerosis: The Asymptomatic Carotid Atherosclerosis Study Group. *Stroke* 1989; **20**: 844–849.
2. CASANOVA Study Group: Carotid surgery versus medical therapy in asymptomatic carotid stenosis. *Stroke* 1991; **22**: 1229–1235.
3. North American Symptomatic Carotid Endarterectomy Trials Collaborators (NASCET). Beneficial effects of carotid endarterectomy in symptomatic patients with high-grade stenosis. *New Engl J Med* 1991; **325**: 445–453.
4. Mayo Asymptomatic Carotid Endarterectomy Study Group. Results of a randomised controlled trial of carotid endarterectomyfor asymptomatic carotid stenosis. *Mayo Clin Proc* 1991; 1992; **67**: 513–518.
5. Hobson RW II, Weiss DG, Fields WS *et al.* and the Veterans Affairs Cooperative Study Group. Efficacy of carotid endarterectomy for asymptomatic carotid stenosis. *New Engl J Med* 1993; **328**: 221–227.
6. European Carotid Surgery Trialists' Collaborative Group: Risk of stroke in the distribution of an asymptomatic carotid artery: The European Carotid Surgery Trailists' Collaborative Group. *Lancet* 1995; **345**: 209–212.
7. Executive Committee for the Asymptomatic Carotid Atherosclerosis Study: Endarterectomy for asymptomatic carotid artery stenosis. *J Am Med Soc* 1995; **273**: 1421–1428.
8. Barnett HJ, Taylor DW, Eliasziw M. Benefit of carotid endarterectomy in patients with symptomatic moderate or severe stenosis. NASCET Collaborators. *New Engl J Med* 1998; **339**: 1415–1425.
9. Randomized trial of endarterectomy for recently symptomatic carotid stenosis: final results of the MRC ECST. *Lancet* 1998; **351**: 1379–1387.
10. Barnett HJM, Meldrum HE, Eliasziw M for the North American Symptomatic Carotid Endarterectomy Trial (NASCET) Collaborators. *Can Med Assoc J* 2002; **166**: 1169–1179.
11. Biller J, Feinberg WM, Castaldo JE *et al.* Guidelines for carotid endarterectomy: a statement for healthcare professionals from a special writing group of the Stroke Council, American Heart Association. *Stroke* 1998; **29**: 554–562.
12. Gorelich PB, Sacco RL, Smith DB, Alberts M *et al.* Prevention of a first stroke: a review of guidelines and a multidisciplinary consensus statement from the National Stroke Association. *J Am Med Assoc* 1999; **281**: 1112–1120.
13. Inzitari D, Eliasziw M, Gates P, Sharpe BL *et al.* for the North American Symptomatic Carotid Endarterectomy Trial Collaborators. The Cause and risk of stroke in patients with asymptomatic internal-carotid artery stenosis. *New Engl J Med* 2000; **342**: 1693–1700.
14. Mineva PP, Manchev IC, Hadjiev DI. Prevalence and outcome of asymptomatic carotid stenosis: a population-based ultrasonographic study. *Eur J Neurol* 2002; **9**: 383–388.
15. Alexandrova NA, Gibson WC, Norris GW. Carotid artero stenosis in peripheral artero disease. *J Vasc Surg* 1996; **23**: 645–649.
16. The United Kingdom Small Aneurysm Trial Participants. Long-term outcomes of immediate repair compared with surveillance of small abdominal aortic aneurysms. *New Engl J Med* 2002: **19**: 1445–1452.
17. Rothwell PM, Slattery J, Warlow CP. Clinical and angiographic predictors of stroke and death from carotid endarterectomy: systemic review. *Br Med J* 1997; **315**: 1571–1577.
18. Ferguson GG, Eliasziw M, Barr HW *et al.* The North American Symptomatic Carotid Endarterectomy Trial: surgical results in 1415 patients. *Stroke* 1999; **30**: 1751–1758.
19. Liapis CD, Kaskisis JD, Kostakis AG. Carotid stenosis. Factors affecting symptomatology *Stroke* 2001; **32**: 2782–2786.
20. Lanzino G, Couture D, Andreoli A *et al.* Carotid endarterectomy: Can we select surgical candidates at high risk for stroke and low risk for perioperative complications. *Neurosurgery* 2001; **49**: 913–924.
21. Goldstein LB, Adams R, Becker K *et al.* AHA Scientific Statement. Primary prevention of ischemic stroke: a statement for healthcare professional from the Stroke Council of the American heart Association. *Stroke* 2001; **32**: 280–299.
22. National Heart, Lung and Blood Institute. *Fact Book Fiscal Year 1996*, Bethesda, Md: US Department of Health and Human Services, National Institute of Health, 1997.
23. Barnett DW, Eliasziw M, Meldrum HE, Taylor DW. Do the facts and figures warrant a 10-fold increase in the performance of carotid endarterectomy on asymptomatic patients? *Neurology* 1996; **46**: 603–608.

24. Sleight SP, Poloniecki J, Halliday AW on behalf of the Asymptomatic Carotid Surgery Trial (ACST) collaborators. *Eur J Vasc Endovasc Surg* 2002; 23: 519–523.

25. Nicolaides AN, Asymptomatic carotid stenosis and risk of stroke: identification of a high risk group (ACSRS): a natural history study. International *Angiology* 1995; 14: 21–23.

26. Cebul RD, Snow RJ, Pine R *et al*. Indications, outcomes, and provider volumes for carotid endarterectomy. *J Am Med Assoc* 1998; 279: 1282–1287.

27. Karp HR, Flanders WD, Shipp CC *et al*. Carotid endarterectomy among Medicare beneficiaries: a statewide evaluation of appropriateness and outcome. *Stroke* 1998; 29: 46–52.

28. Chaturvedi S, Aggarwal R, Murugappan A. Results of carotid endarterectomy with prospective neurologist follow-up. *Neurology* 2000; 55: 769–772.

29. Segal HE, Rummel L, Wu B. The utility of PRO data on surgical volume: the example of carotid andarterectomy. *Am J Publ Hlth* 1993; 79: 1617–1620.

30. Schroeder TV, Moes Gronholdt ML, Sillesen HH. Plaque type can determine the need for asymptomatic carotid intervention: against the motion. In: *The Evidence for Vascular or Endovascular Reconstruction*. RM Greenhalgh (ed). London: Saunders: 2002: 6–11.

31. Nicolaides AN, Shifrin EG, Bradbury A *et al*. Angiographic and duplex grading of internal carotid stenosis: can we overcome the confusion? *J Endovasc Surg* 1996; 3: 158–165.

32. Langsfeld M, Gray-Weale AC, Lusby RJ. The role of plaque morphology and diameter reduction in the development of new symptoms in asymptomatic carotid arteries. *J Vasc Surg* 1989; 9: 548–557.

33. Carr S, Farb A, Pearce WH, Vimini R, Yao JST. Atherosclerotic plaque rupture in symptomatic carotid artery stenosis. *J Vasc Surg* 1996; 23: 755–766.

34. Lusby RJ, Ferrell LD, Ehrenfeld *WK et al.*Carotid plaque hemorrhage : its role in production of cerebral ischemia. *Arch Surg* 1982; 117: 1479–1488.

35. Sitzer M, Mullar W, Siebler W *et al*. Plaque ulceration and lumen thrombus are the main sources of cerebral microemboli in high-grade internal carotid stenosis. *Stroke* 1995; 26: 1231–1233.

36. Hatsukami TS, Ferguson MS, Beach KW *et al*. Carotid plaque morphology and clinical events. *Stroke* 1997; 28: 95–100.

37. Golledge J, Greenhalgh RM, Davies AH. The symptomatic carotid plaque. *Stroke* 2001; 31: 774–781.

38. Carr SC, Farb A, Pearce WH *et al*. Activated inflammatory cells are associated with plaque rupture in carotid artery stenosis. *Surgery* 1997; 122: 757–764.

39. Biasi GM, Sampaolo A, Mingazzini PM *et al*. Computer analysis of ultrasonic plaque echolucency in identifying high risk carotid bifurcation lesions. *Eur J Vasc Endovasc Surg* 1999; 17: 476–479.

40. Geroulakos G, Ramaswami G, Nicolaides A *et al*. Characterization of symptomatic and asymptomatic carotid plaques using high-resolution real-time ultrasonog-raphy. *Br J Surg* 1993; 80: 1274–1277.

41. Biasi GM. Incidence of neurological complications following carotid artery stenting correlated to the characteristics of the plaque composition: preliminary results of the ICAROS study. 27th International Stroke Conference. *Stroke* 2002; 33: 342.

42. Biasi GM. The ICAROS Study Correlating Duplex Plaque Morphology with Periprocedural Complications of CBAS: Current Results and Future Potential. In: *28th Global: Vascular and Endovascular Issues, Techniques and Horizons ™*. 2001: XXIV 6.1–2.

43. Biasi GM, Ferrari SA, Nicolaides AN *et al*. The ICAROS Registry of Carotid Artery Stenting. *J Endovasc Ther* 2001; 18: 46–52.

44. Benade MM, Warlow CP. Costs and benefits of carotid endarterectomy and associated preoperative arterial imaging. *Stroke* 2002; 33: 629–638.

45. Gray WA, White HJ, Barrett DM *et al*. Carotid stenting and endarterectomy. A clinical and cost comparison of revascularization strategies. *Stroke* 2002; 33: 1063–1070.

46. Biasi GM. Is it time to reconsider the selection criteria for conventional or endovascular repair of carotid artery stenosis in the prevention of cerebral ischemia? *J Endovasc Ther* 2001; 8: 339–340.

47. Rothwell PM, Gibson R, Warlow CP. Interrelation between plaque surface morphology and degree of stenosis on carotid angiograms and the risk of ischemic stroke patients with symptomatic carotid stenosis: on behalf of the European Carotid Trialists' Collaborative Group. *Stroke* 2000; 31: 615–621.

48. AbuRahma AF, Wulu JT, Crotty B. Carotid plaque heterogeneity and severity of stenosis. *Stroke* 2000; 33: 1772–1775.

There is no mandate for intervention for asymptomatic carotid disease

Charing Cross Editorial Comments towards Consensus

Asymptomatic carotid procedures are performed all over the world and in some countries very much more frequently than in others. Despite this fact Alison Halliday is able to conclude that no trial has shown that lives or strokes can be saved by stenting asymptomatic carotid artery stenosis, and thus far a high risk group of asymptomatic carotid patients has not been identified to justify either surgery or angioplasty restenting. Nevertheless, Giorgio Biasi's data tend to demonstrate that carotid endarterectomy is not beneficial in asymptomatic patients. This should be understood to be a major statement from Italy where, for years, asymptomatic carotid surgery has been performed frequently. Professor Biasi argues that not all asymptomatic patients are the same, and he argues for the identification of subgroups of high-risk patients based upon carotid plaque morphology.

All would surely agree that until the matter is solved any asymptomatic intervention should be under trial circumstances such as the asymptomatic carotid surgical trial described in the chapter by Alison Halliday.

Roger M Greenhalgh
Editor

Type II endoleaks are clinically unimportant

For the motion

Krassi Ivancev, Nuno Dias,
Martin Malina, Björn Sonesson

Introduction

The definition of type II endoleak is persistent flow in the aneurysm sac through branches without attachment site connection following endovascular aneurysm repair (EVAR).[1] The most common way of diagnosing type II endoleak is by contrast-enhanced spiral-computed tomagraphy (CT) with delayed images. A commonly held opinion is that type II endoleaks are of a benign nature, as opposed to attachment site (type I) endoleaks or endoleaks related to the stent-graft components (type III).[2]

The intention of this chapter is to review the available information in the literature and determine the clinical significance of persistent type II endoleak in the long run.

Prevalence and anatomic origin

A review of the current literature shows reported frequencies of type II endoleak of about 8–24% (Table 1). This variation is most likely explained by the differences in follow-up and the fact that type II endoleaks may resolve spontaneously. Though there are no exact numbers for how often it happens, a spontaneous thrombosis of type II endoleaks has been reported to occur in one-third to half of the patients.[3,5,7,10]

Table 1. Type II endoleak frequency

Reference	No. of patients	Type II endoleaks (%)
Becker[3]	305	14.6
Liewald[4]	160	8.1
Karch[5]	73	8.2
Makaroun[6]	242	23.9
Abraham[7]	116	14.0
Chuter[8]	114	7.9
Hölzenbein[9]	173	15.3
Faries[10]	368	8.9
Van Marrewijk[11]	2463	7.8
Fairman[12]	232	16.8

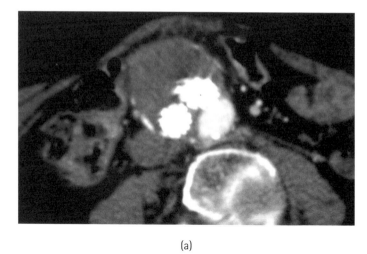

(a)

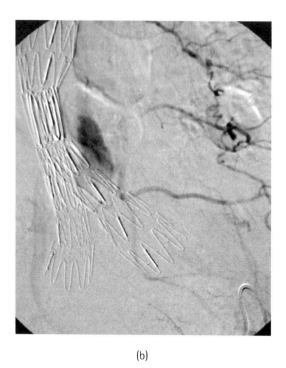

(b)

Figure 1. (a) Contrast-enhanced spiral-CT shows an endoleak in the dorsal aspect of an EVAR-treated AAA. **(b)** Digital subtraction angiography (DSA) with superselective catheterization of an iliolumbar artery shows type II endoleak supplied by multiple lumbar arteries.

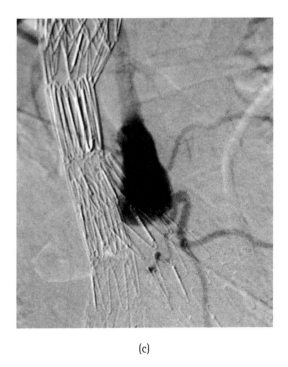

(c)

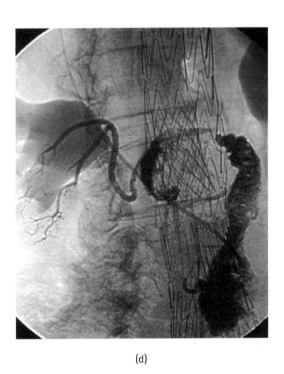

(d)

Figure 1. (c) Translumbar catheterization of the type II endoleak and aneurysmography demonstrates the multiple supply of lumbar arteries. Pressure measurements recorded with PressureWire (RADI Medical System AB, Uppsala, Sweden) demonstrated pulsatile systemic pressure. **(d)** Injection of radio-opaque glue demonstrates the large cavity of the endoleak involving also an accessory renal artery in addition to the previously demonstrated lumbar arteries.

The majority of type II endoleaks are caused by lumbar arteries only, whereas in approximately one-third of the patients the inferior mesenteric artery may also be involved. On rare occasions there is also an involvement of accessory renal arteries. There have been reports suggesting that an enlarged inferior mesenteric artery and multiple lumbar arteries are associated with an increased risk for type II endoleak.[13–14] However, such a claim has not been confirmed by other authors.[15–17] The coagulation status has been suggested to play a role for the occurrence of type II endoleak. Nevertheless, coumadin treatment has been shown not to affect the frequency of type II endoleaks but to contribute to their persistence.[12]

Treatment

Preoperative embolization of lumbar arteries and inferior mesenteric artery has been reported not to decrease the risk for development of type II endoleak.[18] In addition, multiple reports on attempts to close type II endoleak have shown that coil embolization of feeding arteries[5,8] is frequently unsuccessful, owing to recruitment of new collaterals to the perfused aneurysm sac.[19] Furthermore, embolization, especially of the inferior mesenteric artery , may be associated with serious complications, such as colon ischaemia.[20] Laparoscopic clipping of lumbar arteries[21] and translumbar direct puncture into the endoleak[22–24] have been claimed to be the most effective treatment modality available.

Consequences

Aneurysms exposed to type II endoleak usually remain unchanged in size,[13,18,25–27] whereas upon resolution of the endoleak, regardless of whether this is spontaneous or a result of successful treatment, there is a decrease in diameter and volume of the aneurysm sac.[28–29] Enlargement of the aneurysm sac or aneurysm rupture caused by type II endoleak has been anecdotally reported.[30–33]

Discussion

The clinical importance of type II endoleak is directly related to its frequency and consequences. As already mentioned, there are many reports in the literature, according to which its frequency does not exceed 25% of abdominal aortic aneurysms (AAA) undergoing EVAR (Table 1).

In addition, in some of these patients the type II endoleak spontaneously resolves.[3,5,7,10] In the remaining patients, AAA size tends to remain unchanged.[13,18,25–27] The highly limited number of reports on enlargement of aneurysm size and rupture caused by type II endoleak[30–33] suggest that this is a highly unusual event.

The picture becomes even more confused by the fact that it is sometimes difficult to separate so called 'mixed type', i.e. type I or type III plus type II, endoleak, and 'pure' type II endoleak.[8,34] It is possible that some of the reported cases of type II endoleak leading to continuous aneurysm sac pressurization have actually been 'mixed' endoleaks. Direct pressure measurement in the aneurysm sac may help resolve the degree of pressurization caused by type II endoleak. There have been only two reports in the literature claiming that type II endoleak is associated with a systemic or near-systemic pressure.[14,35] However, the pressure measurements in these reports were performed in the leak itself, a fact which can be explained only by a relatively large-sized endoleak.

Personal experience with translumbar pressure measurement in the thrombus of the aneurysm sac has shown that the pressure in successfully excluded AAAs following EVAR does not exceed 20% of the systemic pressure.[36] Similar measurements in aneurysm sacs exposed to type II endoleak have shown a high degree of variation but did not reach the systemic pressure. The only exception from this rule has been a large endoleak associated with the perfusion involving lumbar arteries and an accessory renal artery, where the intrasac aneurysm pressure was systemic. Following intrasac embolization with glue, the leak ceased, the aneurysm decreased in size, and the pressure became consistent with that of a well excluded aneurysm, i.e., below 20% of the systemic pressure (Fig. 1).

Summary

- The frequency of type II endoleak is relatively low, i.e. 20% following EVAR.

- Approximately one-third of type II endoleaks spontaneously resolve.

- The majority of AAA exposed to type II endoleak following EVAR do not increase in size, but remain unchanged.

- There are very few exceptions, with a large endoleak in the presence of the inferior mesenteric artery and/or an accessory renal artery, which may lead to continuous pressurization of the aneurysm sac.

- Type II endoleak can be regarded as clinically unimportant provided that it is not associated with other endoleak, such as type I or III.

References

1. Chaikof EL, Blankensteijn JD, Harris PL et al. Reporting standards for endovascular aortic aneurysm repair. J Vasc Surg 2002; 35: 1048–1060.
2. Veith FJ, Baum RA, Ohki T et al. Nature and significance of endoleaks and endotension: summary of opinions expressed at an international conference. J Vasc Surg 2002; 35: 1029–1035.
3. Becker GJ, Kovacs M, Mathison MN et al. Risk stratification and outcomes of transluminal endografting for abdominal aortic aneurysm: 7-year experience and long-term follow-up. J Vasc Interv Radiol 2001; 12: 1033–1046.
4. Liewald F, Ermis C, Gorich J et al.Influence of treatment of type II leaks on the aneurysm surface area. Eur J Vasc Endovasc Surg 2001; 21: 339–343.
5. Karch LA, Henretta JP, Hodgson KJ et al. Algorithm for the diagnosis and treatment of endoleaks. Am J Surg 1999; 178: 225–231.
6. Makaroun MS, Chaikof E, Naslund T, Matsumura JS. Efficacy of a bifurcated endograft versus open repair of abdominal aortic aneurysms: a reappraisal. J Vasc Surg 2002; 35: 203–210.
7. Abraham CZ, Chuter TA, Reilly LM et al. Abdominal aortic aneurysm repair with the Zenith stent graft: short to midterm results. J Vasc Surg 2002; 36: 217–225.
8. Chuter TA, Faruqi RM, Sawhney R et al. Endoleak after endovascular repair of abdominal aortic aneurysm. J Vasc Surg 2001; 34: 98–105.
9. Hölzenbein TJ, Kretschmer G, Thurnher S et al. Midterm durability of abdominal aortic aneurysm endograft repair: a word of caution. J Vasc Surg 2001; 33 (Suppl 2): S46–54.
10. Faries PL, Brener BJ, Connelly TL et al. A multicenter experience with the Talent endovascular graft for the treatment of abdominal aortic aneurysms. J Vasc Surg 2002; 35: 1123–1128.

11. van Marrewijk C, Buth J, Harris PL *et al.* Significance of endoleaks after endovascular repair of abdominal aortic aneurysms: The EUROSTAR experience. *J Vasc Surg* 2002; 35: 461–473.

12. Fairman RM, Carpenter JP, Baum RA *et al.* Potential impact of therapeutic warfarin treatment on type II endoleaks and sac shrinkage rates on midterm follow-up examination. *J Vasc Surg* 2002; 35: 679–685.

13. Arko FR, Rubin GD, Johnson BL *et al.* Type-II endoleaks following endovascular AAA repair: preoperative predictors and long-term effects. *J Endovasc Ther* 2001; 8: 503–510.

14. Velazquez OC, Baum RA, Carpenter JP *et al.* Relationship between preoperative patency of the inferior mesenteric artery and subsequent occurrence of type II endoleak in patients undergoing endovascular repair of abdominal aortic aneurysms. *J Vasc Surg* 2000; 32: 777–788.

15. Walker SR, Halliday K, Yusuf SW *et al.* A study on the patency of the inferior mesenteric and lumbar arteries in the incidence of endoleak following endovascular repair of infra-renal aortic aneurysms. *Clin Radiol* 1998; 53: 593–595.

16. Gould DA, McWilliams R, Edwards RD *et al.* Aortic side branch embolization before endovascular aneurysm repair: incidence of type II endoleak. *J Vasc Interv Radiol* 2001; 12: 337–341.

17. Petrik PV, Moore WS. Endoleaks following endovascular repair of abdominal aortic aneurysm: the predictive value of preoperative anatomic factors—a review of 100 cases. *J Vasc Surg* 2001; 33: 739–744.

18. Parry DJ, Kessel DO, Robertson I *et al.* Type II endoleaks: predictable, preventable, and sometimes treatable? *J Vasc Surg* 2002; 36: 105–110.

19. Solis MM, Ayerdi J, Babcock GA *et al.* Mechanism of failure in the treatment of type II endoleak with percutaneous coil embolization. *J Vasc Surg* 2002; 36: 485–491.

20. Bush RL, Lin PH, Ronson RS *et al.* Colonic necrosis subsequent to catheter-directed thrombin embolization of the inferior mesenteric artery via the superior mesenteric artery: a complication in the management of a type II endoleak. *J Vasc Surg* 2001; 34: 1119–1122.

21. Wisselink W, Cuesta MA, Berends FJ *et al.* Retroperitoneal endoscopic ligation of lumbar and inferior mesenteric arteries as a treatment of persistent endoleak after endoluminal aortic aneurysm. *J Vasc Surg* 2000; 31: 1240–1244.

22. Baum RA, Carpenter JP, Golden MA *et al.* Treatment of type 2 endoleaks after endovascular repair of abdominal aortic aneurysms: comparison of transarterial and translumbar techniques. *Vasc Surg* 2002; 35: 23–29.

23. Martin ML, Dolmatch BL, Fry PD, Machan LS. Treatment of type II endoleaks with Onyx. *J Vasc Interv Radiol* 2001; 12: 629–632.

24. Schmid R, Gurke L, Aschwanden M *et al.* CT-guided percutaneous embolization of a lumbar artery maintaining a type II endoleak. *J Endovasc Ther* 2002; 9: 198–202.

25. Rhee RY, Eskandari MK, Zajko AB, Makaroun MS. Long-term fate of the aneurysmal sac after endoluminal exclusion of abdominal aortic aneurysms. *J Vasc Surg* 2000; 32: 689–696.

26. Czermak BV, Fraedrich G, Schocke MF *et al.* Serial CT volume measurements after endovascular aortic aneurysm repair. *J Endovasc Ther* 2001; 8: 380–389.

27. Resch T, Ivancev K, Lindh M *et al.* Persistent collateral perfusion of abdominal aortic aneurysm after endovascular repair does not lead to progressive change in aneurysm diameter. *J Vasc Surg* 1998; 28: 242–249.

28. Liewald F, Ermis C, Gorich J *et al.* Influence of treatment of type II leaks on the aneurysm surface area. *Eur J Vasc Endovasc Surg* 2001; 21: 339–343.

29. Ermis C, Kramer S, Tomczak R *et al.* Does successful embolization of endoleaks lead to aneurysm sac shrinkage? *J Endovasc Ther* 2000; 7: 441–445.

30. White RA, Donayre C, Walot I, Stewart M. Abdominal aortic aneurysm rupture following endoluminal graft deployment: report of a predictable event. *J Endovasc Ther* 2000; 7: 257–262.

31. Dattilo JB, Brewster DC, Fan CM *et al.* Clinical failures of endovascular abdominal aortic aneurysm repair: incidence, causes, and management. *J Vasc Surg* 2002; 35: 1137–1144.

32. Hinchliffe RJ, Singh-Ranger R, Davidson IR, Hopkinson BR. Rupture of an abdominal aortic aneurysm secondary to type II endoleak. *Eur J Vasc Endovasc Surg* 2001; 22: 563–565.

33. White RA, Walot I, Donayre CE *et al.* Failed AAA endograft exclusion due to type II endoleak: explant analysis. *J Endovasc Ther* 2001; 8: 254–261.

34. Amesur NB, Zajko AB, Orons PD, Makaroun MS. Embolotherapy of persistent endoleaks after endovascular repair of abdominal aortic aneurysm with the ancure-endovascular technologies endograft system. *J Vasc Interv Radiol* 1999; 10: 1175–1182.

35. Baum RA, Carpenter JP, Cope C *et al.* Aneurysm sac pressure measurements after endovascular repair of abdominal aortic aneurysms. *J Vasc Surg* 2001; 33: 32–41.

36. Sonesson B, Dias N, Malina M *et al.* Intra-aneurysm pressure measurements in successfully excluded abdominal aortic aneurysms following endovascular repair. *J Vasc Surg* (in press).

Type II endoleaks are clinically unimportant

Against the motion
Geoffrey H White

Introduction and overview

Retrograde endoleak from lumbar and other collateral vessels behaves differently from other types of endoleak and has been classifed separately as type II endoleak.[1-6]

The identification of this form of endoleak track may relate not only to the anatomy but also to the diligence, special techniques, and skill used to demonstrate it.[1,6] This aspect is exemplified by the fact that endoleak may be missed on computed tomography (CT) scan imaging done when there is poor contrast enhancement of the blood (particularly with non-helical CT scanners), or if the CT scan images are obtained only in the early phase when contrast fills the graft lumen but has not yet reached or filled the retrograde endoleak channel.

High resolution duplex scanning may identify endoleak in some cases where it has not been demonstrated on CT scanning. On all imaging studies, it may be extremely difficult to differentiate the exact source of endoleak, or to be sure that there is not a co-existent element of type I (periprosthetic channel) endoleak in some patients who also have continued filling of the lumbar or inferior mesenteric arteries (Figs 1 and 2). There should be a high index of suspicion when an endoleak of apparent type II form is associated with aneurysm pulsatility or growth.

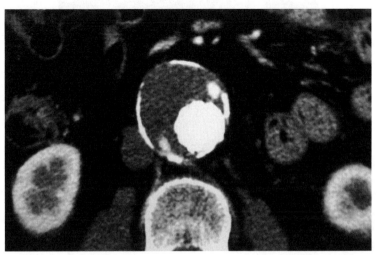

Figure 1. CT scan appearance of endoleak. Typical CT scan appearance suggesting type II endoleak. There is contrast within the AAA sac in continuity with several lumbar arteries and adjacent the inferior mesenteric artery.

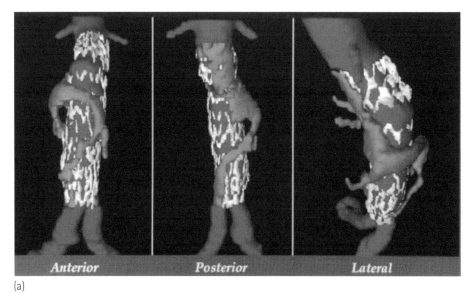

(a)

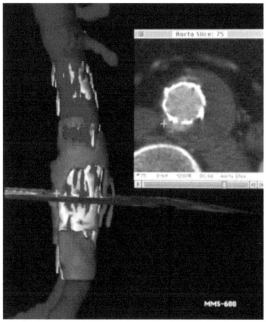

(b)

Figure 2. Apparant type II endoleak as a marker for type I endoleak. Three-dimensional reconstruction of the CT scan images from the same patient as Fig. 1 demonstrates that this is, in fact, a case of proximal attachment site type I endoleak, which causes bloodflow in the sac (the flow via the patent lumbar arteries and the inferior mesenteric artery is outflow from the proximal leak).

It had previously been presumed that type II endoleak was not graft-related and that its occurence was not associated with an error in patient assessment or graft deployment, nor with device failure. Recent information now suggests that the incidence of type II endoleak is higher with certain graft designs;[7-9] if this is true then there may be implications for future device development. Such differences in incidence may be partly explained by variations in imaging protocols, but it has been postulated that this phenomenon may also be related to differences or variations in the transmission of pressure to the aneurysm sac by graft wall movements or oscillations,[2] by porous grafts,[10] or by pressure transmission through semi-liquid thrombus which is sealing the graft.[5] These factors may be related to graft materials and design; there are many factors which may influence the incidence of type II endoleaks (Table 1).

Although the prognosis of type II endoleak appears to be relatively favourable during the first 12–18 months,[4] there is now ample evidence that it also results in continued pressurization of the sac,[11] and sometimes in aneurysm growth.[12] The long-term effects remain unknown.

It is possible that in some cases persistent retrograde perfusion of the aneurysm sac may also have secondary effects on the biological reactions within the aneurysm thrombus, the geometry of the aneurysm sac, or the graft wall, any of which could result in late deleterious alterations in graft function and integrity. There have now been reports of late rupture of aneurysms due to type II endoleaks in a few cases (see below), and a parallel may be drawn to ruptures of abdominal aortic aneurysms (AAA) treated by surgical ligation and exclusion[13] or by induced thrombosis.[14]

Until further data are available, there is reason for continuing caution with regards to the outcome of persistent or uncorrected type II endoleak.

Table 1. Factors which may influence the incidence of type II endoleak

1. Patient-related or anatomic factors
   a. Preoperative number of patent lumbar vessels
   b. Patency or occlusion of the inferior mesenteric artery
   c. Size of any patent collateral vesels
   d. Distribution of thrombus within the AAA sac
   e. AAA size, shape, flow channel, wall calcification
   f. Thrombotic factors / use of anticoagulants
   g. Haemodynamics (cardiac output, hypertension, etc)

2. Device design factors
   a. Graft porosity
   b. Graft fabric thickness
   c. Attachment system (self-expanding vs balloon)
   d. Device wall support (fully suported vs partial
   e. Graft configuration (tube vs bifurcated vs aortoiliac))
   f. Graft configuration (short trunk vs long trunk)
   g. Graft flexibility and pulsatility / graft wall movements

3. Device physics and haemodynamics
   a. Transmission of pressure through the device to the AAA sac
   b. Graft fabric compliance and oscillations
   c. Graft wireform/stent recoil and compliance
   d. Longitudinal graft movements
   e. Graft twist or torque
   f. Presence or absence of sac inserts

Definition: type II endoleak

Type II endoleak is a condition occuring after endovascular graft repair of aneurysms defined by the presence of persistent blood flow into the aneurysm sac from patent branch vessels.[2] For an AAA, this is typically retrograde flow via lumbar arteries or the inferior mesenteric artery. (This does not include, however, lumbar perfusion resulting from connection to the main flow lumen by type I or type III endoleak.) Rarely the median sacral artery or a patent accessory renal artery may be implicated. The situation may be dynamic or changeable; flow may be retrograde alone, or there may be an element of to-and-fro flow from one branch to another (e.g. retrograde inflow to AAA sac from the inferior mesenteric artery with established outflow via a lumbar artery). In complex cases the situation has been described as similar to an arteriovenous fistula, with convoluted pathways of flow.

Background information from open repair of AAA

During open repair operations for AAA it is almost always necessary to oversew several patent lumbar arteries, and often also the inferior mesentric artery. It is logical to presume, then, that a high percentage of endovascular AAA cases would also have patent lumbar arteries immediately after endograft implantation and in the early postoperative period. These may be demonstated by obtaining delayed angiographic views on the completion angiogram, or by injection of contrast into the sac by a catheter left *in situ* to monitor pressure within the sac (Fig. 3). The process of exclusion of the aneurysm sac by an endoluminal graft results in early closure of most of these channels; imaging by ultrasound or CT scan within several days of the procedure shows persistent channels in a minority of cases. It is not known why some seal spontaneously and others do not.

The observation that exclusion of an aneurysm (even by surgical ligation) does not necessarily protect against rupture was proven in Resnikoff's report of experience with non-resective treatment of AAA wherin 17 patients of a total of 831 required intraoperative ligation of collaterals, and during follow-up a further 17 (2%) of aneurysm sacs remained patent on duplex scanning at intervals between 5 and 103 months.[13] Fourteen of these patients received treatment; four were for sac rupture and three for pain. Patients with rupture had exhibited no shrinkage of the aneurysm and continued blood flow within the sac on duplex studies (a condition similar to many patients with persistent type II endoleak).

Aims of endovascular repair of AAA

The major aims of AAA surgery are to prevent rupture of the aneurysm, and also to prevent other complications (e.g. compression of adjacent structures or arterial emboli) of an untreated growing aneurysm. Ideally, with endovascular grafting technique, these aims would be assured by achieving the following process:

1. inflow to the sac is excluded by the endovascular graft;
2. patent lumbar arteries close by a process of thrombosis;
3. there is no blood flow within the sac;
4. the pressure within the sac reduces and is maintained at a low level;
5. the AAA sac contents thrombose and consolidate or fibrose;
6. the AAA sac shrinks.

In the early days of endovascular grafting experience, it was assumed that this would be the 'normal' process after implantation of an endograft within the AAA sac. Follow-up studies with ultrasound and CT scanning have demonstrated, however,

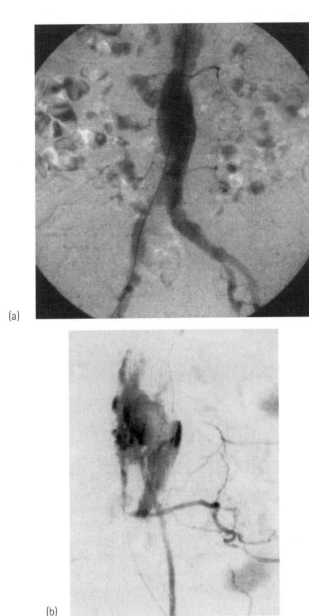

(a)

(b)

Figure 3. Patent lumbar arteries at the time of endovascular graft implantation.
(a) Angiogram done prior to endograft implant demonstrates the presence of several patent lumbar arteries.
(b) An angiogram done through a catheter left in the AAA sac after the endograft procedure demonstrates contrast in the sac and flow via the lumbar arteries which have not occluded at this early stage.

that lumbar arteries (and sometimes the inferior mesentric artery) remain open in a proportion of cases. The occurence of type II endoleak was initially considered to be non-graft dependant, but accumulating data reveal that the incidence is different with different designs of endograft.[7,8] Opinion and evidence are starting to favour the concept that type II endoleak does depend on graft design to some extent,[9] (Tables 2 and 3) and this complication may be regarded in this sense as a failure of the device to achieve AAA exclusion, rather than as a purely patient-related phenomenon.

Table 2. Evidence that type II endoleak may be device-dependant

Incidence of type II endoleak in core-lab reports of FDA phase II studies		
Graft type	Discharge/1 month	6 months
Lifepath	5%	2%
Ancure	48%	21%
AneuRx	48%	18%
Excluder	38%	17%

FDA: Food and Drug Authority

Table 3. Evidence that type II endoleak may be device-dependant

Incidence of type II endoleak in a single-centre experience		
Graft type	n	type II endoleak*
Ancure	43	30%
Talent	114	17%
AneuRx	37	16%
Zenith	29	3.4%
Endologix	24	4.2%

* From CT scan and angiogram at 1 month
Reproduced from: Ref. 7.

Difficulty in differentiating type II endoleak from other causes of endoleak

One of the major ways in which type II endoleak is 'significant' in clinical practice is in the abnormalities it presents on intraoperative and postoperative monitoring of device results. Bloodflow in the AAA sac is detected usually by duplex ultrasound, CT scan or magnetic resonance imaging (MRI). Type II endoleak appears as an abnormality on these studies, denoting incomplete exclusion of the AAA sac wall and contents from the pressure effects and biological effects of flowing blood. In clinical practice, an 'abnormal' finding or report for follow-up studies is always less than satisfactory.

In addition to this underlying abnormal finding, there may be an added clinical difficulty in that it can be difficult or impossible to differentiate this form of endoleak from other types that require more urgent treatment. For example, if type I (attachment site) endoleak is present but is misinterpreted as type II because of non-diagnostic appearance on imaging, then requisite management by secondary endograft, extension cuff or other techniques may be delayed or ignored, possibly resulting in aneurysm rupture.

Aneurysm growth with type II endoleak

The effect of type II endoleaks on changes in the AAA sac size and volume is variable. Usually the aneurysm sac will remain stable or enlarge slowly,[12] but in some cases the aneurysm may shrink.[15] The latter effect probably depends upon pressure from the endoleak being localized or compartmentalized to its point of entry, rather than being transmitted throughout the sac. Chronic type II endoleaks tend to increase both AAA size and volume, both of which may be regarded as parameters of unsuccessful treatment.[16] Reports from core-lab monitored FDA phase II trials of several devices have proven that persistent type II endoleaks result in non-shrinkage of the sac in the large majority of cases.

Intuitively, both the treating surgeon and the patient prefer to find that the aneurysm is getting progressively smaller on follow-up studies; if not there is always a doubt as to the true effectiveness of the treatment, and the security of AAA repair. In addition, continued growth of the AAA may increase the risk of rupture.

Aneurysm sac pressures remain high with type II endoleak

Pressure in the AAA sac may be measured at the time of graft implant and also later during transfemoral angiography of endoleak channels or by translumbar approach. Studies of the pressures associated with type II endoleaks have consistently shown that pressure remains high. Baum *et al.* found 'near systemic pressures' within the aneurysm sacs of patients with type II endoleaks when investigated by translumbar puncture with associated angiogram and presure measurement.[11,17]

In addition, pulsatile waveforms were recorded. Coil embolization rapidly brought down the pressure within the sac to the 25–30 mmHg range in a model,[18] but embolization in clinical practice is not always successful and it is not yet clear whether embolized endoleaks remain closed. These haemodynamic measurements have influenced some to recommend early treatment (after as little as 3 months) of persistent type II endoleaks.[15,19]

Furthermore, in benchtop model experiments, Redd *et al.* showed that AAA sac pressure in the presence of type II endoleak is strongly influenced by the characteristics of the collaterals feeding or draining the aneurysm sac.[18] Pulsatility of the sac was eliminated if the sac pressure remained less than diastolic pressure; however, when type II endoleak resulted in sac pressure exceeding diastolic pressure, pulsatility returned to the aneurysm.

Pressure transmission through thrombosed type II endoleaks

The majority of type II endoleaks close eventually, usually within 6–12 months. Presumably this closure is by a process on thrombosis. Ohki and co-workers have demonstrated in a bench-top model that pressure transmission to the AAA sac can continue through a thrombosed type II endoleak; this pressure transmission is more likely with an endoleak channel which is short in length and of wide diameter.[20] The applicability of this bench model to the clinical situation is uncertain, but it does raise the prospect of recurrrent or continuing pressurization of the AAA sac after endoleak resolution.

Pressure transmission to the sac has now been noted in clinical type II endoleaks that have sealed spontaneously, presumably by a mechanism of transmission via thrombus.[21] It is not known how effective is the barrier formed by the thrombus within a closed lumbar artery, and it is possible that this is variable according to anatomic and haematological factors. Perhaps this may be one explanation for the phenomenon of endotension.[22]

Aneurysm rupture associated with type II endoleak

Although rare, aneurysm rupture has been reported in association with type II endoleak in a number of patients.[23-27] This is not surprising, given the prior experience which demonstrated the possibility of rupture following surgical ligature exclusion of aneurysms.[13]

In addition, analysis of data from the Eurostar registry also showed an increased relative risk of AAA rupture in patients who have had type II endoleak,[28] although this may not be an independant variable.

In recent updates on the EUROSTAR Registry data, Harris reported an association between type II endoleak and subsequent AAA rupture.[28-30] Of 421 patients with documented type II endoleak, there were nine (2.1%) instances of AAA rupture at follow-up of a mean 14.7 months.[30] In eight of these nine cases there was said to be co-existent type I endoleak, whereas of 164 patients with isolated type II endoleak, rupture occured in one (0.6%). Thus they concluded that type II endoleak in isolation is relatively benign, but they considered it possible that persistent type II endoleak represents a marker for type I endoleak.

Continuing activity in the AAA sac due to bloodflow from type II endoleak

The thrombus within an aneurysm sac is an active environment. In some cases, a thrombolytic reaction has been documented and this may lead to formation of a hygroma-like fluid sac and aneurysm growth.[31] Biochemical, inflammatory and immunological reactions continue after endovascular grafting, and it is quite likely that these may be influenced or activated by continuing blood flow from a type II endoleak. The biological activity and pressure profiles may have secondary deleterious effects on the implanted device, or influence growth of the aortic neck and the sac.

Higher frequency of follow–up imaging in patients with type II endoleak

Patients with type II endoleak are usually submitted to increased follow-up CT and ultrasound imaging studies, with resultant implications for cost and radiation exposure. In particular, angiography is often required for accurate diagnosis of persistent endoleaks and to assist in the planning of interventions.

High incidence of interventions for type II endoleak

Further evidence that type II endoleak is indeed clinically significant can be gained from the fact that almost all clincans who practice endovascular grafting believe that this form of endoleak should be treated in certain circumstances[17,19,20] (Table 4). Type II endoleaks remain one of the highest 'predictors' of secondary interventions in the Eurostar Registry experience.[30] The current difficulty is in identifying which patients with type II endoleaks do require interventions (Figs 4 and 5), because of a real or perceived ongoing risk of AAA rupture. These may include type II endoleak in association with the following:

1. symptomatic aneurysm;
2. pulsatile AAA;
3. AAA sac enlargement > 5mm;
4. persistence of the endoleak for longer than 6 or 12 months;
5. transmission of pressure from the endoleak to the sac (if this can be measured);
6. large volume endoleak;
7. type II endoleak in a large AAA.

Table 4. Treatment options for type II endoleak

1. Observation
2. Percutaneous transfemoral interventions
   - catheter access via iliac or mesenteric branches
   - embolization by coils, pledgets, liquid glues, etc
3. Percutaneous translumbar embolization
   - direct translumbar puncture of AAA sac
   - pressure measurement and embolization
4. Laparoscopic ligation
5. Open laparotomy and ligation
6. Conversion to open repair of the AAA by graft replacement

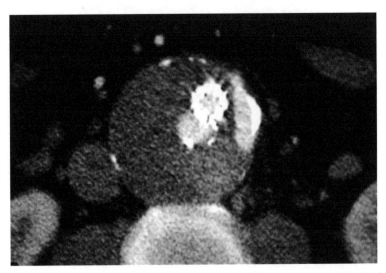

Figure 4. Type II endoleak from the inferior mesenteric artery. There is contrast within the AAA sac in continuity with the ostium of the inferior mesenteric artery.

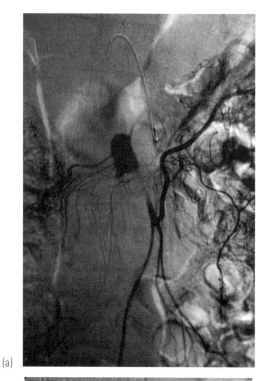

(a)

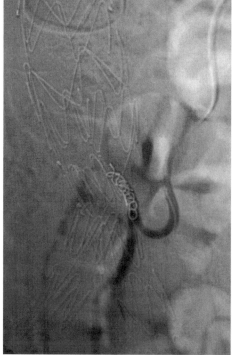

(b)

Figure 5. Treatment of type II endoleak by percutaneous coil embolization.
(a) Angiography done via a selective catheter in the superior mesenteric artery, demonstrating collateral flow via the inferior mesenteric artery causing endoleak. (b) Because of persistence of this endoleak for more than 12 months, and associated enlargement of the AAA sac, the endoleak channel was successfully closed by percutaneous transvascular coil embolization technique. Coils are seen in the inferior mesenteric orifice, with abolishment of bloodflow into the aneurysm sac.

In other situations, most would favour observation, with the expectation that the endoleak channel may close. Observation is usually continued for an interval of 6–12 months, particularly when the aneurysm is small and stable or shrinking, and there are no symptoms attributed to the AAA.

Conclusions

Type II endoleaks are difficult to predict, prevent or treat, and most appear to be relatively benign in behaviour.[32] Nevertheless they remain clinically significant, since those that do not seal may lead to AAA enlargement, sac pressurization and increased risk of rupture. The long-term outcome will only be learnt by many years of follow-up; it is not clear whether some sealed endoleaks may continue to transmit pressure through thrombus, or to contribute to endotension by intermittent flow. Diagnosis of type II endoleak may be difficult to confim, particularly with respect to differentiating the more dangerous type I or type III endoleaks.

It appears that a conservative approach is justified for the majority of side-branch endoleaks and those that do close spontaneously may prove to be clinically insignificant, but most clinicians favour treatment in circumstances of AAA growth, symptoms or when there is long-term persistence of these channels because of significant concerns regarding the associated systemic arterial pressures and pulsatile waveforms within the aneurysm sac.

Summary

Type II endoleak is clinically significant for the following reasons:

- Type II endoleak represents failure to completely exclude blood flow from the AAA sac.

- Type II endoleak may be difficult to differentiate from other forms of endoleak.

- Type II endoleak may produce high pressure within the AAA sac.

- Type II endoleak may produce pulsatile waveforms within the AAA sac.

- Type II endoleak may prevent AAA consolidation and shrinkage.

- Type II endoleak may cause AAA growth and rupture.

- Type II endoleak leads to increased follow-up imaging studies and may require angiography.

- Type II endoleak leads to secondary interventions in many cases.

- Type II endoleak may cause haematological, immunological and biochemical reactions within the aneurysm sac.

- Type II endoleak may cause late deleterious effects on the aneurysm and the device.

- Type II endoleak may be a predictor of poor clinical outcome in the long term.

References

1. White GH, Yu W, May J *et al*. Endoleak as a complication of endoluminal grafting of abdominal aortic aneurysms: Classification, incidence, diagnosis and management. *J Endovasc Surg* 1997; 4: 152–168.

2. White GH, May J, Waugh RC, Yu W. Type I and type II endoleak: A more useful classification for reporting results of endoluminal AAA repair. *J Endovasc Surg* 1998; 5: 189–191.

3. Wain RA, Marin ML, Ohki T *et al*. Endoleaks after endovascular graft treatment of aortic aneurysms: classification, risk factors, and outcome. *J Vasc Surg* 1998; 27: 69–80.

4. Resch T, Ivancev K, Lindh M *et al*. Persistent collateral perfusion of abdominal aortic aneurysm after endovascular repair does not lead to progressive change in aneurysm diameter. *J Vasc Surg* 1998; 28: 242–249.

5. White GH, May J, Waugh RC *et al*. Type III and type IV endoleak: Towards a complete definition of bloodflow in the sac after endoluminal repair of AAA. *J Endovasc Surg* 1998; 5: 305–309.

6. Goodman MA, Lawrence-Brown M, Prendergast F *et al*. "Retroleak" –Retrograde branch filling of the excluded aneurysm. (letter) *J Endovasc Surg* 1998; 5: 37837-9.

7. Fairman RM, Velazquez OC, Carpenter JP. How are type II endoleaks related to endograft design? *Program Book. Vascular Endovascular Issues Techniques Horizons 28th Symposium*, Vol 28: VI 5.1, 2001.

8. White GH, Yu W, Johari A. Type II endoleak is dependant on device design: Evidence from the Lifepath AAA graft trials (abstr). *J Endovasc Ther* 2002; 9: S19.

9. Gupta NY, Makaroun MS. Endoleak behaviour is graft specific. In: Veith FJ, Baum RA (eds). *Endoleaks and Endotension*. New York: Marcel Dekker Inc. 2003.

10. Sanchez, LA, Faries PL, Marin ML *et al*. Chronic intra-aneurysmal pressure measurement: An experimental method for evaluating the effectiveness of endovascular aortic aneurysm exclusion. *J Vasc Surg* 1997; 26: 222–230.

11. Baum RA, Carpenter JP, Cope C, Golden MA *et al*. Aneurysm sac pressure measurements after endovascular repair of abdominal aortic aneurysms. *J Vasc Surg* 2001; 33: 32–41.

12. Armon MP, Yusuf SW, Whitaker SC, Gregson RH, Wenham PW, Hopkinson BR. Thrombus distribution and changes in aneurysm size following endovascular aortic aneurysm repair. *Eur J Vasc Endovasc Surg* 1998; 16: 472–476.

13. Resnikoff M, Darling R, Chang BB *et al*. Fate of the excluded abdominal aortic aneurysm sac: long-term follow-up of 831 cases. *J Vasc Surg* 1996; 24: 851–855.

14. Schanzer H, Papa MC, Miller CM. Rupture of surgically thrombosed abdominal aortic aneurysm. *J Vasc Surg* 1985; 2: 278–280.

15. Franco TJ, Zajko AB, Federle MP, Makaroun MS. Endovascular repair of abdominal aortic aneurysm with the Ancure endograft: CT follow-up of perigraft flow and aneurysm size at 6 months. *J Vasc Intervent Radiol* 200; 11: 429–435.

16. Arko FR, Rubin GD, Johnson BL *et al*. Type II endoleaks following endovascular AA repair: preoperative predictors and long-term effects. *J Endovasc Ther* 2001; 29: 292–308.

17. Baum RA, Cope C, Fairman RM, Carpenter JP. Translumbar embolization of type II endoleaks after endovascular repair of abdominal aortic aneurysms. *J Vasc Intervent Radiol* 2001; 12: 111–116.

18. Redd D *et al*. Experimental AAA flow model for evaluation of aortic sac pressure with type II endoleak. *SCIVR* 2001.

19. Solis MM, Hodgson KJ. Endoleaks and endotension: the Springfield experience. In: Veith FJ, Baum RA (eds). *Endoleaks and Endotension*. New York: Marcel Dekker Inc. 2003.

20. Mehta M, Ohki T, Veith FJ *et al*. All sealed endoleaks are not the same: a treatment strategy based on an ex vivo analysis. *Eur J Vasc Endovasc Surg* 2001; 21: 541–544.

21. Darling RC, Ozsvath K, Chang BB *et al*. The incidence, natural history, and outcome of secondary intervention for persistent collateral flow in the excluded abdominal aortic aneurysm. *J Vasc Surg* 1999; 30: 968–976.

22. White GH, May J, Waugh R *et al*. Endotension: An explanation for continued AAA growth after successful endoluminal repair. *J Endovasc Surg* 1999; 6: 308–315.

23. Politz JK, Newman VS, Stewart MT. Late abdominal aortic aneurysm rupture after AneuRx repair: A report of three cases. *J Vasc Surg* 2000; 31: 599–606.

24. White RA, Donayre C, Walot I, Stewart M. Abdominal aortic aneurysm rupture following endoluminal graft deployment: report of a predictable event. *J Endovasc Ther* 2000; 7: 257–262.

25. Hinchcliffe RJ, Singh-Ranger R, Davidson IR, Hopkinson BR Rupture of an abdominal aortic aneurysm secondary to type II endoleak. *Eur J Vasc Endovasc Surg* 2001; 22: 563–565.

26. Bade MA, Ohki T, Cynamon J, Veith FJ. Hypogastric artery aneurysm rupture after endovascular

graft exclusion with shrinkage of the aneurysm: Significance of endotension from a 'virtual' or thrombosed type II endoleak. *J Vasc Surg* 2001; **33**: 1271–1274.

27. Ohki T, Veith FJ *et al.* Late abdominal aortic aneurysm rupture after endorepair. *J Vasc Surg* 2001; **33**: 599–606.

28. Harris PL, Vallabhaneni SR, Desgranges P, Becquemin JP, van Marrewijk C, Laheij RJ. Incidence and risk factors of late rupture, conversion, and death after endovascular repair of infrarenal aortic aneurysms: the EUROSTAR experience *J Vasc Surg* 2000; **32**: 739–749.

29. Vallabhaneni SR, Harris PL. Lessons learnt from the EUROSTAR registry on endovascular repair of infrarenal aortic aneurysms. *Eur J Radiol* 2001; **39**: 34–41.

30. Leheij RJF, Buth J, Harris PL *et al.* Need for secondary interventions after endovascular repair of abdominal aortic neurysms. Intermediate term follow-up results of a European collaborative registry (EUROSTAR). *Br J Surg* 2000; **87**: 1666–1673.

31. Risberg B, Delle M, Eriksson E *et al.* Aneurysmal sac hygroma: a cause of endotension. *J Endovasc Ther* 2001; **8**: 447–453.

32. Chuter TAM. Opinions on Endoleaks. In: Veith FJ, Baum RA (eds). *Endoleaks and Endotension*. New York: Marcel Dekker, Inc. 2003.

Type II endoleaks are clinically unimportant

Charing Cross Editorial Comments towards Consensus

Geoffrey White classified these endoleaks and argues the view that type II endoleak represents a failure to exclude blood flow completely from the aneurysm sac. He states that such an endoleak may produce high pressure thus preventing shrinkage and cause increase in diameter and rupture. The most damning comment he makes is that a type II endoleak may be a marker for other forms of endoleak, poor graft performance and poor clinical outcome.

Krassi Ivancev has none of it! He stresses that approximately a third of type II endoleaks resolve spontaneously and that the majority of aneurysms with type II endoleak do not increase in size. He regards such an endoleak as clinically unimportant provided that it is not associated with an endoleak such as type I or type III.

This is a very important debate and the significance of type II endoleaks remains a little hazy despite these giants throwing light upon it.

Roger M Greenhalgh
Editor

Several commercially available systems render emergency aneurysm repair an option for at least 50% of ruptures

For the motion

Frank J Veith, Takao Ohki, Evan C Lipsitz

Introduction

This discussion involves the management of ruptured infrarenal abdominal aortic aneurysms (AAA) and ruptured aortoiliac aneurysms. By definition a ruptured AAA is one in which the wall of the aneurysm contains a hole or a vent through which blood has leaked and is present outside the aneurysm wall. This discussion does not consider the treatment of so-called 'acute aneurysms' which present with pain and even hypotension, but which show no evidence of blood outside the aneurysm wall.

Why should endovascular graft repair of ruptured AAAs be considered?

Unlike elective AAA in which open surgery can be performed with a less than 5% operative mortality and a reasonably low morbidity, the open surgical treatment of ruptured AAA carries an operative mortality in the 50% range (35–70%).[1-6] This persists despite all the technical and other adjunctive improvements that have been suggested. Moreover, the morbidity of open surgery for ruptured AAA remains high. Thus endovascular repair of ruptured aneurysms offers considerable room for improvement.

Why has endovascular aneurysm repair (EVAR) not been used more?

In view of the poor results of open surgery for ruptured AAA, one may fairly ask why has EVAR not been used more. One reason is that in the early days of EVAR, it took time to make the measurements required for endografting, and it took additional time to procure the appropriate graft or grafts. The second reason is that all surgeons have traditionally advocated the need in ruptured AAA patients to gain rapid aortic control, usually by clamp placement proximal to the aneurysm at the infrarenal or supracoeliac level. This mandated emergency laparotomy.

It turns out that both these factors are not necessarily obstacles to EVAR. In 1994, we and others first began to treat ruptured AAA with endovascular grafts.[7-9] This was possible because the Montefiore and Nottingham groups had endografts that could be prepared rapidly and they were used to treat a wide variety of patients with ruptured AAA. It also was apparent in these early patient experiences that at least some ruptured AAA patients remained stable or at least viable long enough for the endovascular grafting procedure to be successfully performed. EVAR was proven feasible.

Methods

Hypotensive haemostasis

In the past, it has been noted that restricting blood transfusions and other fluid resuscitation was an effective way to control haemorrhage and improve treatment outcomes in patients who were bleeding. This was noted with patients who had upper gastrointestinal bleeding in the 1940s and subsequently those who had a variety of other conditions including vascular trauma.[10-12] In the mid-1990s, we made the observation that restricting fluid resuscitation could also be effective in the ruptured aneurysm setting, and we coined the term 'hypotensive haemostasis.'[13-14] By that we

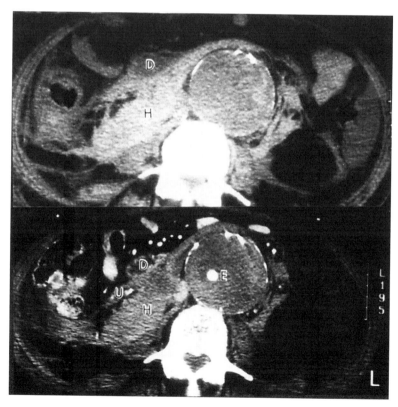

Figure 1. CT scan preoperatively (upper) and 4 days after insertion of an aorto-unifemoral graft (MEGS) (lower). Postoperatively all contrast was contained within the graft and the ruptured AAA was excluded. Note resolution of the retroperitoneal haemorrhage (H). D is the duodenum and U is the ureter containing contrast.

mean aggressively restricting all fluid resuscitation in ruptured AAA patients as long as they remain conscious and able to talk and move. We accept a reduction in arterial systolic blood pressure to the 50–70 mmHg range and still minimize fluid resuscitation, as difficult as that can sometimes be. However, by doing so, bleeding will temporarily cease and time will be available to perform an endovascular graft repair (Figs 1 and 2).

Supracoeliac balloon control

Although hypotensive haemostasis can be an effective method to temporarily control bleeding in many ruptured AAA patients, it can sometimes fail with cardiovascular collapse. Moreover, if patients are anaesthetized with concomitant loss of their sympathetic nervous system compensation for a reduced blood volume, they frequently undergo cardiovascular collapse. In these circumstances emergency aortic control proximal to the rupture site becomes mandatory. As detailed in the Current Montefiore ruptured AAA management protocol section which follows, placement under fluoroscopic control of a guidewire via a brachial or femoral access site in the

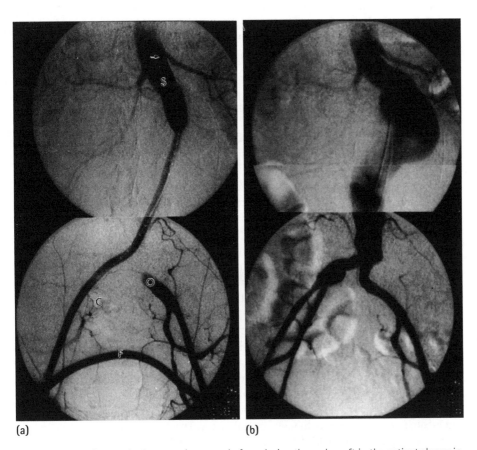

(a) (b)

Figure 2. A: arteriogram in the operating room before placing the endograft in the patient shown in Fig. 1. At this time the patient's blood pressure was 50 mmHg. Note there is no contrast outside the lumen of the aorta and the aneurysm because of the hypotension. B: completion arteriogram after placement of an aorto-unifemoral endovascular graft, an occluder (O) in the left common iliac artery and coils (C) in the right hypogastric artery. A femorofemoral bypass (F) has also been performed. S is the proximal Palmaz stent. The arrow points to the top of the graft.

supracoeliac aorta should be carried out under <u>local</u> anaesthesia. This enables angiographic evaluation of the patient's arterial anatomy to determine suitability for endovascular grafting. More important, this guidewire can be used to enable rapid placement of a large (14 Fr) sheath (Cook Inc.) through which a large compliant balloon can rapidly be inserted to occlude the supracoeliac aorta.[13-17]

Appropriate grafts

The original endovascular grafts that were used to treat ruptured AAA were fabricated or assembled by surgeons so that they could be quickly inserted in the ruptured aneurysm setting.[7-9;18-19] However, subsequently a variety of commercially made grafts have been employed. Most of these have been of the modular bifurcated variety, although some ruptured AAA patients have been treated with unibody devices. A key requirement is that a large inventory of devices be on hand so that anatomic variations can be properly managed and the adverse events that inevitably occur can be dealt with. Maintaining such a large inventory of devices can be expensive, particularly if modular bifurcated devices are to be used.

For this reason, there are clear advantages to using a unilateral aortoiliac or aortofemoral endograft in conjunction with contralateral iliac occlusion and a femorofemoral bypass, and much of the early EVAR for rupture experience employed devices with this configuration. Such devices can be unibody or modular. They offer the additional advantage that the aneurysm will be largely depressurized once the graft is deployed.

Current Montefiore ruptured AAA management protocol

Most centres require ruptured AAA patients to be stable enough to undergo a computed tomographic (CT) scan to confirm the rupture and allow a decision to be made that the patient is a suitable endovascular graft candidate. We do not adhere to that requirement although approximately half of our ruptured AAA patients have had a CT scan performed either in our own institution or elsewhere.

Our current ruptured AAA management protocol is as follows: once a presumed diagnosis of a ruptured AAA is made,[20] the patient is rapidly transported to the operating room which must have full digital fluoroscopy capacity (OEC, model #9800), a radiolucent movable operating table and a large inventory of endovascular supplies (catheters, guidewires, sheaths, stents and endovascular grafts). As the patient is being prepared for the procedure, fluid is restricted as outlined above. Intravenous and intra-arterial lines are placed. Tubes are placed in the bladder and stomach. The patient is positioned, prepared and draped with the right arm extended and the right antecubital fossa, lower chest, abdomen and thighs exposed. The fluoroscope is placed on the patient's left side. Under local anaesthesia, a 5 Fr sheath is placed percutaneously in the right brachial or femoral artery. Through this sheath a catheter and guidewire are manipulated into the supracoeliac aorta. Using a pigtailed catheter in the suprarenal aorta, an abdominal aortogram is performed with posteroanterior and oblique views to define the aneurysm neck and iliac artery anatomy. A decision is made whether the patient is suitable for endovascular repair or will require an open repair. This decision is based on a number of factors including the patient's anatomy and the type of endograft available.

If an <u>open repair</u> is required, the guidewire is replaced in the supracoeliac aorta. Anaesthesia is induced and the open repair performed in a standard fashion. If the patient has a cardiovascular collapse, a 14 Fr sheath is placed over the guidewire followed by a 33- or 40-cm compliant balloon (Meditech). Under fluoroscopic control the balloon is placed and inflated in the infrarenal neck of the aneurysm, if it is long enough. Balloon inflation is monitored fluoroscopically using dilute contrast to fill the balloon until the aorta is occluded. If the proximal neck is short, the balloon is placed and inflated in the supracoeliac aorta. In this position every effort must be made to minimize balloon inflation time and to obtain infrarenal clamp control as soon as possible. Systemic heparin is administered when the aorta is occluded.

If an <u>endovascular repair</u> is to be performed, it may in some instances be carried out under local anaesthesia.[21] However, we have found that ruptured AAA patients move about on the operating table, making accurate fluoroscopic localization and graft deployment difficult. We have therefore chosen general anaesthesia in most of our ruptured AAA patients. Large sheath (14 Fr) and balloon placement is only carried out if required by the patient's cardiovascular collapse, since these manoeuvres can damage the brachial artery and the presence of the inflated balloon can complicate placement of the endograft.

Results

Montefiore experience with EVAR for rupture

Since 1994 we have used endovascular techniques to treat 35 patients with ruptured AAA. In the first 12 cases, endovascular graft repair was performed only in patients who were considered prohibitive risks for open repair because of a hostile abdomen, medical co-morbidities or both. All these patients had preoperative CT scans although several were haemodynamically unstable at the time of their repair.[9,13]

In 1996 we adopted the current management protocol described above. With two exceptions when staff and facilities were unavailable, all patients with ruptured AAA seen by our service between 1996 and the present were managed according to this protocol. These 23 patients plus the original 12 patients constitute our total experience.[13,14] Of these 35 patients, six had unsuitable anatomy for EVAR. All six survived their open operation. Only two required suprarenal balloon control.

The remaining 29 ruptured aneurysm patients were acceptable for EVAR and had an endograft placed. Although 24 of these patients received a Montefiore Endovascular Grafting System (MEGS)* aortounifemoral graft (Fig. 2B),[9,13,14] the six remaining patients were treated with a commercially available graft (two Corvita tubes, four AneuRx bifurcates). Of the 29 patients undergoing EVAR for rupture, 25 survived and were discharged from the hospital with their aneurysm excluded. Only eight of the 29 patients undergoing EVAR for rupture required balloon control during their procedure. Two of the 25 survivors required evacuation of their perianeurysmal haematoma because of abdominal compartment syndrome. One surviving patient developed a late (1 year) type I endoleak which was successfully treated by placement of a second MEGS graft. There have been no other endoleaks although one patient required open conversion for endotension with an enlarging painful aneurysm.

---

*To be commercialized by Vascular Innovation Inc., Perrysberg, Ohio

Other experience with EVAR for rupture

Increasing numbers of EVAR for rupture are being performed throughout the world using a variety of grafts, mostly commercially available. We are in the process of summarizing the results of these procedures. Although it is too early to say with certainty, and although there clearly is case selection in the performance of these procedures, we have the impression that operative mortality is considerably below the 35–70% range reported for open ruptured AAA repair. Clearly EVAR for rupture avoids many of the problems which are associated with open ruptured AAA repair and which contribute to the high mortality associated with this procedure. These problems include increased blood loss associated with release of tamponade, retroperitoneal dissection and inadvertent venous injury; injury to other retroperitoneal structures including the duodenum and the ureters; hypothermia associated with hypotension and laparatomy and the impaired blood coagulability common in the ruptured AAA setting.

Summary

- Hypotensive haemostasis with fluid restriction is effective in many patients with a ruptured AAA and is helpful in the management of this entity.

- Fluoroscopically monitored proximal aortic balloon control can be obtained under local anaesthesia. It is an advantageous method whether the definitive repair is performed open or with an endograft.

- Proximal aortic control is only required in one-third of patients with a ruptured AAA provided hypotensive haemostasis is used.

- EVAR is feasible for rupture.

- Preliminary results give promise that EVAR for rupture will lower morbidity and mortality.

- Several presently available or soon to be available commercial endografting systems render emergency EVAR a BETTER option for at least 50% of ruptures.

- The case FOR the motion is conclusively made.

References

1. Johansen K, Kohler TR, Nicholls SC *et al. Ruptured* abdominal aortic aneurysm: the Harbor view experience. *J Vasc Surg* 1991; 13: 240–247.
2. Gloviczki P, Pairolero PC, Mucha P. Ruptured abdominal aortic aneurysms: repair should not be denied. *J Vasc Surg* 1992; 15: 851–859.
3. Marty-Ane CH, Alric P, Picot MC *et al. Ruptured* abdominal aortic aneurysm: influence of intraoperative management on surgical outcome. *J Vasc Surg* 1995; 22: 780–786.
4. Darling RC, Cordero JA, Chang BB. Advances in the surgical repair of ruptured abdominal aortic aneurysms. *Cardiovasc Surg* 1996; 4: 720–723.
5. Dardik A, Burleyson GP, Bowman H *et al.* Surgical repair of ruptured abdominal aortic aneurysms in the state of Maryland: factors influencing outcome among 527 recent cases. *J Vasc Surg* 1998; 28: 413–423.

6. Noel AA, Gloviczki P, Cherry KJ Jr. *et al*. Ruptured abdominal aortic aneurysms: the excessive mortality rate of conventional repair. *J Vasc Surg* 2001; 34: 41–46.

7. Marin ML, Veith FJ, Cynamon J *et al*. Initial experience with transluminally placed endovascular grafts for the treatment of complex vascular lesions. *Annl Surg* 1995; 222: 1–17.

8. Yusuf SW, Whitaker SC, Chuter TA *et al*. Emergency endovascular repair of leaking aortic aneurysm. *Lancet* 1994; 344: 1645.

9. Ohki T, Veith FJ, Sanchez LA *et al*. Endovascular graft repair of ruptured aorto-iliac aneurysms. *J Am Coll Surg* 1999; 189: 102–123.

10. Andresen AFR. Management of gastric hemorrhage. *NY State J Med* 1948; 48: 603–611.

11. Shaftan GW, Chiu CJ, Dennis C, Harris B. Fundamentals of physiologic control of arterial hemorrhage. *Surgery* 1968; 58: 851–856.

12. Bickell WH, Wall MJ Jr, Pepe PE *et al*. Immediate versus delayed fluid resuscitation for hypotensive patients with penetrating torso injuries. *N Engl J Med* 1994; 331: 1105–1109.

13. Veith FJ, Ohki T. Endovascular approaches to ruptured infrarenal aorto-iliac aneurysms. *J Cardiovasc Surg (Torino)* 2002; 43: 369–378.

14. Ohki T, Veith FJ. Endovascular grafts and other image guided catheter based adjuncts to improve the treatment of ruptured aortoiliac aneurysms. *Annl Surg* 2000; 232: 466–479.

15. Hesse FG, Kletschka HD. Rupture of abdominal aortic aneurysm: control of hemorrhage by intraluminal balloon tamponade. *Annl Surg* 1962; 155: 320–322.

16. Hyde GL, Sullivan DM. Fogarty catheter tamponade of ruptured abdominal aortic aneurysms. *Surg Gyn Obstet* 1982; 154: 197–199.

17. Greenberg RK, Srivastava SD, Ouriel K *et al*. An endoluminal method of hemorrhage control and repair of ruptured abdominal aortic aneurysms. *J Endovasc Ther* 2000; 7: 1–7.

18. Yusuf SW, Whitaker SC, Chuter TAM *et al*. Early results of endovascular aortic aneurysm surgery with aortouniiliac graft, contralateral iliac occlusion, and femorofemoral bypass. *J Vasc Surg* 1997; 25: 165–172.

19. Yusuf SW, Hopkinson BR. It is feasible to treat contained aortic aneurysm rupture by stent-graft combination? In: Greenhalgh RM (ed). *Indications in Vascular and Endovascular Surgery*. London: Saunders; 1998: 153–165.

20. Veith FJ. Emergency abdominal aortic aneurysm surgery. *Comp Ther* 1992; 18: 25–29.

21. Lachat ML, Pfammatter T, Witzke HJ *et al*. Endovascular repair with bifurcated stent-grafts under local anaesthesia to improve outcome of ruptured aortoiliac aneurysms. *Eur J Vasc Endovasc Surg* 2002; 23: 528–536.

Several commercially available systems render emergency aneurysm repair an option for at least 50% of ruptures

Against the motion
Philip Davey, Lesley Wilson,
Carol Nevin, Dominic Fay,
Eric LG Verhoeven, John Rose,
Michael G Wyatt

Introduction

It is widely accepted that abdominal aortic aneurysm (AAA) may be successfully managed by either conventional open surgery or by endovascular repair (EVAR) in selected cases. Dramatic advances made in the elective treatment of AAA over the past 50 years have resulted in perioperative mortality rates of less than 7% following open surgery. Initial experiences show that EVAR can produce similar results and we await a formal comparison and evaluation of the two treatment modalities for elective AAA repair (UK EVAR trials). Unfortunately, this significant improvement in elective outcome has not been witnessed in the case of ruptured AAA and a recent meta-analysis [1] demonstrated that while there has been a gradual reduction in ruptured AAA mortality of 3.5% per decade over the last 50 years, the pooled overall operative mortality is still in the region of 40%. Clearly, there is a need for improved management strategies in ruptured AAA and these may well incorporate the use of a modified endovascular approach.

There is little doubt that the principles of EVAR are particularly attractive in the case of AAA rupture. Avoidance of laparotomy and the use of local anaesthesia (in selected cases) confer a marked physiological advantage over open surgery in an already dire situation.[2] Nevertheless the urgency associated with ruptured AAA repair results in little or no time being available to gather the required morphological information (aneurysm suitability and graft-sizing) prior to EVAR. Furthermore, the requirement of a permanently available on-call endovascular team with access to the appropriate facilities for EVAR is a significant obstacle in most centres.

Endovascular techniques for ruptured aortic aneurysm

Following a clinical diagnosis of rupture, the patient is resuscitated with permissive hypotension, prepared as for open repair and as haemodynamic stability permits, assessed for EVAR. A subsequent pre-operative CT scan or an on-table angiogram is used to determine the anatomical suitability of the ruptured AAA for EVAR. If adverse ruptured AAA morphology is demonstrated, open repair is performed without delay.

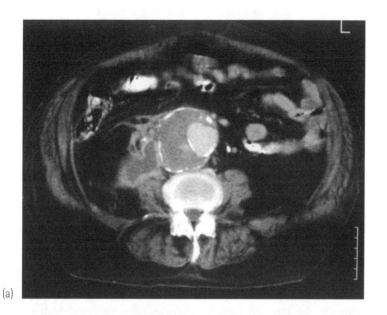

(a)

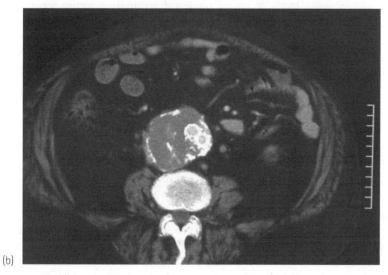

(b)

Figure 1. CT scans showing the preoperative (a) and 1-year (b) CT appearances of a patient treated for ruptured AAA using a bifurcated Vanguard® aortic stent-graft. Note the complete resloution of the extra-aortic haematoma on the 1-year scan.

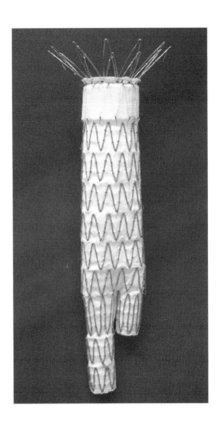

Figure 2. Example of a commercially available bifurcated stent-graft for the treatment of ruptured AAA (Zenith ®).

For those proceeding to EVAR, several options are available. Initially, an intra-aortic balloon can be inserted over a stiff guidewire to allow initial control of proximal haemorrhage in the event of patient deterioration during the stent-graft insertion.[3,4] Alternatively, immediate graft deployment and sealing of the rupture has also shown to be effective[5,6] The graft type may be either aorto-uni-iliac, which effects a quicker proximal seal, or a bifurcated modular system (Fig. 1) that avoids the additional procedures (crossover grafting) associated with a aorto-uni-iliac repair. At present, approximately 90% of elective procedures performed with commercial devices utilize bifurcated systems (Fig. 2).

Evidence

The first case report of successful EVAR following ruptured AAA was by Yusuf *et al.* in 1994.[7] They described the use of a aorto-uni-iliac system with femorofemoral crossover graft for the treatment of a ruptured AAA in a haemodynamically stable 61-year-old man. However, it was not until 2001 that the same centre published their 6-year results of EVAR for ruptured AAA in a series of only 20 patients.[5] Limited patient recruitment was attributed mainly to the unfulfilled requirement of an experienced and available endovascular team and highlights a major problem in the implementation of EVAR as a first-line option in the treatment of ruptured AAA. Unfavourable ruptured AAA anatomy on CT imaging also prohibited EVAR, but the report does not include details of the number of patients turned down due to such anatomical unsuitability. Interestingly, 50% (10/20) of the cases treated in this series had what was considered by the authors to be 'adverse anatomical morphology' (Table 1).

The Montefiore group remain ardent supporters of EVAR for ruptured AAA. Their initial series of EVAR in 12 ruptured aortoiliac aneurysms (six true, six false, 1993–1998) reported a low morbidity and a 16% mortality rate.[4] Nevertheless, no data is provided regarding the 35 ruptured AAA admissions turned down for EVAR during the study. In addition, only four of these EVAR procedures were for true ruptured AAA. Endovascular repair was performed in all cases using the MEG (Montefiore Endovascular Graft) system, a 'home-made' non-commercial hybrid graft composed of a proximal balloon-expandable stent sutured to an expanded polytetrafluoroethylene (ePTFE) segment for distal anastomosis. The device is aorto-uni-iliac, requiring insertion of a contralateral 'occluder' segment and surgical femorofemoral crossover. The Ivancev-Malmo endoprosthesis is similar. It was used in the successful EVAR of the three ruptured AAA series reported by Greenberg et al. in 2000.[8] Neither of these devices is commercially available at the time of writing.

In 1996 the Montefiore group instituted a modified treatment regime for all ruptured AAA admitted to their hospital, proposing EVAR as first-line therapy. All patients diagnosed with ruptured AAA were taken to the operating theatre and an on-table angiogram performed to assess anatomical feasibility for repair with the MEG system. Exclusion criteria included a proximal neck diameter > 28 mm, a neck length < 12 mm and long iliac artery occlusions. The mortality rate for this study was 9.7% and in the latter 19 cases of ruptured AAA, following revision of their treatment protocol, six patients (32%) were deemed unsuitable for EVAR and converted to open repair.[3] In a more recently reported series, Yilmaz et al. quote comparable EVAR-eligibility rates for 'acute' AAA of 69% but admit to using a custom-specified two-part aorto-uni-iliac Talent system.[6] The study includes no mention of limiting anatomical criteria for stenting and the study population includes both frank ruptures and symptomatic AAA.

Lee et al. have recently reported a more realistic estimation of EVAR-eligibility in ruptured and symptomatic AAA using commercially available devices.[9] In a 10-year review of their AAA admissions, 83 patients were identified as having either ruptured AAA (42), or symptomatic AAA (41). Only 28 (10 ruptured AAA) were stable enough for CT imaging. With allowance for 'considerable latitude' in the determination of anatomical suitability and adjunctive procedures (Table 1) only 46% (10/28) of these aneurysms would have been suitable for EVAR using one of the two currently available FDA-approved stent-graft systems (AneuRx and Ancure, both bifurcated devices). This compared with an elective EVAR-eligibility of 74%. This observed difference is explained by the significantly wider and shorter proximal necks identified in the ruptured and symptomatic groups.

Verhoeven et al. have recently presented a series of EVAR procedures performed in acute AAA patients utilizing local anaesthetic techniques. In their 4-year study (1998–2001), 163 patients with acute AAA were assessed. EVAR was considered if both a stent-graft and an endovascular team were available. Of the 47 cases meeting these criteria, only 16 patients were anatomically suitable (see Table 1) for EVAR using commercially available endografts (Vanguard, Talent or Zenith Trifab), an acute AAA EVAR-eligibility rate of 34%.[10]

Van Sambeek et al. offer further evidence suggesting a current limited suitability of ruptured AAA for EVAR. During a 6-month period in 2001, 22 consecutive patients were admitted with an acute AAA. Six haemodynamically unstable patients

Emergency aneurism repair – a 50% option with commercial systems • **Against the motion** • MG Wyatt et al.

150

Table 1. Review of current data regarding EVAR in acute AAA (CTA, computed tomographic angiography; CIA, common iliac artery; NR, not reported)

Group	Year	Total no. of acute AAA admissions	No. assessed for EVAR (rupture AAA:sAAA)	No. of AAA declined EVAR	Imaging technique	Anatomical inclusion critera	EVAR-mortality rate	EVAR-eligibility rate	Ref. no.
Hinchliffe et al.	1994–2000	?	20 (20:0)	?	Spiral CTA (17) OTA (2)	Neck diameter < 32 mm Neck length > 15 mm Angulation < 60° CIA < 22 mm	45%	?	5
Ohki et al.	1993–1998	47	12 (12:0)	?	Spiral CT	Neck diameter 20–28 mm	16%	?	4
Veith et al.	1996–2002	19	13 (13:0)	6	OTA	Neck diameter < 28 mm Neck length > 12 mm No long iliac artery occlusion	9.7%	68%	3
Yilmaz et al.	2001	26	18 (17:1)	8	CT	NR	17%	69%	6
Greenberg et al.	2000	?	3 (3:0)	?	Spiral CT	NR	0%	?	8
Lee et al.	1991–2001	83	28 (10:18)	15	CT	Neck diameter 18–26 mm Neck length > 15 mm Angulation < 60°	–	47%	9
Verhoeven et al.	1998–2001	163	47 (32:15)	31	CT	Neck length > 15 mm Angulation < 60° CIA < 20 mm	6%	34%	10
Van Sambeek et al.	2001	22	16 (10:8)	10	CT	NR	0%	37.5%	11

proceeded immediately to open repair whereas the remaining 16 cases underwent CT imaging with a view to possible EVAR. Of these, only six patients (five Excluder and one Zenith) were stented, an eligibility rate of 37.5%.[11]

Conclusion

The introduction of EVAR has revolutionized the management of patients with elective AAA. More recently the technique has been applied to patients presenting with both ruptured and other acute AAAs. Several centres have reported excellent eligibility rates and significantly reduced perioperative mortality results using 'home made' devices. Nevertheless, there are no data to support the motion that 'several commercially available systems render emergency aneurysm repair an option for at least 50% of ruptures'.

Randomized controlled trial?

Yes definitely.

Summary

- Conventional open repair in ruptured AAA is associated with high mortality.

- Specialist centres are reporting vastly improved results with EVAR for ruptured AAA as opposed to open surgery.

- High EVAR-eligibility rates in ruptured AAA are only currently achievable with specially constructed hybrid grafts or custom-specified devices that are not commercially available.

- More realistic rates for EVAR-eligibility in ruptured AAA with the presently available commercial devices lie between 30 and 40%.

- Further advances in endovascular technology are needed if the potential benefits of EVAR in ruptured AAA are to be realized.

- The proposed EVAR study comparing EVAR with open repair in ruptured AAA would allow further evaluation of this approach to management.

References

1. Bown MJ, Sutton AJ, Bell PRF, Sayers RD. A meta-analysis of 50 years of ruptured abdominal aortic aneurysm repair. *Br J Surg* 2002; **89**: 714–730.
2. Hinchliffe RJ, Hopkinson BR. Ruptured abdominal aortic aneurysm: Time for a new approach. *J Cardiovasc Surg* 2002; **43**: 345–347.
3. Veith FJ, Ohki T. Endovascular approaches to ruptured infrarenal aortoiliac aneurysms. *J Cardiovasc Surg* 2002; **43**: 369–378.
4. Ohki T, Veith FJ, Sanchez LA *et al.* Endovascular graft repair of ruptured aortoiliac aneurysms. *J Am Coll Surg* 1999; **189**: 102–113.

5. Hinchliffe RJ, Yusuf SW, Macierewicz JA *et al.* Endovascular repair of ruptured abdominal aortic aneurysm-a challenge to open repair? Results of a single centre experience in 20 patients. *Eur J Vasc Endovasc Surg* 2001; **22**: 528–534.

6. Yilmaz N, Peppelenbosch N, Cuypers PWM *et al.* Emergency treatment of symptomatic or ruptured abdominal aortic aneurysms: the role of endovascular repair. *J Endovasc Ther* 2002; **9**: 449–457.

7. Yusuf SW, Whitaker SC, Chuter TAM, Wenham PW, Hopkinson BR. Emergency endovascular repair of leaking aortic aneurysm. *Lancet* 1994; **344**: 1645.

8. Greenberg RK, Srivastava SD, Ouriel K *et al.* An endoluminal method of hemorrhage control and repair of ruptured abdominal aortic aneurysms. *J Endovasc Ther* 2000; **7**: 1–7.

9. Lee WA, Huber TS, Hirniese CM *et al.* Eligibility rates of ruptured and symptomatic AAA for endovascular repair. *J Endovasc Ther* 2002; **9**: 436–442.

10. Verhoeven ELG, Prins TR, van den Dungen J *et al.* Endovascular repair of acute abdominal aortic aneurysms under local anaesthesia with bifurcated graft systems: a feasibility study. *J Endovasc Ther* 2003; (in press).

11. van Sambeek MRHM, van Dijk LC, Hendriks JM. Endovascular versus conventional open repair of acute abdominal aortic aneurysm. *J Endovasc Ther* 2002; **9**: 443–448.

Several commercially available systems render emergency aneurysm repair an option for at least 50% of ruptures

Charing Cross Editorial Comments towards Consensus

The Montefiore experience is substantial and the authors speak from experience.

The opposition is also enthusiastic for endovascular aneurysm repair and the Newcastle centre have given a balanced assessment. Their contention is that at present there are no data to support the motion that commercially available systems render emergency aneurysm repair an option for at least 50% of ruptures. The opposition does stress that the reports from New York are given without details of those patients that were turned down for the procedure. The opposition is as potentially enthusiastic about endovascular aneurysm repair for rupture as New York but say that the proof is not yet there. They call for a randomized control trial. This is a very British approach but Frank Veith and his group are also very supportive of such approach seeking the evidence where it is missing.

Both groups give the subject 'a good shake' and highlight the problems which currently exist.

Roger M Greenhalgh
Editor

Suprarenal fixation of stent-grafts is a disadvantage

For the motion
D Raithel

Introduction

Endovascular aneurysm repair (EVAR) has become an alternative method to open surgery in elected abdominal aortic aneurysms.

A wide variety of aortic stent-grafts are under investigation, and the optimal design is not yet known. A significant design consideration is the secure fixation of the proximal part of the stent-graft to avoid migration and to prevent especially proximal type-I endoleaks.[1,2]

During the early development of endografts for EVAR, aortic aneurysms with a neck under 20-15 mm were excluded from endoluminal treatment. Therefore, bare-spring-graft components extending 15 mm or more proximal to the Dacron-graft fabric were developed in order to treat these patients, especially with larger aortic necks (over 28 mm).

The philosophy was, that with this supra-/transrenal fixation a more reliable management of those aneurysms with shorter, angulated and/or large aortic necks would be possible. There was, however, the awareness of the potential risk of renal infarctions and also renal artery occlusions, up to the development of renal insufficiency. Among this group of endografts with suprarenal fixation are the *Quantum*, *Talent* and *Zenith* grafts. *Endologix* and *Vanguard* provide the possibility of both supra-, and infrarenal fixation (Table 1).

Ancure, *AneuRx*, *Excluder* and *Lifepath* only work with infrarenal fixation. To achieve a secure long-term attachment of these aortic endografts, hooks or fixation crimps have been used for the *Ancure* device and the *Lifepath* system, respectively. These two grafts remain in place without migration, by these fixation systems.

Table 1. Different designs

Suprarenal fixation
Quantum, Talent, Zenith
Infrarenal fixation
Ancure, AneuRx, (Chuter), Excluder, Lifepath
Supra-/Infrarenal fixation
Endologix, Vanguard

Nuremberg experience

Between August 1994 and August 2002, 748 infrarenal aortic aneurysms were treated endovascularly. We operated on 681 men and 67 women with a mean age of 70.1 years, using 154 tubes, 591 bifurcated grafts and three mono-iliac systems. The mean diameter of the aneurysms treated was 50.1 mm.

Table 2 shows the different types of devices.

Table 2. Devices used in Nuremberg

Ancure 1994	Lifepath 1999
AneuRx 1997	Quantum 2002
Chuter 1994	Talent 1996
Endologix 1999	Vanguard (Mintech) 1994/96
Excuder 1998	Zenith 1998

Results

Endoleakage rate

The endoleakage rate in 280 *unibody* grafts was 18.9% (Table 3). In this series, the endoleakage rate of 180 bifurcated *Ancure* devices was 15% (mostly type II); with 98 *Endologix* devices it was 25%.

Table 3. Unibody devices: endoleakage

Device	Primary	Secondary	Total
Unibody (280)	40 (14.3%)	13 (4.6%)	53 (18.9%)
Ancure (180)	20 (11.1%)	7 (3.9%)	27 (15%)
*Chuter (2)	1 (50%)	0	1 (50%)
Endologix (98)	19 (19.4%)	6	25 (25.5%)

*Numbers too small

Modular systems (n = 311) had a higher endoleakage rate with 28.5% (Table 4). The highest endoleakage rate was seen with the *Vanguard/Mintec* system, with 49%. The *AneuRx* system had a leakage rate of 28.1%, the *Lifepath* 5.4%, and the *Zenith* graft 29.7%.

Table 4. Modular devices: endoleakage

Device	Primary	Secondary	Total
Modular (311)	53 (17.0%)	36 (11.5%)	89 (28.5%)
AneuRx (57)	9 (15.8%)	7 (12.3%)	16 (28.1%)
*Excluder (6)	2 (33%)	0	2 (33%)
Lifepath (37)	2 (5.4%)	0	2 (5.4%)
*Quantum (13)	1 (7.7%)	0	1 (7.7%)
Vanguard/MinTec (98)	21 (21.4%)	17 (17.3%)	48 (49.0%)
Zenith (101)	18 (17.8%)	12 (11.9%)	30 (29.7%)

*Numbers too small

The proximal type I endoleakage rate of the 748 grafts was 4.9% (Table 5). Comparing 220 grafts with suprarenal fixation to 528 grafts with infrarenal fixation, the endoleakage rate was 5% and 7%, respectively.

Table 5. Proximal type I endoleak

Fixation	Primary	Secondary	Total
Suprarenal (220)	5 (2.3%)	6 (2.7%)	11 (5.0%)
Infrarenal (528)	16 (3.0%)	7 (1.3%)	23 (7.0%)
Total (748)	21 (2.8%)	13 (1.8%)	36 (4.9%)

Conversions

Due to the fact, that the first series of the *Mintec/* later *Vanguard* devices had a relatively high rate of stent fractures or suture breaks, we had a high re-do surgery and conversion rate (Table 6). The primary conversion rate was 2.9%, the secondary conversion rate 5.5%: a total of 8.4% of conversions.

Out of 63 conversions, about 52% were attributable to failures of the tube grafts.

Table 6. Conversion

Primary	22	2.9%
Secondary	42	6.0%
Total	63	8.4%

The conversion rate was highest with the *Vanguard* (*Mintec*) devices. Furthermore, modular systems had a higher conversion rate than unibody systems (7.4% versus 2.5%).

Of all 63 conversions, only seven were due to a proximal type I endoleak (Table 7). Of these seven proximal endoleaks which led to conversion, three occurred in patients with a *Vanguard* device and suprarenal fixation, and two in the *Zenith* series.

Table 7. Indication for conversion (n = 63) 8.4%

Indication	Primary (intraoperative)	Within 24 h	Secondary
Graft misplacement	6	3	1
Device defect	6	–	1
Type I endoleak			
proximal	–	1	6
distal	–	–	22
Type II endoleak	–	–	1
Type III endoleak	–	–	3
Graft thrombosis body	–	1	2
Iliac artery perforation	8	2	–
Distal secondary aneurysm	–	–	2

Renal infarctions

With 11.1%, we had a relatively high renal-infarction rate (n = 82): 3.1% were anticipated infarcts (covering pole artery), while 8% were unexpected renal infarcts (n = 59).

The renal infarction rate was highest (22%) in patients treated with the *Zenith* graft

(Table 8); 15 patients had a total unilateral renal infarction (four *AneuRx*, four *Vanguard*, seven *Zenith*). With 23.2%, suprarenal fixation had a higher renal infarction rate than the infrarenal fixation (6.6%).

Table 8. Renal infarction: devices

	Total	Infarcts n	%
Ancure Guidant	224	18	8.0
AneuRx Medtronic	58	10	17.2
Chuter	3	–	0*
Endologix	100	7	7.0
Excluder Gore	6	–	0*
Lifepath Edwards	37	2	5.4
Vanguard/Mintec BSc.	205	23	11.2
Zenith Cook	101	22	22.0
Quantum	13	–	0*

*Numbers too small

Thrombi

Due to the systems used in large aortic necks (> 28 mm), we found thrombi in the follow-up CT scans of seven patients with a *Zenith* graft. In two patients, this problem led to a trash foot. This seems to be a problem with larger devices, especially those with suprarenal fixation.

Evidence

Since August 94, the Vascular Clinic at the Nuremberg hospital has treated 748 patients with infrarenal aortic aneurysms via the endovascular route. The 30-day mortality rate was 0.5%. We have been using 10 different devices including grafts with infra- and devices with suprarenal fixation.

Analysing these results, there was no benefit using grafts with the possibility of suprarenal fixation for EVAR. The total primary type I endoleakage rate in our series was 4.9%. Comparing the grafts with suprarenal fixation to those with infrarenal fixation, there was no significant difference in both series, with 5% versus 7% endoleakage. A further aspect is, that this group of grafts with infrarenal fixation includes a high share of grafts from the first series. Both aspects, that of the learning curve and the fact, that the first-generation devices were associated with a high failure rate due to suture breaks, and others, need to be considered here.[1-3]

The success of endoluminal stent-grafts is critically dependent on the optimal proximal fixation of the graft.

Grafts such as the *Ancure* device with hooks or the *Lifepath* system with so-called fixation crimps have the advantage of an optimal proximal fixation, even in short angulated necks. We have treated many aortic aneurysms with short necks (1 cm or below) with the *Ancure* device and dispose of follow-up results of these devices since 1994.

Makaroun *et al.* have also not seen any significant difference comparing the *Ancure* device with the *Excluder*.[4]

Resch *et al.* have shown in experimental studies, that hooks and barbs improved the fixation of self-expandable stents and that balloon dilatation of the proximal stent after deployment might increase fixation further.[5]

Bernhard *et al.* have analysed the literature regarding ruptured abdominal aortic aneurysms after EVAR.[6] They found 47 post-endograft AAA ruptures; 27 were due to a type I endoleak, two to type II, and 11 to type III endoleaks. In four patients, a leak was present, but the source was not reported. In three patients the cause was not reported. Of the 27 post-endograft ruptures due to type I endoleakage, only 12 were due to a proximal-attachment endoleak. These data show clearly, that the frequency of proximal type I endoleaks leading to rupture is very low, and this does not necessarily suggest, that suprarenal fixation should be attempted.

In the literature, the incidence of renal failure was reported to range from 4% to 6.2%. In those patients, early renal complications included migration or occlusion of stent-grafts (17% vs 32%) and renal atheroembolism.[7] This cannot be confirmed in our series. The rate of renal infarctions (followed up by CT-scans) was in 220 patients with suprarenal fixation 23.2%, in 528 patients with infrarenal fixation in contrast only 6.6%. Furthermore, the renal infarction rate with the *Zenith* graft (suprarenal fixation) was very high with 22% (Table 8).

The *AneurRx* graft showed an infarction rate of 17.2%, compared with the renal infarction rate with the *Ancure* device of 8% and the *Lifepath* device of 5.4%.

These data document that the potential risk of impairing renal function increases with the transrenal attachment and complex reconstructions. Optimal proximal fixation with hooks/fixation crimps is a key to safety (Fig. 1).

In the long-term follow-up there might even be an improvement of the results of infrarenal fixation, since in our patient population there is a great portion of devices of the first generation which had yielded markedly worse results in our series.[2,8]

Our data show that suprarenal fixation is associated with more problems (at least in our series) than EVAR with infrarenal fixation.

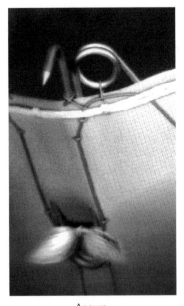

Ancure

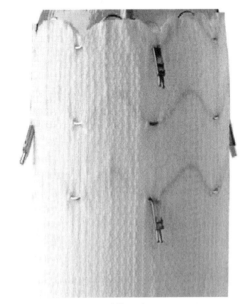

Lifepath

Figure 1. The potential risk of compromising renal function increases with transrenal attachment and complex reconstructions. Optimal proximal fixation with hooks/fixation crimps is the key to safety.

Summary

- Nuremberg data document no significant difference in proximal type I endoleaks comparing infrarenal to suprarenal fixation.

- The conversion rate due to proximal type I endoleaks was very low after EVAR with infrarenal fixation.

- The renal infarction rate after EVAR using infrarenal fixation was more than three times lower than with suprarenal fixation.

- Infrarenal fixation shows optimum results in grafts with hooks or fixation crimps.

References

1. Raithel D. Which industry-made endovascular grafts are best for abdominal arotic aneurysm repair and why? In: *Perspectives in Vascular Surgery.* Gloviczki P (ed). New York, Stuttgart: Thieme, 1999: Vol 12, No.1.

2. Beebe HG. Late failures of devices used for endovascular treatment of abdominal aortic aneurysm: What have we learned and what is the task for the future? In: *Perspectives in Vascular Surgery* Gloviczki P (ed). New York, Stuttgart: Thieme, 2001: Vol 14, No. 1: 29–46.

3. Laheij RJF, van Marrewijk CJ, Bluth J *et al.* The influence of team experience on outcomes of endovascular stenting of abdominal aortic aneurysms. *Eur J Vasc Endovasc Surg* 2002; 24: 128–133.

4. Makaroun M, Zaiko A. Endoleaks following endovascular aortic aneurysm repair: Clinical significance and treatment modalities. In: *Perspectives in Vascular Surgery.* Gloviczki P (ed). New York, Stuttgart: Thieme, 2000: Vol 13, No 1, pp. 1–14.

5. Resch T, Malina M, Lindblad B *et al.* The impact of stent design on proximal stent-graft fixation in the abdominal aorta: An experimental study. *Eur J Vasc Endovasc Surg* 2000; 20: 190–195.

6. Bernhard VM, Mitchell RS, Matsuma JS *et al.* Ruptured abdominal aortic aneurysm after endovascular repair. *J Vasc Surg* 2002; 35: 1157–1162.

7. Izzedine H, Koskas F, Cluzel P *et al.* Renal function after aortic stent-grafting including coverage of renal arterial ostia. *Am J Kidney Dis* 2002; 39: 730–736.

8. Raithel D. Which endograft is best? *Endovascular Today* 2002; 1: 40–43.

Suprarenal fixation of stent-grafts is a disadvantage

Against the motion
Michael MD Lawrence-Brown,
James B Semmens

Introduction

This defence of suprarenal fixation of endografts represents the work and experience of many individuals who have published and contributed to the research, development and evolution of the Zenith Endoluminal Graft since 1994.

The purpose of endoluminal grafting is to provide a secure durable conduit through and across a chiasm of dilated artery that is prone to burst from the pressure on the wall within it. Endoluminal grafting for abdominal aortic aneurysm (AAA) has provided an attractive alternative to open aneurysm repair because it is much less invasive, with reduced stress upon the patient – if it is successful and durable.[1-3]

Paradoxically, thoracic grafts, which are of greater diameter than infrarenal endografts, may be more stable to a degree. Straight endoluminal grafts, which have only a small diameter differential, are rarely feasible in the infrarenal aorta, but they are the primary design of thoracic stent-grafts.[4] Due to the lateral forces, thoracic grafts seem more likely to be displaced from both proximal and distal ends, depending on the wall contact in each landing zone.[5] However, infrarenal grafts appear much more likely to be displaced than thoracic grafts, and the displacement will tend to occur at the proximal end.

A tube within a tube of the same diameter offers little resistance to flow and is therefore, not prone to dislodgment unless there is a curve when the centre of the force acts to dislodge each end of the tube in the direction of the force vector (Figs 1a, 1b). In contrast, a tube that narrows in diameter resists the current and behaves as a windsock or sea-anchor. An aortoiliac graft is such a tube. A bifurcated aorto-bi-iliac graft is also such a tube and additionally maybe be subject to an oscillating moment if there is differential flow between the two run-offs. Every beat of the heart pulses against this resistance – forty million times a year – and will continue to act to dislodge until this event occurs, or the graft becomes so firmly encased in the body that it no longer needs to serve as a bridge on its own, and this may take years.

Cardiac output increases with activity and will increase the drag on a bifurcated graft. Blood pressure usually also increases with activity, particularly in the elderly, and adds to the activity effect of cardiac output. Therefore, attachment design at the proximal end and patient selection must take into account a safety margin to accommodate for a peak value for the forces acting on an endoluminal graft.

A more detailed assessment of the forces acting on an endograft used computa-

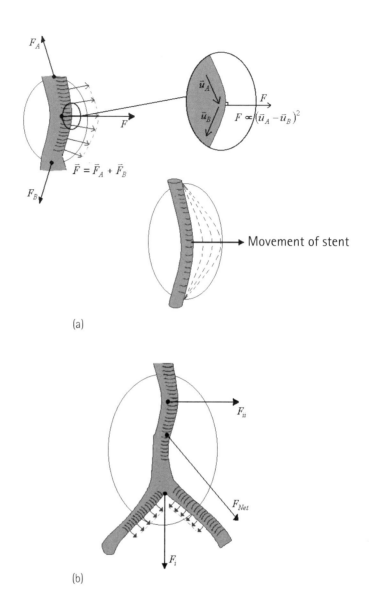

(a)

(b)

Figure 1. Forces acting upon a stent graft.
Figure 1a: On a constant diameter artery, the force will be constant along all points of the wall. Force F is the resultant force of all the velocity changes, ie the curvature and narrowing of the tube. The magnitude of the force (F) will increase as the curvature increases. Fa and Fb are the reaction forces that are required to balance force F. Over time, the cyclic action of the stresses on the stent will tend to move it until the wall of the aneurysm supports it. This will stress the joint at the proximal and distal points. The place of least resistance will be displaced. The maximum point of movement and stress per unit force, is in the centre of the tube or centre of the force. [2]
Figure 1b: The force acting on the bifurcation is a result of the change of velocity of the fluid at that point. The net force (F_{net}) acting on the stent is the sum of the forces acting on the bifurcation (F_i) and the force acting on the curvature (F_{ii}) of the stent.[2]

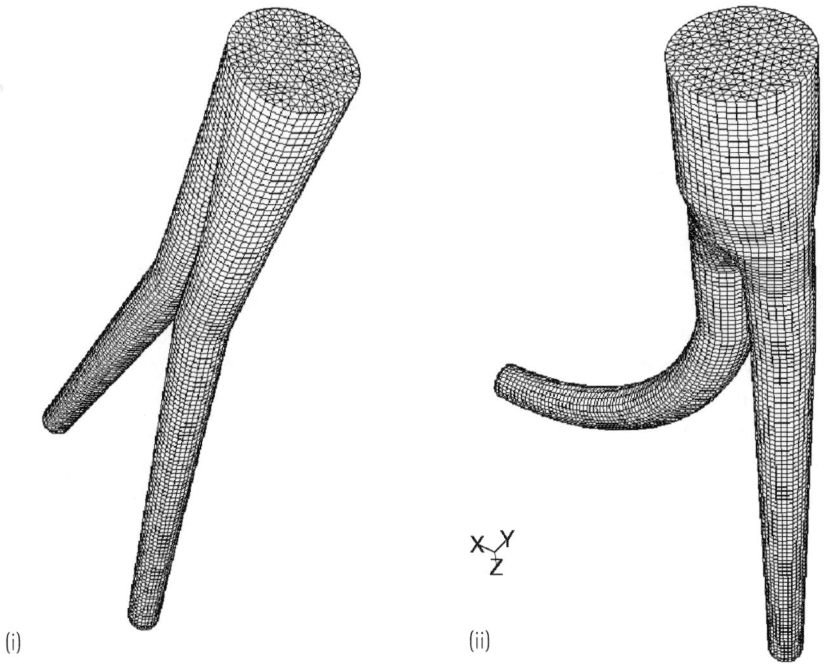

Figure 1c. (i) The 'flat' computational domain (ii) The 'bent in the plane' domain illustrates the techniques of computational fluid dynamics.[5]

tional fluid dynamics (CFD) to solve the equations of fluid motion on a mathematical grid that typically takes the shape of the object of interest.[5] As an example of the gridding process, the CFD grids used to compute the forces on the Zenith graft are shown in Fig.1c. CFD models were constructed of the force on an endoluminal graft due to the steady, turbulent flow of blood through the graft. Two different configurations of bifurcated endoluminal grafts, a straight lie and curved lie, and two sizes of grafts were studied. The forces on the graft depended more on the size rather than the curvature of the graft. For the large, straight, symmetrical design, the maximum downward 'windsock' force (i.e. the force required to detach the proximal end of the graft) was 8 Newton (N), while the small graft was subject to a maximum downward force of 3.8 N. In the curved graft, the maximum downward force for the large graft was approximately 9 N, while the curved small graft was subject to a force of 5.1 N. Comparing these downward forces with the 5 to 6 N that is required for displacing the proximal end of a unbarbed stent suggests that stent-graft migration may be partly due to this 'windsock' force.

For the curved grafts, both the large and small grafts generated a sideways force of 1.3 and 1.5 N, respectively and are small by comparison. These lateral forces act to move the distal and proximal ends of the graft from their required positions within the aneurysm. Side forces on the curve add to the drag forces on the proximal end and provide an upward displacement force from the distal landing zone. Overall, forces on an infrarenal bifurcated graft are greater than for tube grafts, especially in terms of drag on the proximal attachment zone.

Adequate endoluminal wall contact

Should movement/migration occur so that the defect is no longer spanned, then the graft is as useful as a ladder or bridge that is too short (Fig. 2). Flow within an AAA after the insertion of an endoluminal graft implies pressure to a varying degree. Absence of flow does not assure absence of pressure because they are different parameters. The size of an AAA is not determined by imaging the flow current, but by measuring the diameter from wall to wall because of laminated thrombus. Placing a short tube in the middle of an AAA in the channel of laminated thrombus is no less useful than a graft that spans 99.9% of the distance from one landing zone to another. In other words, any movement that shifts a graft from 360 degrees wall contact breaks the pressure seal, fails the primary purpose and endangers the patient. While infection is undoubtedly a cause of pressure build-up, and hygroscopic pressure may be a cause of 'endotension', pressure within an aneurysm sac must be considered to be arterial pressure. Exposure to aortic pressure is either primary failure that may be unrecognized because of the presence of laminated thrombus and mere channel lining or secondary failure from migration and graft durability.

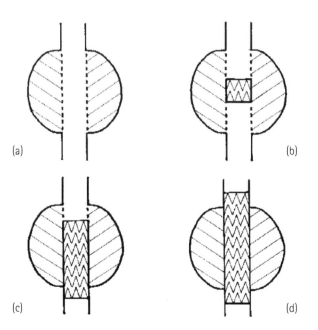

Figure 2. Only (d) below provides adequate aneurysm protection from pressure, while all may provide a similar image for the flow patterns on contrast angiography (or CT)

Obtaining a secure hold

There has been an increasing use of suprarenal fixation during endoluminal repair of AAA to provide secure proximal fixation in an area of the aorta that is less likely to dilate or contain atheroma (Fig. 3a).[2,3,6,7] Suprarenal fixation provides the facility of secure fixation in a stable and secure region of the aorta. Fixation is different from

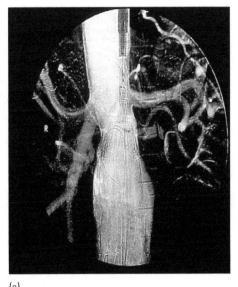
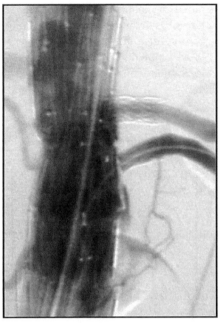

(a)   (b)

Figure 3a. Neck with stent fixation across renal artery to show quality of the aorta.
Figure 3b. Fenestration to increase secure wall contact.

seal, but inadequate fixation may break the seal. The recent developments in design, which allow modular building and fenestration, have provided a greater number of treatment options for patients with more complex neck morphology (Fig. 3b).[8] These options necessarily require secure attachment or run the risk of vital vessel occlusion secondary to migration.

The position of an open stent-wire close to or across the orifice of the renal artery

The position of an open stent-wire close to or across the orifice of the renal artery has caused concern about the potential effects on renal blood flow and altered renal function. The possible disadvantages of suprarenal fixation are:

1. Occlusion or adverse reduction of flow of renal vessels by strut.
2. Occlusion of renal vessel by intimal hyplerplasia induced by strut.
3. Occlusion or adverse reduction of flow by particular build-up on strut.
4. Occlusion of vessel origin by moving diseased intima (plague/thrombus) into or across the vessel during deployment.
5. Dilation of the stented area or extension of the AAA by the radial force of the stent.
6. Fracture and breakage of the stent – namely barbs or hooks.
7. Difficulty in dealing with the anchor stent if graft explanation required.

To address the concerns regarding suprarenal fixation and the effect of a wire crossing an orifice, an understanding of the blood and flow properties are also required to complement the knowledge base of patient outcomes that suggest the practice is safe and effective. Quantitative mathematical and computational analysis have been also used to determine the impact of a stent-wire on renal artery blood flow as a function of the relative size of the wire to the opening diameter of the vessels under conditions simulating a normal and stenosed artery (Fig. 4, Tables 1 and 2).[3,9]

0.46 mm diameter stent wire

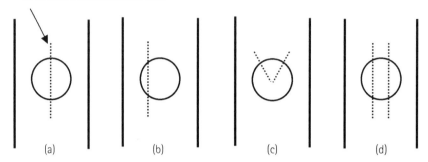

Figure 4. Stent-wire configurations used in the experiments: (a) central stent-wire, (b) off-centre stent-wire at 1/4 spacing, (c) V-shaped stent-wire at the centre, and (d) two stent-wires at 1/3 spacing. Note that the stent-wires have a finite thickness, *d*, so it is the central axis of the stent-wires that is taken as the representative line for each stent-wire.[4]

Table 1. Summary of computational results

	Percentage decrease in side artery arm flow rate with stent-wire (%)			
	7 mm side artery arm		3 mm side artery arm	
	1 m/s (2.31 litre/min)	0.2 m/s (0.462 litre/min)	1 m/s (0.424 litre/min)	0.2 m/s (0.0848 litre/min)
Central stent-wire	6.8	6	6	8
Off-centre stent-wire at 1/4 spacing	4.9	2.9	8.4	6.5

Table 2. Summary of experimental results on the effect of flow through a renal artery due to the presence of stent-wires in front of the renal artery entrance

	Percentage decrease in side-artery arm flow rate with stent cases (%)			
	7 mm side artery arm		3 mm side artery arm	
	1 m/s (2.31 litre/min)	0.2 m/s (0.462 litre/min)	1 m/s (0.424 litre/min)	0.2 m/s (0.0848 litre/min)
Central stent-wire	0.89–1.06 ± 0.1 av = 0.95 ± 0.1	0.47–0.53 ± 0.36 av = 0.51 ± 0.36	1.08–1.99 ± 0.41 av = 1.45 ± 0.41	1.53–2.62 ± 0.78 av = 1.90 ± 0.78
Off-centre stent-wire at 1/4 spacing	0.53–0.72 ± 0.1 av = 0.60 ± 0.1	Negligible	0.6–1.04 ± 0.41 av = 0.81 ± 0.41	0.65–1.56 ± 0.78 av = 1.20 ± 0.78
V-shaped stent-wire at the centre	0.74–0.85 ± 0.1 av = 0.79 ± 0.1	Negligible	1.74–2.25 ± 0.41 av = 1.94 ± 0.41	1.64–2.95 ± 0.78 av = 2.28 ± 0.78
Two stent-wires at 1/3 spacing	1.26–1.42 ± 0.1 av = 1.33 ± 0.1	0.71–0.93 ± 0.36 av = 0.82 ± 0.36	3.37–5.06 ± 0.41 av = 4.11 ± 0.41	6.03–6.62 ± 0.78 av = 6.35 ± 0.78

Of particular interest is the phenomenon of vortex shedding, where, depending on the flow rates, vortices can be shed by the stent-wire at time intervals that are small relative to the blood pulse timescale. Vortex shedding can decrease the drag of the wire on the fluid and may assist the flow of blood into the arteries (Fig. 5).[5]

Turbulence in fluid dynamics refers to the propensity of fluids to form a cascade of eddies (whirlpools of fluid) of all different sizes and is called vortex shedding. The number of eddies is, usually, inversely proportional to the size of the eddy. So there are only a few, very large eddies and a large number of small eddies. The intriguing

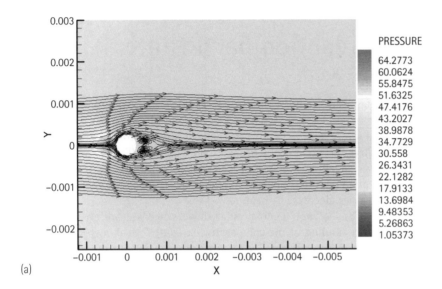

(a)

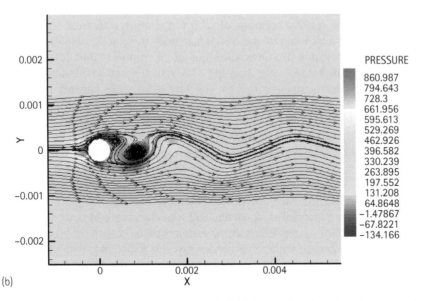

(b)

Figure 5a. A streamline and pressure contour plot of the flow past the wire, where the pressure is in units of Pascals and the pressure has been set relative to a background reference pressure.
Figure 5b. A modified magnification of the flow shown in Fig. 5a: a streamline and pressure colour contour plot of the flow past the wire clearly show the vortices shed by the wire. Here the pressure is in units of Pascals and has been set relative to the reference pressure.

and, from the engineer's point of view, frustrating aspect of turbulence is that the smallest eddies can dramatically affect the large scale motion of the flow, a bit like the 'tail wagging the dog'. The size of these 'tail' eddies is usually much smaller than the smallest grid volume that can be created with current computer technology. So, it is necessary to model this 'sub-grid' turbulence with a specifically designed turbulence model. Vortex shedding may partly explain why the observed flow reduction is less than the mathematically and computationally fluid dynamically calculated expectation. The sheer thinning properties of blood would be expected to further benefit flow (Figs 5a, 5b).[5]

Intimal reaction particulate adherence

The experimental results indicate that for all the stent-wire configurations tested (see Fig. 4), the presence of stent-wire(s) had a minimal effect on the blood flow rate through a renal artery with most flow rates decreasing by around 1%. This was true provided that there was no build-up of material on the wire (Figs 6a, 6b). When material build-up was 'encouraged' to occur, then decreases in flow rate of up to 40% were observed. The numerical and analytic methods used, indicated that the flow rates would, in most cases, decrease by around 3–10%.[4]

Pre-clinical testing of new endovascular devices needs a variety of methodologies plus an understanding of the comparative strengths, weaknesses and error susceptibility of each method. Durability is an issue in testing for the longer term and this requires some accelerated testing methods, which is not possible in vivisection experiments. While live experiments will continue to have a place in assessing the biological response to the foreign body and/or the induced stress response, the value of theoretical mathematical calculations, computational modelling and bench modelling and the relative accuracy of each to the other with cross-testing validity of the results is important to the development of these technologies. The importance of the observation of vortex shedding into a confined conduit is unknown. It may enhance flow by reducing drag but also activate platelets. Indefinite prophylactic anti-platelet treatment might be considered for these patients to reduce the possibility of adhesion forming upon stent-wires. The composition of the wire may be a variable.

The results of the study confirm that the flow interference by isolated or widely spaced traversing inert wires has little effect on the flow through medium sized vessels.

The likelihood of intimal hyperplasia across an orifice is related to the proximity of the struts of the stent to each other. Those that are close together, such as in braided or small aperture expanded mesh stents, will provide a scaffold upon which intimal hyperplasia may link across. Whereas, occlusion is unlikely with the widely separated single wires of a Z-stent with relatively few crowns. Experience with 170 cases over 6 years has not shown any deterioration in biochemical renal function measured by creatinine levels, and no renal artery occlusions following the procedure. The argument therefore for placing open stents across the renal arteries is that the risk of renal impairment when the renal artery orifices are normal are less than the risks to the patient of an insecure proximal fixation or an open operation.

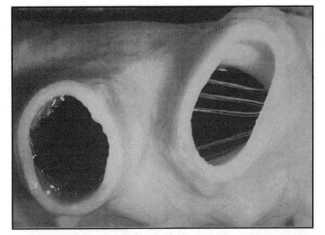

(a)

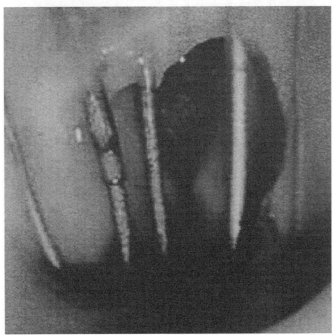

(b)

Figure 6a. Stents and vessel origins. On the left – a balloon-expandable stent in the orifice. On the right, a z-stent across the orifice.
Figure 6b. Intimal reaction to stent crossing an orifice in a growing pig.

The use of serum creatinine as a measurement of renal function

Transrenal manipulation, with or without transrenal fixation is associated with some risk of renal embolization. Measurement of serum creatinine is part of the standard short- and long-term follow-up protocol to monitor any changes in renal function. Patients admitted for endoluminal repair are often elderly, and it is inappropriate to compare an older person's renal function with the reference intervals derived from younger subjects. Aging affects some routinely measured biochemical parameters and serum creatinine is speculated to be one of them. Knowledge of age-related variation in serum creatinine is required for the clinical interpretation of renal function following both endoluminal grafting for AAA and renal artery intervention for renal substance preservation.

Alterations in renal structure and function and in creatinine metabolism are associated with normal aging. Walser (1987)[10] has shown that the normal aging process is

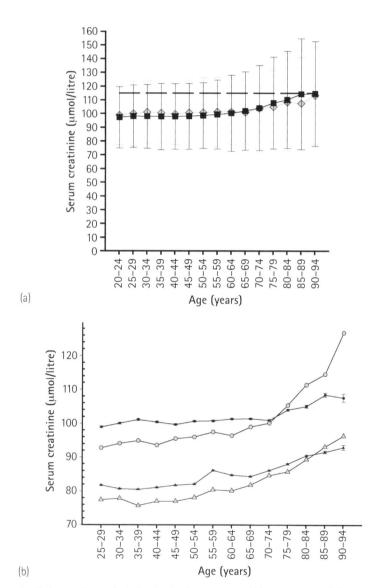

(a)

(b)

Figure 7a. Reference intervals derived using Bhattacharya (▲)and Hoffmann (■) method (mean±2SD). Both methods give similar reference intervals and both demonstrated an increase in serum creatinine with age. Current reference value for serum creatinine is represented by the dotted line.[11]

Figure 7b. Comparison of serum creatinine derived using the Bhattacharya method and the Busselton study (●) in male (■) and female (▲) plotted against age. Each mean calculated from the Bhattacharya method is accompanied by a standard error. Serum creatinine increases steadily in male and female with age. Both studies indicate an increase in serum creatinine with age.[11]

associated with a decline in renal creatinine excretion. The effect of age on serum creatinine is not well defined and it is not common practice to quote reference intervals by age. Current reporting practice provides a single current reference interval irrespective of age. In a recent report, it was shown that serum creatinine concentrations increase with age (Figs 7a,b).[11] These findings question the appropriateness of current practice which uses a single reference interval to interpret serum creatinine.

Strength of attachment with different anchor stents

Pull-out experiments have been performed using harvested pig aortas to examine the stability and durability of stents after deployment (Fig. 8).[2] The method employed a simple spring force measuring device to pull on the deployed stent until it started to move and become detached. It was used to compare covered stents with stents on the outside and no hooks, covered stents with stents on the inside and no hooks, and covered stents attached by an anchor stent with hooks. The force required to pull out and displace a non-hooked stent was 5–6 N (600Gml) compared with 40–50 N for the hooked stents. This meant that up to 10-times the force is required to dislodge a graft by straightening the hooks. A sutured anastomosis has a rupture force around 125 N and this may involve arterial tear. Stapled anastomoses have been proposed and are expected to have the pull-down strength of a sutured anastomosis. Some workers object to penetration of the arterial wall, but this has to be balanced against the danger of migration, and has not been a problem for the authors to date. Understanding the forces acting within the pressurized aorta, and upon the stent-graft, and how they may affect the ongoing performance of the stent-graft is important for lasting effective exclusion of the aneurysm. Investigation of the forces acting on a stent-graft have shown that they may be close to the force threshold required to dislodge the stent-graft when relying on radial attachment alone.

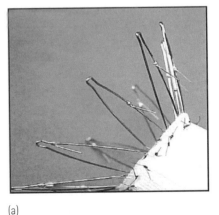

(a)

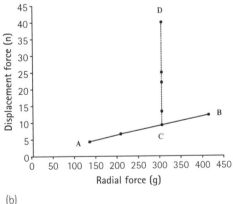

(b)

Figure 8. (a) Anchor stent of the Zenith graft. (b) Experiment demonstrating increasing pull-out force with increasing radial force along A to B. Increasing pull-out force required with increasing strength of hook attachment (C – D). The relationship of C – D is independent of the position along A – B.[2]

Precautions and adjunct measures

Deal with renal stenosis before putting struts across the narrowed orifice – avoid unnecessary manoeuvres in the renal artery vicinity – such as dragging devices across the orifice.

Alternatives

1. Accept possible migration and deal with it as an independent event.
2. Develop secure fixation below.

There is an infrarenal device in Australia and there are guidelines that govern its usage. Experience with the infrarenal device stable-mate in Australasia is that it was used in only 2% (15 of 764) endografts for 2001 in cases of endoluminal repair.

Clinical problems in practice

1. Non-adherence to guidelines (Fig. 9).[12]
2. Progressive dilatation of the aorta.
3. Psychological effect on a patient from additional procedures.
4. Infection risk with redo procedures.
5. Removal of graft.

Will changing clinical practice affect the need for suprarenal fixation?

1. Should we treat small aneurysms with tube grafts prophylactically?
2. How do you balance technical advantage/disadvantage with best medical practice.

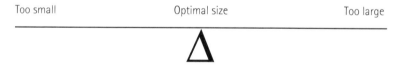

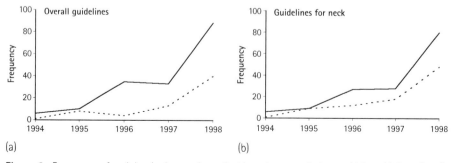

Figure 9. Frequency of endoluminal procedures that have been carried out within guidelines (----) and outside guidelines (——) for A: all and B: neck.[12]

The need for secure proximal fixation with endoluminal grafting for AAA

Success and durability of endoluminal grafting depends primarily on a proximal secure attachment and seal. Endoleaks, especially proximal endoleaks, are not only evidence of failure, but also increase the risk of rupture because an endoleak with significant in-flow and no out-flow may create a higher mean pressure in the aneurysm chamber than in the lumen of the aorta that increases the potential for expansion and rupture of the aneurysm. Secure proximal attachment and seal are dependent on patient selection (aneurysmal anatomy) and graft design.

Summary

- The definite consequences of stent-graft migration and the need for secure proximal fixation of an endoluminal graft for AAA outweighs any potential disadvantage and risk of impairing renal function.

References

1. Lawrence-Brown MMD, Hartley D, MacSweeny S, The Perth Endoluminal Bifurcated Graft System – Development and Early Experience. *J Cardiovasc Surg* 1996; 4: 706–712.
2. Lawrence-Brown MMD, Semmens JB, Hartley DE *et al.* How is durability related to patient selection and graft design with endoluminal grafting for abdominal aortic aneurysm? In: *Durability of Vascular and Endovascular Surgery*. RM Greenhalgh (ed). London: Saunders, 1999: 375–385.
3. Lawrence-Brown MMD, Semmens JB, Stanley BM *et al.* Endoluminal building of the aortic grafts for abdominal aortic aneurysm disease. In: *Vascular and Endovascular Opportunities*. R M Greenhalgh, JT Powell, AWM Mitchell (eds). London: Saunders, 2000: 249–261.
4. Lawrence-Brown MMD, Sieunarine K, Van Schie G *et al.* Hybrid open-endoluminal technique for repair of thoracoabdominal aneurysm involving the celiac axis. *J Endovasc Surg* 2000; 7: 513–519.
5. Liffman K, Lawrence-Brown MMD, Semmens JB *et al.* Analytical modelling and numerical simulation of forces in an endoluminal graft. *J Endovasc Ther* 2001; 8: 358–371.
6. Lawrence-Brown MMD, Sieunarine K, Hartley D *et al.* Should an anchor stent cross the renal artery orifices when placing an endoluminal graft for abdominal aortic aneurysm? In *Indications in Vascular and Endovascular Surgery*. RM Greenhalgh (ed). London: Saunders, 1998: 261.
7. Lawrence-Brown MMD, Semmens JB, Hartley DE. The Zenith endoluminal stent-graft system: suprarenal fixation, safety features, modular components, fenestration and custom crafting. In *Vascular and Endovascular Surgical Techniques* 4th edn. RM Greenhalgh, JP Becquemin, A Davies *et al.* (eds). London: Saunders, 2001: 219–223.
8. Stanley B, Semmens JB, Lawrence-Brown MMD *et al.* Fenestration in endovascular grafts for aortic aneurysm repair: new horizons for preserving blood flow in branch vessels. *J Endovasc Ther* 2001; 8: 16–24.
9. Liffman K, Lawrence-Brown MMD, Semmens JB *et al.* Supra-renal fixation: the effect of an endoluminal stent wire on renal blood flow. *J Endovasc Ther* (in press).
10. Walser M. Creatinine excretion as a measure of protein nutrition in adults of varying age. *J Parenteral Enteral Nutr* 1987; 11(Suppl): 735–785.
11. Tiao J, Semmens JB, Maserai J, Lawrence-Brown MMD. The effect of age on serum creatinine levels in an aging population: relevance to vascular surgery. *Cardiovasc Surg* 2002; 10: 445–451.
12. Stanley B, Semmens JB, Mai Q *et al.* Evaluation of patient selection guidelines for endoluminal grafting of aneurysm of the abdominal aorta with the Zenith graft: the Australasian experience. *J Endovasc Ther* 2001; 8: 457–464.

Suprarenal fixation of stent-grafts is a disadvantage

Charing Cross Editorial Comments towards Consensus

'It *is* a disadvantage', says Dieter Raithel because in his considerable experience of various stent-graft systems, he reports a 22% renal infarction rate using the Zenith system, which uses suprarenal fixation.

It is therefore appropriate that Michael Lawrence-Brown and colleague's experience is with the Zenith system which they swear by.

Dieter Raithel recommends a type of endoluminal device which does not have suprarenal fixation because of concern of renal infarction.

The opposition is quite clear that suprarenal fixation is required and it is without the disadvantage of renal infarction. Their main argument for using suprarenal fixation is the avoidance of migration and the proper fixation, which takes account of considerable longitudinal forces.

It will be interesting to hear if case selection or technique of deployment can explain the differences with respect to the kidney complication.

Roger M Greenhalgh
Editor

Open surgery is no longer required for aortic arch occlusive disease

For the motion

Hero van Urk, Marc RHM van Sambeek, Lucas C van Dijk, Jan W Kuiper

Introduction

Occlusive arterial disease of the supra-aortic vessels, like innominate, subclavian, common carotid and vertebral arteries, is not a common feature of patients with atherosclerotic disease.

If atherosclerotic disease is the cause of stenosis or occlusion in these vessels, it is usually seen in patients with extensive generalized atherosclerosis. Other causes are fibromuscular dysplasia, Takayasu's disease, post-radiation arteritis and trauma. Chronic costoclavicular compression syndrome may cause stenosis by external compression, but may also lead to aneurysmal dilatation with mural thrombus formation, which in turn can cause distal (micro)emboli. Occlusion of the left subclavian artery frequently results in the angiographic phenomenon of reversed flow or 'subclavian steal', but seldom leads to the typical symptoms of 'subclavian steal syndrome' and consequently only seldom needs therapy.

Until fairly recently, treatment of symptomatic stenoses and/or occlusions of supra-aortic vessels was based upon vascular surgical reconstructions, including endarterectomy, transposition, interposition of autologous or synthetic grafts, or bypass surgery. However, since the early 1980s percutaneous transluminal angioplasty (PTA) and other catheter procedures have been introduced. Since the early 1990s these techniques have gradually replaced the open surgical reconstructions. Nowadays, in the 21st century it can be stated that open surgery is outdated and no longer required for the majority of occlusive disease of the supra-aortic vessels. It must be admitted, however, that the evidence for supremacy of one method over the other is lacking: no prospective controlled clinical trials have been conducted or reported that show either better long-term results or fewer complications. The rarity of these lesions will probably also preclude such trials in the future. The current approach of preferential use of endovascular techniques should be considered as a natural development and a logical consequence of the global trend towards less invasive surgery.

Surgical reconstruction

Surgical reconstruction of supra-aortic vessels became popular in the early 1960s, after the introduction of local tromboendarterectomy by Crawford and DeBakey in

1962[1] and carotid-subclavian transposition by Parrot in 1964.[2] The advantage of these operations was that they could be performed by an extrathoracic approach, thus avoiding many of the disadvantages of transthoracic surgery. The accompanying morbidity and mortality of open thoracic surgery in those days was often prohibitive and consequently, these 'major' operations were seldom attempted.

In the ensuing years many extrathoracic techniques became available, including a variety of extra-anatomical approaches with graft interpositions, but the simple carotid-subclavian transposition remained the most favoured procedure.[3,4]

An extensive review of the various surgical options was published in 1982 by Criado,[5] who subsequently became one of the most prominent protagonists of endovascular surgery.

Open surgical reconstructions will remain the treatment of choice for a variety of situations in which not only the supra-aortic vessels, but also the aortic arch or aortic valves are affected. Extracorporeal circulation with or without deep hypothermia is mandatory in those cases and with the current knowledge and available catheter-based instrumentation it seems unlikely that this will easily be replaced. However, percutaneous aortic valve replacement is already available for clinical use in very high-risk patients. Congenital malformations, like the aberrant origin of the right subclavian artery (A. subclavia lusoria, sometimes presenting as dysphagia lusoria) still requires surgical correction when indicated, albeit in combination with endovascular occlusion of the origin.

Extrathoracic surgical reconstructions carry the risk of iatrogenic lesions to the adjacent structures, like brachial plexus, vagal and phrenic nerves, subclavian and other veins, and thoracic lymph duct. Pneumo- and haematothorax are sometimes considered to be part of the procedure, but can cause much discomfort to the patient. Wound healing is usually not a problem in the neck region but the few exemptions should not be neglected.

Endovascular options

In 1980 PTA was almost simultaneously introduced by Bachman[6] and Mathias et al.[7] As the disease is too rare to allow large single-author or single-institution series, the literature over the ensuing two decades reports only small series and case histories, the largest series being the personal experience of Mathias, (46 patients) reported in 1993.[8]

A nice overview of the literature was presented by Gonzales et al. in 2002, describing a total of 226 patients with total occlusions divided over 31 publications.[9] The technical success rates in these reports vary widely from 0 to 100%. The success rates are higher for stenotic lesions than for total occlusions, and the addition of stenting to PTA (either primary stenting or on indication) results in more than a 90% technical success.[10]

Technical considerations

Morphology of the lesion and local anatomy need to be considered before an intervention can be planned. Eventually, the experience of the performing team is decisive for the approach, the materials, the safety and the final results.

The approach can be via the brachial artery or the femoral artery; sometimes both approaches are desirable in order to have optimal control of the procedure and different options for visualizing the lesion as well as the result. If a brachial approach means that the brachial artery at the end of the procedure should be closed surgically because of its small diameter, this should not be considered a reason to cancel this approach. On the contrary: good teamwork between interventional radiologist and endovascular surgeon should easily solve this problem, to the benefit of the patient.

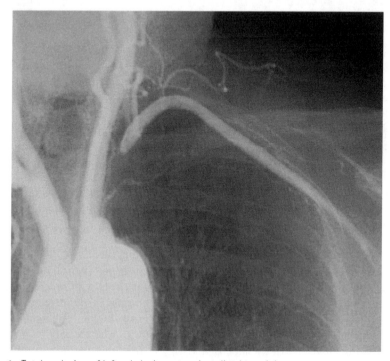

Figure 1. Total occlusion of left subclavian artery just distal to origin.

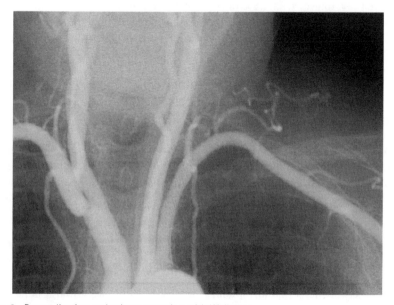

Figure 2. Recanalization and primary stenting with Wallstent.

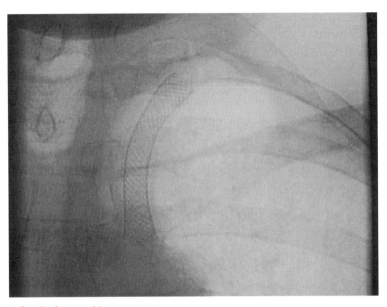

Figure 3. Detail of stent without contrast.

Similar to PTA and stenting of the carotid bifurcation, the use of cerebral protection devices should be considered as well as the choice between primary or secondary stenting, and the potential need for predilatation. In patients with severe stenosis or occlusion of the left subclavian artery, in which the flow in the cerebral artery is either continuously or intermittently reversed (subclavian steal phenomenon), the danger of cerebral embolization is less likely than in cases with forward flow. Primary stenting is probably the safest endovascular way to treat these lesions. Neurological complications are not reported in a single case in the reports mentioned by Gonzales,[9] but in the series that included innominate artery lesions serious neurological complications are to be expected in 4.5% in addition to 'minor' complications in 7%.[8,11–14]

Serious neurological complications are to be avoided at any cost. Cerebral protection devices (distal balloon occlusion, filters, or reversal of antegrade flow may be helpful in reducing the risk of cerebral embolization. Reversed flow cannot be used for origo lesions, neither can filters be used in such cases because the guidewires that need to be used for these devices (0.014–0.018) are too thin. The usefulness of these devices will have to be determined by prospective controlled series; such series do not exist at this time.

Consequently, the decision on how to treat a subclavian or innominate artery lesion remains a matter of personal preference, based on personal experience and will depend on the morphology and localization of the lesion, the flow conditions and the presenting symptoms. If a surgical procedure clearly appears to be the safest way to treat a lesion, no surgeon or interventionalist should refrain from resorting to this option.

Long-term efficacy

As in all other locations that are suitable for PTA and stenting, ostial lesions should be treated by primary stenting. Ostial lesions should be considered mainly as a disease of the aortic wall; consequently, exact positioning of the stent is required. Usually this can be achieved better with balloon-expandable stents that with self-expending stents, but the newest versions of the latter (with less foreshortening during expansion) allow more precise positioning in the origin of the artery.

Long-term patency is threatened by acute thrombosis, in-stent restenosis caused by intimal hyperplasia, and (in the case of balloon-expandable stents) by external compression of the stent. Although the newest stent generation, the drug-eluting stents, may have an improved long-term patency as a result of less intimal hyperplasia and less constrictive remodelling, these beneficial effects will have to be proven by prospective clinical trials. At the present time, such series do not exist. Acute stent thrombosis may be reduced by treatment with platelet aggregation inhibitors like aspirin and clopidogrel. Although virtually all patients are treated with one of these medications or both, the evidence for this regimen is not available and this practice is entirely derived from the published experience with coronary stents.

Summary

- Stenotic disease of the supra-aortic vessels is relatively rare compared with atherosclerotic disease of the lower limbs. When present, the indications for therapy are limited.

- Transthoracic surgical reconstructions have all the drawbacks of major vascular surgery; extrathoracic surgical reconstructions are more patient-friendly and have a proven long-term efficacy.

- All open surgical procedures carry the inevitable risk of perioperative complications due to damage of the adjacent structures.

- Endovascular treatment is less invasive and more patient-friendly than surgery. Immediate technical success rates are high. Complication rates are low. Long-term efficacy is good.

- No randomized controlled series are available to compare surgical reconstruction with endovascular intervention; nor are cost-benefit analysis studies.

- Notwithstanding the lack of scientific evidence, it can be stated that endovascular treatment of supra-aortic stenotic disease is the treatment of choice in the 21st century.

References

1. Crawford ES, DeBakey ME *et al*. Segmental thrombo-obliterative disease of the great vessels arising from the aortic arch. *J Thorac Cardiovasc Surg* 1962; **43**: 38–43.
2. Parrot JD. The subclavian steel syndrome. *Arch Surg* 1964; **88**: 661–665.
3. Crawford ES *et al*. Occlusion of the innominate, common carotid and subclavian arteries: long term results of surgical treatment. *Surgery* 1983; **94**: 781–791.
4. Mannick JA. Extrathoracic operations for lesions of the vessels arising from the aortic arch. In: *Indications in Vascular Surgery*. Greenhalgh RM (ed). London: Saunders, 1988: 63–69.
5. Criado FJ. Extrathoracic management of aortic arch syndrome. *Br J Surg* 1982; **69** (suppl): 45–51.
6. Bachman DM, Kom RM. Transluminal dilatation for subclavian steal syndrome. *Am J Roentgenol* 1980; **135**: 995–996.
7. Mathias KD, Steiger J *et al*. Perkutane katheter angioplastie der Arteria subclavia. *Dtsch Med Wochenschr* 1980; **105**: 16–18.

8. Mathias K, Luth I, Haarmann P. Percutaneous transluminal angioplasty of proximal subclavian artery occlusions. *Cardiovasc Intervent Radiol* 1993; **16**: 214–218.

9. Gonzales A, Gil-Peralta *et al*. Angioplasty and stenting for total symptomatic atherosclerotic occlusion of the subclavian or innominate arteries. *Cerebrovasc Dis* 2000; **13**: 107–113.

10. Reekers JA. Subclavian artery stenosis is best managed by PTA and stent. In: *The Evidence For Vascular And Endovascular Reconstruction*. Greenhalgh RM (ed). Saunders, 2002: 101–105.

11. Ingall RL, Lambert D *et al*. Percutaneous transluminal angioplasty of the innominate, subclavian and axillary arteries. *Eur J Vasc Surg* 1990; **4**: 591–595.

12. Sharma S, Kaul U, Rajani M. Identifying high-risk patients for percutaneous transluminal angioplasty of subclavian and innominate arteries. *Acta Radiol* 1991; **32**: 381–385.

13. Hebrang A, Maskovic J, Tomac B. Percutaneous transluminal angioplasty of the subclavian arteries: long-term results in 52 patients. *Am J Roentgenol* 1992; **156**: 1091–1094.

14. Korner M, Baumgartner I *et al*. PTA of the subclavian and innominate arteries: long-term results. *Vasa* 1990; **28**: 117–122.

Open surgery is no longer required for aortic arch occlusive disease

Against the motion

Edouard Kieffer

Preliminary remarks

The comparison between conventional and endovascular surgery for the treatment of occlusive disease of the supra-aortic trunks is difficult, mainly because most of the authors reporting endovascular treatment do not use the widely accepted reporting standards, as published by the SVS/ISCVS.

Besides, the number of patients in these studies is usually small and/or the follow-up is short. Finally, techniques are evolving and most authors would now agree that the best results are obtained by angioplasty and stenting, a recently introduced adjunct, making the series available for study rather rare at the moment.

A well-organized multicentre prospective randomized study would be an optimal mean to solve the problem. It would, however, need a large number of patients. Besides the number of patients treated for occlusive disease of the supra-aortic trunks is not so important.

The decision as to which treatment is best is thus influenced by numerous factors that cannot be controlled at the moment.

Lesions

Let us not mix oranges and apples. Lesions subjected to conventional and endovascular surgery are not the same. Endovascular surgery is advisable in short, stenotic, mostly atherosclerotic lesions. It is not suitable for occlusions or extensive lesions, as seen in a fairly large number of patients with atherosclerosis and in most patients with Takayasu's disease or radiation arteritis.

In our 1995 study of 148 patients with atherosclerotic lesions of the innominate artery,[1] 18 (12%) had occlusions while 136 (88%) had stenosis. However, the lesion was limited to the proximal portion of the innominate artery in 104 (73%) patients, the mid-portion in only nine patients and the distal portion in 21 patients. One would agree that only these nine lesions (6%) were ideal indications for endovascular surgery. In addition, in 13 patients (8.8%), the innominate artery and the left common carotid artery originated from a common trunk of the transverse aortic arch with a risk of embolization in the left common carotid artery during angioplasty and stenting of the innominate artery.

Similarly, in a non-reported study[2] of 163 patients who underwent subclavian-to-common carotid transposition to treat lesions of the subclavian artery in our Department from 1980 to 1995, 43 (26%) had an occlusion of the subclavian artery a recognized difficulty in angioplasty and 49 (30%) had an associated lesion of the ipsilateral vertebral artery that deserved a specific treatment at the time of operation (trans-subclavian endarterectomy or separate transposition of the vertebral artery to the common carotid artery). Besides, 42 patients (25.8%) had a stenosis of the ipsilateral carotid bifurcation, that was treated surgically during the same session.

Early results

For lesions amenable to both therapies, early results are roughly the same.

In the nine patients with stenosis of the mid-portion of the innominate artery, our mortality and major (neurological and cardiac) morbidity was 0%.

In the 39 patients in the isolated (i.e. without simultaneous carotid endarterectomy) stenosis of the subclavian artery not affecting the origin of the artery and the take-off of the vertebral artery, there was one death from pulmonary complications (2.5%) and no major morbidity.

However, endovascular treatment has the distinct advantage over conventional surgery of saving general anaesthesia, incision, pain and money. Yet, it is not without potential complications, including death,[3] and subclavian artery rupture.[4]

Late results

Despite more advanced lesions, late results are definitely better for conventional surgery.

The anatomical durability of transternal innominate artery and transcervical subclavian artery reconstruction is much better than the durability of endovascular surgery (Tables 1–3).

Conclusions

For most lesions of the subclavian artery, conventional surgery remains the treatment of choice, because of its universal applicability, low mortality and morbidity rates combined with excellent late patency rates. Isolated proximal lesions of the subclavian artery are best treated through a cervical approach, by subclavian-to-carotid transposition with or without ostial endarterectomy of the vertebral artery. One may have to resort to alternative extrathoracic techniques (crossover bypass, carotid-to-distal subclavian artery bypass or carotid-to-axillary artery bypass) in cases with inoperable occlusive disease of the common carotid artery or extensive lesions of the subclavian and axillary arteries (as seen in Takayasu's disease).

At present, we would advocate endovascular surgery for short, stenotic lesions of the subclavian artery in those rare patients unfit for surgery through a cervical approach. Among this group are most patients with the coronary-subclavian steal syndrome.[18]

In patients fit for surgery, lesions of the innominate artery are best treated through a transthoracic approach. Partial sternotomy and modern perioperative care allow

Table 1. Cumulative primary patency rates for surgical reconstruction of the subclavian artery

Author [reference]	Period	No of patients	Technique	Lost to follow-up (%)	Mean follow-up (months)	Cumulative primary patency rates (%)	
						5 years	10 years
Sandmann[5]	77–85	72	SCT	12.5	46	95	NA
Edwards[6]	67–93	175	SCT	3	46	99	99
Perler[7]	79–89	31	CSB	0	42	92	83
Branchereau[8]	79–85	97	Misc	6.3	54.5	92.5	86.4
Vitti[9]	68–90	124	CSB	NA	91.5	94	94
AbuRahma[10]	78–98	52	CSB	NA	92.4	96	92
Krestschmer[11]	75–98	84	SCT	9.5	73	100	100
Petit[2]	80–95	163	SCT	11.8	73	98.4	98.4

SCT : Subclavian to carotid transposition; CSB : Carotid to subclavian bypass; NA : Not available; Misc: Miscellaneous

Table 2. Cumulative primary patency rates for surgical reconstruction of the intrathoracic great vessels

Author [reference]	Period	No of patients	Artery	Lost to follow-up (%)	Mean follow-up (months)	Cumulative primary patency rates (%)	
						5 years	10 years
Kieffer[1]	74–93	148	IA	7	77	98.4	96.3
Berguer[12]	81–96	100	Misc	8	51	94	88
Azakie[13]	60–97	94	IA	0	92	99	97
Rhodes[14]	88–98	58	Misc	14	45	80	NA

IA : Innominate artery; NA : Not available; Misc: Miscellaneous

Table 3. Patency rates for endovascular treatment of supra-aortic trunk lesions

Author [reference]	Period	No of arteries	SAT	Lesions		Technical success (%)	Lost to follow-up (%)	Mean follow-up (months)	Restenoses (%)	Cumulative primary patency rates (%)		
				O	S					1 year	3 years	5 years
Sullivan[15]	93–97	66	SCA	10	56	93.9	11	12.9	4.5	90	84	NA
		7	IA	0	7	100.0						
Rodriguez-Lopez[16]	91–95	70	SCA	17	53	96.0	NA	13	10	73	NA	NA
Krestschmer[11]	75–98	127	SCA	NA	NA	91.3	5	37	19	85	80	70
Amor[3]	94–02	89	SCA	13	76	93.3	14.5	42	19	88	75	NA
Ruebben[17]	93–96	8	IA	0	8	100.0	0	17	0	100	NA	NA

SCA: Subclavian artery; IA: Innominate artery; NA: Not available safe performance of innominate artery endarterectomy or aorto-innominate bypass in the majority of patients.

A trans-sternal approach may be contraindicated by technical problems (previous sternotomy with multiple coronary bypasses or postoperative mediastinitis, massive mediastinal irradiation) or, more commonly, for general reasons (age over 80 years, advanced uncorrectable heart disease, respiratory insufficiency). In such cases, in the presence of an innominate artery stenosis, endovascular surgery is in competition with transcervical surgery. However, we would advocate a cervical approach to perform innominate artery angioplasty and stenting,[17,19] avoiding embolization into the right common carotid.

Summary

- Although a multicentre prospective randomized study would be the optimal means to solve the problem, it has many difficulties.

- Lesions subjected to conventional and endovascular surgery are not the same: endovascular surgery takes care of short, stenotic lesions whereas conventional surgery adresses all types of disease, including long and occlusive lesions.

- For lesions amenable to both therapies, early results are roughly the same. Endovascular surgery has the advantages of saving general anaesthesia, incisions, pain and money.

- Despite more advanced lesions, late results are definitely better for conventional surgery.

- For most lesions of the subclavian and innominate arteries, surgery remains the treatment of choice.

References

1. Kieffer E, Sabatier J, Koskas F, Bahnini A. Atherosclerotic innominate artery occlusive disease: early and long-term results of surgical reconstruction. *J Vasc Surg* 1995; 21: 326–337.
2. Petit MD. Transpositions sous-clavio-carotidiennes: résultats à long terme. Thèse, Paris, 1996.
3. Amor M, Eid-Lidt G, Wilentz J. Subclavian artery stenting. In: Amor M, Bergeron P, Mathias K, Raithel D (eds). *Carotid Artery Angioplasty and Stenting.* Torino: Minerva Medica, 2002: 255-260.
4. Lin PH, Bush RL, Weiss VJ *et al.* Subclavian artery disruption resulting from endovascular intervention: treatment options. *J Vasc Surg* 2000; 32: 607–611.
5. Sandmann W, Kniemeyer HW, Jaeschock R *et al.* The role of subclavian-carotid transposition in surgery for supra-aortic occlusive disease. *J Vasc Surg* 1987; 5: 53–58.
6. Edwards WH Jr, Tapper SS, Edwards WH Sr *et al.* Subclavian revascularization: a quarter century experience. *Ann Surg* 1994; 219: 673–678.
7. Perler BA, Williams GM. Carotid-subclavian bypass: a decade of experience. *J Vasc Surg* 1990; 12: 716–723.
8. Branchereau A, Magnan PE, Espinoza H, Bartoli JM. Subclavian artery stenosis: hemodynamic aspects and surgical outcome. *J Cardiovasc Surg* 1991; 32: 604–612.
9. Vitti MJ, Thompson BW, Read RC *et al.* Carotid-subclavian bypass: a twenty-two-year experience. *J Vasc Surg* 1994; 20: 411–418.
10. AbuRahma AF, Robinson PA, Jennings TG. Carotid-subclavian bypass grafting with polytetrafluoroethylene grafts for symptomatic subclavian artery stenosis or occlusion: a 20-year experience. *J Vasc Surg* 2000; 32: 411–419.

11. Krestschmer G, Sautner T, Domenig C *et al.* Subclavian artery stenosis is best managed by PTA and stent: against the motion. In: Greenhalgh RM (ed). *The Evidence for Vascular or Endovascular Reconstruction.* London: Saunders, 2002: 106–116.

12. Berguer R, Morasch MD, Kline RA. Transthoracic repair of innominate and common carotid artery disease: immediate and long-term outcome for 100 consecutive surgical reconstructions. *J Vasc Surg* 1998; **27**: 34–42.

13. Azakie A, Mc Elhinney DB, Higoshima R *et al.* Innominate artery reconstruction. *Ann Surg* 1998; **228**: 402–410.

14. Rhodes JM, Cherry KJ, Clark RC *et al.* Aortic-origin reconstruction of the great vessels: risk factors of early and late complications. *J Vasc Surg* 2000; **31**: 260–269.

15. Sullivan TM, Gray BH, Bacharach JM *et al.* Angioplasty and primary stenting of the subclavian, innominate, and common carotid arteries in 83 patients. *J Vasc Surg* 1998; **28**: 1059–1065.

16. Rodriguez-Lopez JA, Werner A, Martinez R *et al.* Stenting for atherosclerotic occlusive disease of the subclavian artery. *Ann Vasc Surg* 1999; **13**: 254–260.

17. Ruebben A, Tettoni S, Muratore P. Feasibility of intraoperative balloon angioplasty and additional stent placement of isolated stenosis of the brachiocephalic trunk. *J Thorac Cardiovasc Surg* 1998; **115**: 1316–1320.

18. Hallisey MJ, Rees JH, Meranze SG. Use of angioplasty in the prevention and treatment of coronary-subclavian steal syndrome. *JVIR* 1995; **6**: 125–129.

19. Queral LA, Criado FJ. The treatment of focal aortic arch branch lesions with Palmaz stents. *J Vasc Surg* 1996; **23**: 368–375.

Open surgery is no longer required for aortic arch occlusive disease

Charing Cross Editorial Comments towards Consensus

Hero van Urk argues that endovascular therapy is more patient-friendly and a major operation is avoided. Is there another argument?

There are no randomized controlled trials and therefore no data.

Professor Kieffer has a very large experience of approaching the aortic arch for surgical reconstruction with outstanding results and very low recurrence rate.

It is likely that in time more people will be able to offer the endovascular treatment then be able to reproduce Professor Kieffer's experience.

The question really arises for the patient who could choose between the two, either excellent open reconstruction or excellent endovascular repair. At the present time there simply is insufficient evidence to give a firm answer. Certainly the trend is towards endovascular but this does not make it right. In time there may be more facts available on which to make a robust decision.

R M Greenhalgh
Editor

Endografting for thoracic aneurysm has replaced the need for open surgery

For the motion

Jason T Lee, Rodney A White

Introduction

Determining the indications for repair of thoracic aortic aneurysms (TAAs) and other surgical diseases of the thoracic aorta presents a challenging problem for cardiothoracic and vascular surgeons. The incidence of TAAs and acute and chronic type B dissections is estimated to be as high as 10 cases per 100000 people per year, and occurs more commonly in the elderly and more medically debilitated.[1] The natural history of untreated disease includes progressive expansion, increasing risk of rupture, and ultimately death, with 2-year survival rates of less than 30%.[1,2]

Traditional surgical treatment involves aortic graft replacement via a left thoracotomy and has been found to improve survival in comparison with medical therapy.[3] Despite dramatic advances in the technical expertise for performing these complex thoracic aortic surgical repairs, open surgery is complicated by operative mortality rates ranging between 8 and 20% for elective cases and up to 60% for emergency operations.[3–6] Survivors of an open operation further suffer from morbidity rates of almost 50% related to renal, intestinal and spinal cord ischaemia that substantially limit functional recovery and long-term survival.[7]

With the successful development of endovascular stent-grafts to treat abdominal aortic aneurysms (AAAs), a concomitant effort to adapt this technology to the treatment of descending thoracic aneurysms and type B dissections has demonstrated promising results. Proposed advantages of the endograft approach include shorter operative time, decreased need for general anaesthesia, lack of aortic cross-clamp time, avoidance of cardiopulmonary bypass, and avoidance of major thoracic or thoracoabdominal incisions. Most reported series, including our own, have documented the high technical success of this technology, along with major reductions in morbidity and mortality.[8–20]

The improvements in patient outcome are even more encouraging when we take into account the fact that most of the patients in the early experience treated with endografts had already been rejected for open surgical repair because of significant co-morbid medical illnesses. We herein describe our technique for thoracic endografting and provide evidence that endografting is a safe, successful, and viable option for many patients with thoracic aneurysms and other related diseases of the thoracic aorta.

Technique and illustration

All patients referred for endovascular repair of thoracic aortic pathology at our institution are prospectively enrolled into FDA-approved Investigational Devices Exemption trials. All protocols as well as the pre- and postoperative surveillance and imaging are in compliance with the Institutional Review Board of our institution. The diagnoses are confirmed using spiral computed tomography (CT)-angiography including three-dimensional (3-D) reconstruction in a computerized interactive environment utilizing Preview software (Medical Media Systems, West Lebanon, NH, USA).

Procedures are performed in a specially designed endovascular suite equipped with ceiling-mounted fluoroscopy capable of digital subtraction angiography. All patients are placed in the supine position with arterial blood pressure monitors and prepared for possible thoracotomy and cardiopulmonary bypass. Under local anaesthetic with minimal intravenous sedation, the common femoral artery is exposed and isolated using Roummel tourniquets. If the vessel is too small to accommodate the introducer sheath, the common iliac artery is reached via retroperitoneal approach while converting to general anaesthetic. Through a transverse arteriotomy, 0.025 Microvina or 0.035 Amplatz super-stiff wires are introduced via appropriately sized sheaths and guided up to the aortic arch.

We routinely utilize intravascular ultrasound (IVUS) to confirm the anatomy, specifically the diameter and length of the proximal neck, as well as post-deployment to verify optimal placement of the stent-graft. We oversize the proximal neck by 10-20% and preferentially have used the self-expanding AneuRx and Talent (Medtronic AVE, Santa Rosa, CA, USA) devices, and more recently, the Gore Thoracic Excluder device (WL Gore, Inc, Flagstaff AZ, USA). Contrast angiography is kept to a minimum during the procedure and used after the deployment to evaluate for the presence of an endoleak.

At the completion of the procedure, the patient is observed overnight in the intensive care unit and then transferred to the surgical ward for an average length of stay of 3 days. Follow-up spiral CTs are obtained immediately after the operation, after 1 month, 3 months, 6 months, and annually thereafter. Figures 1 and 2 demonstrate two patients with serial 3-D images of a successfully excluded thoracic aneurysm and the mid-term imaging follow-up.

Evidence

Thoracic aneurysms

Since 1992 there have been 13 reported series worldwide of patients undergoing endovascular treatment of TAAs.[8-20] Although the patient populations are obviously very diverse and there is some amount of selection bias that cannot be avoided because this is an evolving technology, the overall results are favourable. A summary of the raw data from the trials (only the cases of thoracic aneurysms are included) is presented in Table I.

The treatment of TAAs with several prototype endovascular devices in multiple worldwide centres has met with high technical success. Some of the earlier studies[10,11,14] which did not achieve at least 90% technical success, acknowledge that the failures occurred early in their experience, when patient selection criteria and technical expertise were not as streamlined as they are currently. One controlled investigation directly compared open versus endovascular repair and found 30-day

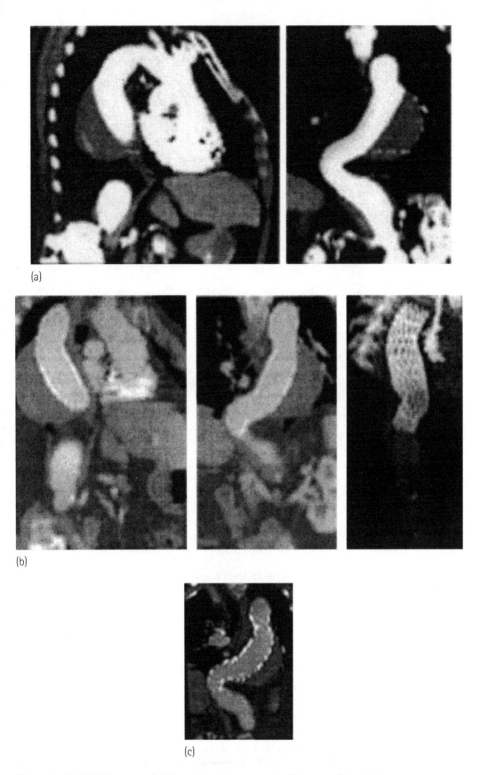

(a)

(b)

(c)

Figure 1. Serial 3-D images of a 9.3 cm thoracic aneurysm with successful exclusion seen on postoperative CT and regression of the aneurysm to 7.2 cm after 14 months. TAA thrombus volume also decreased from 353 to 218cc as the aneurysm regressed.

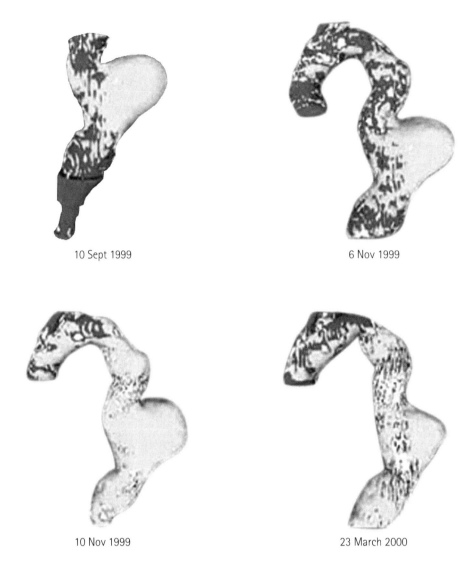

10 Sept 1999

6 Nov 1999

10 Nov 1999

23 March 2000

Figure 2. Sequential reconstructions of 10-cm TAA after exclusion. By 4-month follow-up, total aneurysm volume decreased from 616 to 442 cc.

mortality was decreased from 31% to 10%, and that there was significantly decreased intervention time, hospital stay, and rate of neurological impairment.[9]

In order to demonstrate superiority over the traditional repair, one would have to show that short- and long-term survival is improved in a randomized trial. Such a trial will be difficult to perform given the ethics and high morbidity and mortality associated with the disease process as well as open repair. Only the large series from Stanford has enough follow-up time to estimate actuarial survival rates, which allows for useful comparison.[10,21] The Stanford group reported 81% survival at 1-year follow-up and 73% after 2 years. This is compared with traditional open surgery, where the actuarial survival rates are estimated to be 70% at 5 years and 40% at 10 years of *survivors* of the open repair.[2,3,22,23] Combining the fact that most of the patients who

Table 1. Comparison of 13 series of thoracic aneurysms treated with endovascular devices. Other morbidity refers to cardiopulmonary, renal, infectious and neurological complications. Endoleaks include those found during follow-up CT scanning and requiring secondary intervention for resolution.

Series	Device	No of patients	Success	Paralysis	Other morbidity	Length of stay (days)	30-Day mortality	Endoleak
Dake[8] '92–'94	Home-made	13	100%	0%	0%	4.8	0%	15%
Ehrlich[9] '97	Talent	10	100%	0%	10%	6	10%	20%
Mitchell[10] '92–'97	Home-made	103	73%	3%	25%	8	9%	24%
Temudom[11] '97–'98	Vanguard Gore	14	78%	0%	14%	2.9	14%	14%
Grabenwoger[12] '96–'99	Talent Gore	21	100%	0%	9.5%	9.8	9.5%	5%
Taylor[13] '97–'00	AneuRx Gore	23	100%	0%	4.3%	4	8.7%	13%
Greenberg[14] '93–'97	Cook	25	88%	4%	n/a	n/a	25%	12%
Bortone[15] '99–'00	Gore	11	100%	0%	9%	n/a	9%	0%
White[16] '97–'99	AneuRx	16	94%	6%	6%	5	12%	12%
Won[17] '94–'99	Tae-woong	11	100%	0%	9%	n/a	0%	0%
Cambria[18] '96–'01	Cook Gore	18	100%	0%	28%	n/a	5.5%	21%
Thompson[19] '00–'01	Gore	26	100%	0%	23%	5	4%	8%
Totaro[20] '00–'01	Gore	7	100%	0%	0%	10	0%	30%

underwent stent-graft repair had already been turned down for open repair and yet had similar mid-term survival, a case can certainly be made that the long-term survival will be at least as good with endografting versus open surgery.

Paralysis is one of the most feared complications of open thoracic aortic repair and previously occurred in 20–30% of cases, but has improved recently to 8–15% with numerous adjunctive advances in spinal cord protection.[24,25] Interestingly, there has been a gratifying lack of spinal cord ischaemic events with thoracic endografting, and in the few series that have reported paralysis those patients also had concomitant open aortic interventions at the same time.[10,14] This suggests that the neurological complications after thoracic aortic surgery are more related to the aortic cross-clamp time and hypoperfusion during circulatory arrest and cardiopulmonary bypass. Placing a thoracic stent across even a long segment of thoracic intercostals does not appear to lead to significant paraplegia in the reported series.

Acute and chronic dissections

Further indications of the utility of thoracic endografting are its applicability to numerous other disease entities in the thoracic aorta, including acute and chronic type B dissections, penetrating ulcers, and rupture from all causes.[26–30] The current indications for open repair of type B dissections include uncontrollable hypertension, persistent pain, expanding aneurysm, or end organ ischaemia. Acute dissection leads to 36–72% mortality within 48 hours if left untreated, and even operative therapy is associated with 50–70% mortality.[26] It is no wonder there has been keen interest in utilizing less invasive endovascular grafting for these critical patients, and early small series report lower rates of mortality of 16–28%.[26,27] Stent-graft coverage of the proximal entry site of a type B dissection in theory should limit the extent of the dissection, obliterate the flow into the entry tear, and promote thrombosis of the false lumen.[16,28]

Figures 3 and 4 demonstrate the successful repair and mid-term follow-up of an acute dissection recurring after chronic thoracoabdominal dissection with thoracic and abdominal aneurysm formation that we treated utilizing staged thoracic and aortic endograft devices in a symptomatic 83-year-old man.

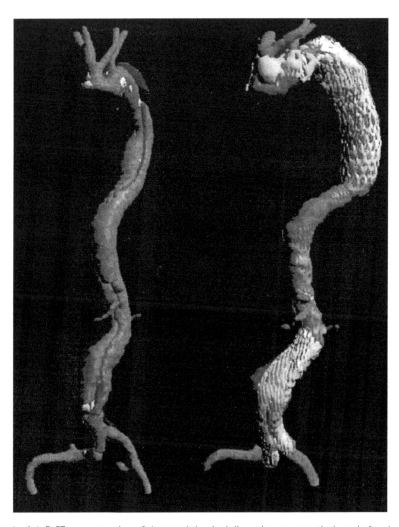

Figure 3. A 3-D CT reconstruction of thoracoabdominal dissection preoperatively and after 1-year follow-up demonstrating a reconstituted true lumen following the deployment of the devices.

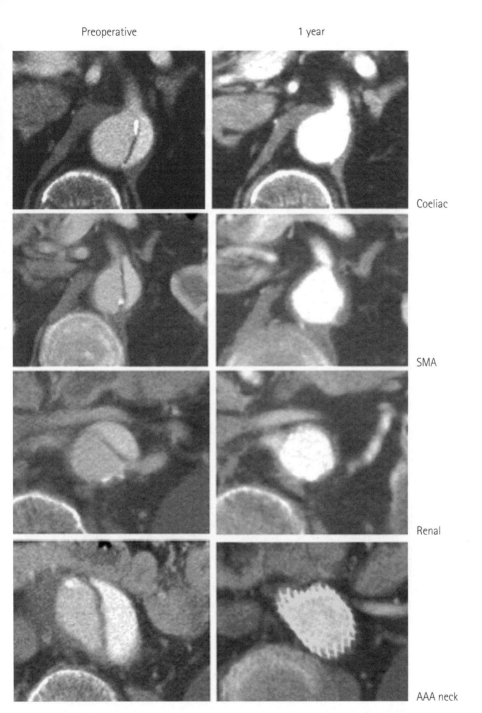

Figure 4. Axial CT images perpendicular to the centerline of the flow lumen at the coeliac artery, superior mesenteral artery (SMA), lowest renal artery, and the neck of abdominal portion of the thoracoabdominal dissection prior to the procedure and 1 year following treatment.

Coeliac

SMA

Renal

AAA neck

Endografting for thoracic aneurysm has replaced open surgery • **For the motion** • JT Lee, RA White

Conclusions

The feasibility, safety, and at least mid-term efficacy of thoracic endografting has been delineated in numerous series. The morbidity and mortality associated with the endovascular repair of thoracic aneurysms appear to be significantly less than conventional operative treatment. Not only is there reduced mortality, but the associated morbidity, such as paraplegia, renal failure, cardiac complications and pulmonary compromise, is substantially reduced because of the avoidance of a general anaesthetic and large incision and the associated shorter hospital stay and quicker recovery. Other promising endeavours include the treatment of other devastating diseases of the thoracic aorta including acute and chronic dissections, ulcerating plaques, and acute rupture. Even at this early state of this technology, where results are affected by the rapid evolution of the technology in extremely high risk patients, the dramatic improvements in acute survival and reduced morbidity and mortality makes this approach a very appealing alternative to surgery. In many patients, thoracic endografting is the only alternative that can be offered as surgery is often denied to these prohibitively high-risk lesions.

Summary

- Open surgical repair of thoracic aneurysms and dissections is associated with high rates of morbidity and mortality, especially in the acute setting.

- Endografting of the thoracic aorta is technically feasible and successful.

- Endografting affords significantly lower morbidity and mortality for acute presentations of aneurysms, dissections and ruptures when compared with traditional open repair.

- Long-term follow-up is still required to understand the natural history of the disease as well as the consequences of unique endovascular complications.

- A randomized, prospective trial will be difficult to perform given the high morbidity and mortality associated with open repair.

- Thoracic endografting provides the only alternative for many high-risk patients who are denied conventional surgery because of the known morbidity and mortality.

References

1. Bickerstaff LK, Pairolero PC, Hollier LH *et al.* Thoracic aortic aneurysms: a population-based study. *Surgery* 1982; **92**: 1103–1108.
2. Crawford ES, DeNatale RW. Thoracoabdominal aortic aneurysm: observations regarding the natural course of the disease. *J Vasc Surg* 1986; **3**: 578–582.
3. Svensson LG, Crawford ES, Hess KR, Coselli JS, Safi HJ. Experience with 1509 patients undergoing thoracoabdominal aortic operations. *J Vasc Surg* 1993; **17**: 357–370.
4. Safi HJ, Miller CC III, Subramaniam MH *et al.* Thoracic and thoracoabdominal aneurysm repair using cardiopulmonary bypass, profound hypothermia, and circulator arrest via left side of the chest incision. *J Vasc Surg* 1998; **28**: 591–598.
5. Golden MA, Donaldson MC, Whittemore AD, Mannick JA. Evolving experience with thoracoabdominal aortic aneurysm repair at a single institution. *J Vasc Surg* 1991; **13**: 792–797.

6. Cox GS, O'Hara PJ, Hertzer NR *et al.* Thoracoabdominal aneurysm repair: A representative experience. *J Vasc Surg* 1992; **15**: 780–788.

7. Rectenwald JE, Huber TS, Martin TD *et al.* Functional outcome after thoracoabdominal aortic aneurysm repair. *J Vasc Surg* 2002; **35**: 640–647.

8. Dake MD, Miller DC, Semba CP *et al.* Transluminal placement of endovascular stent-grafts for the treatment of descending thoracic aortic aneurysms. *N Engl J Med* 1994; **331**: 1729–1734.

9. Ehrlich M, Grabenwoeger M, Cartes-Zumelzu F *et al.* Endovascular stent graft repair for aneurysms on the descending thoracic aorta. *Ann Thorac Surg* 1998; **66**: 19–25.

10. Mitchell RS, Miller DC, Dake MD *et al.* Thoracic aortic aneurysm repair with an endovascular stent graft: the "first generation". *Ann Thorac Surg* 1999; **67**: 1971–1974.

11. Temudom T, D'Ayala M, Marin ML *et al.* Endovascular grafts in the treatment of thoracic aortic aneurysms and pseudoaneurysms. *Ann Vasc Surg* 2000; **14**: 230–238.

12. Grabenwoger M, Hutschala D, Ehrlich MP *et al.* Thoracic aortic aneurysms: treatment with endovascular self-expandable stent-grafts. *Ann Thor Surg* 2000; **69**: 441–445.

13. Taylor PR, Gaines PA, McGuinness CL *et al.* Thoracic aortic stent grafts—early commercial experience from two centres using commercially available devices. *Eur J Vasc Endovasc Surg* 2001; **22**: 70–76.

14. Greenberg R, Resch T, Nyman U *et al.* Endovascular repair of descending thoracic aortic aneurysms: an early experience with intermediate-term follow-up. *J Vasc Surg* 2000; **31**: 147–156.

15. Bortone AS, Schena S, Mannatrizio G *et al.* Endovascular stent-graft treatment for diseases of the descending thoracic aorta. *Eur J Card Thor Surg* 2001; **20**: 514–519.

16. White RA, Donayre CE, Walot I *et al.* Endovascular exclusion of descending thoracic aortic aneurysms and chronic dissections: Initial clinical results with the AneuRx device. *J Vasc Surg* 2001; **33**: 927–934.

17. Won JY, Lee DY, Shim WH *et al.* Elective endovascular treatment of descending thoracic aortic aneurysms and chronic dissections with stent-grafts. *J Vasc Interv Radiol* 2001; **12**: 575–582.

18. Cambria RP, Brewster DC, Lauterbach SR *et al.* Evolving experience with thoracic aortic stent graft repair. *J Vasc Surg* 2002; **35**: 1129–1136.

19. Thompson CS, Gaxotte VD, Rodriguez JA *et al.* Endoluminal stent grafting of the thoracic aorta: initial experience with the Gore Excluder. *J Vasc Surg* 2002; **35**: 1163–1170.

20. Totaro M, Mazzesi G, Marullo AGM *et al.* Endoluminal stent grafting of the descending thoracic aorta. *Ital Heart J* 2002; **3**: 366–369.

21. Fann JI, Miller DC. Endovascular treatment of descending thoracic aortic aneurysms and dissections. *Surg Clin NA* 1999; **79**: 551–574.

22. DeBakey ME, McCollum CH, Graham JM. Surgical treatment of aneurysms of the descending thoracic aorta. *J Cardiovasc Surg* 1978; **19**: 571–576.

23. Pressler V, McNamara JJ. Thoracic aortic aneurysm: natural history and treatment. *J Thorac Cardiovasc Surg* 1980; **79**: 489–498.

24. Safi HJ, Campbell MP, Ferreira ML *et al.* Spinal cord protection in descending thoracic and thoracoabdominal carotid aneurysm repair. *Semin Thorac Cardiovasc Surg* 1998; **10**: 41–44.

25. Hamilton IN, Hollier LH. Adjunctive therapy for spinal cord protection during thoracoabdominal aortic aneurysm repair. *Semin Thorac Cardiovasc Surg* 1998; **10**: 35–39.

26. Dake MD, Kato N, Mitchell RS *et al.* Endovascular stent-graft placement for the treatment of acute aortic dissection. *N Engl J Med* 1999; **340**: 1546–1552.

27. Nienaber CA, Fattori R, Lund G *et al.* Non-surgical reconstruction of thoracic aortic dissection by stent-graft placement. *N Engl J Med* 1999; **340**: 1539–1545.

28. White RA, Donayre C, Walot I *et al.* Regression of a descending thoracoabdominal aortic dissection following staged deployment of thoracic and abdominal aortic endografts. *J Endovasc Ther* 2002; **9**: II-92-II-97.

29. Kos X, Bouchard L, Otal P *et al.* Stent-graft treatment of penetrating aortic thoracic aortic ulcers. *J Endovasc Ther* 2002 ; **9**: II-25-II-31.

30. Alric P, Berthet JP, Branchereau P *et al.* Endovascular repair for acute rupture of the descending thoracic aorta. *J Endovasc Ther* 2002; **9**: II-51-II-59.

Endografting for thoracic aneurysm has replaced the need for open surgery

Against the motion
Wilhelm Sandmann, Klaus Grabitz, Tomas Pfeiffer, Dimitris-Solon G Georgopoulos

Introduction

The spontaneous course of descending thoracic aortic aneurysm leads to rupture depending on the size of the aneurysm and associated risk factors;[1] therefore an aggressive approach has been advised,[2] especially for aneurysms of and over 6 cm maximal diameter.[3,6] Transthoracic open repair has become the method of choice since the publication of DeBakey and Cooley in 1953[4] until Volodos *et al.* reported their first experience with endografting in 1991.[5] Since then the number of publications reporting favourable results with endovascular stent-grafting has increased significantly while reports on conventional repair have nearly disappeared or appeared as historical controls for comparison with endografting or are only mentioned in publications dealing mainly with replacement not only of the thoracic but of the thoracoabdominal aorta. Does this observation mean, that endovascular grafting has replaced open surgery?

Evidence

The answer to this question has to take several aspects into consideration. Clouse *et al.*[6] have estimated the incidence rate of descending thoracic aortic aneurysms (TAA) to be 10.4 per 100 000 persons years, which is substantially lower than for aneurysms in the infrarenal position (AAA). Therefore the overall number of publications reporting either about open repair or endovascular stent-grafting in the thoracic location is rather small and does not allow valid statistical conclusions concerning the indication for treatment and the superiority of one technique over the other.

Contrary to reports about open treatment the number of cases treated with the endovascular method is small, because the technical feasibility is limited and endografts can only be applied in selected patients, although in some centres it is extensively practised.

Are studies about open repair and endovascular stent-grafting comparable?

This means, that statistical analysis on an intention-to-treat protocol is not possible. In the reported series of conventional repair one finds regularly a large spectrum of aetiologies and anatomical locations of aneurysms which are not identical to reports on endovascular stent-grafting. Authors in favour of endovascular stent technology compare their results with open surgery, but the publications they refer to appeared a long time previously,[2,7,8] and in this aspect a distorted picture is created. Although endografting is a rather new technology and comparison with historical series of open repair seems appropriate, in order to compare the same level of experience during the time the technique is evolving, one must keep in mind, that open repair has also made progress since 1991. As we have to take care of the patient of today and not of yesterday, assessment of the efficacy and efficiency of both methods only makes sense, if techniques and modalities of today are compared.

Another problem, which makes comparison of the two techniques difficult, arises because of the large variety of indications and aetiologies, which are included in the various studies. In order to show an impressive quantity of cases, aetiologies such as acute and chronic dissection, remaining or newly developed descending aneurysms in patients treated for type A dissection, mycotic aneurysms, penetrating ulcers, atherosclerotic aneurysms, contained rupture, traumatic disruption, post-surgical aneurysms after replacement for thoracic coarctation, and anastomotic aneurysms have been included into the reports about endovascular stent-grafting.[9–24]

A similar case-mix can be observed concerning the size, and extention of the aneurysm as well as the length of aortic involvement and replacement. Short and small distal arch aneurysms, extensive descending aneurysms reaching out to the coeliac axis, short segmental aneurysms in the middle of the descending aorta are mixed with aneurysms located in the distal descending thoracic aorta only and with type I thoracoabdominal aneurysms. Of course, the same is true for publications on conventional repair, especially if the value of adjuncts to avoid cardiac complications and spinal cord injury are compared. These series often include elective, urgent and emergency cases in the same statistical package.[8,25]

The data from the current literature do not allow statistical conclusions of scientific value. Not a single study comparing the two treatment modalities for the same anatomical location and aetiology has been published. For example, in patients with atherosclerotic aneurysms located in the middle part of the descending thoracic aorta, which is the most frequent location and easier to deal with for both techniques, a prospective randomized study could be performed but, due to the very small number of patients treated in single centres, assessment would be only feasible by multicentre prospective studies.

Another important aspect is the length of the aortic segment being replaced or excluded, because this relates directly to the risk of paraplegia and renal failure. Appropriate information is lacking in most of the endovascular and open studies.

Risk of open repair

Additionally, comparative evaluation becomes complicated, because authors in favour of endografting describe their patients as being 'very sick' and 'at significant' risk if exposed to open surgery.[11,17,20,24] The reason for underlining the high risk is understandable, because the use of a new, attractive but most probably less efficient method can only be explained, if many more patients could benefit from the new method than from the old one. By pointing out the severity of the sickness of their patients the authors generate the impression, that their patients could only tolerate endovascular grafting and would not have survived open surgery repair.

Surprisingly, patients in whom the procedure failed technically and had to be converted to open surgery, survived open repair despite a long torture of endovascular trying. It is a general phenomenon today, that endovascular treatment is justified by claiming the inoperability for and contraindication to open repair. The reader, who is familiar with the evolution of aneurysm surgery from personal experience, asks himself whether in earlier times only healthy patients were exposed to open surgery. However, it can be assumed, that the health status of the patients treated by one of the two modalities is not significantly different, as has been shown for the treatment of infrarenal aortic aneurysms classifying patients according to the American Society of Anaesthesiology in the Registry of the German Society of Vascular Surgery.[26]

So if comparison of the two techniques should become possible in the future, the cohort should have the same aetiology, location, extension and even symptomatology of the aneurysm so that early, mid-term and late results can be evaluated.

Dissection and dissecting aneurysm – a special case

With the advent of endovascular techniques obviously a new era has begun. Indications for treatment of TAA have been created, which did not exist before. For example, a localized dissection at the descending thoracic aorta from trauma, leading or not to contained rupture of the descending aorta in a polytraumatized patient was only rarely treated with the open technique, because the spontaneous course leads to healing through fibrotic tissue and heavy calcification. The patient remains asymptomatic and only many years later can a chronic circumscript aneurysm be accidentally detected due to heavy calcification. Very rarely this type of aneurysm becomes symptomatic and requires surgery. Taking into consideration this benign course, endovascular grafting is not justified and could eventually result in tetraplegia as has been described lately by Kasirajan *et al.*[13]

The optimal treatment of acute type B dissection is non-operative.[27, 28] In the majority of patients some kind of dilatation of the false lumen will develop, if thrombosis does not occur. Complications such as intrapleural bleeding from rupture, remaining heavy pain from progressing dissection and severe ischaemia are indications for open repair. In a stable patient open repair is not only unnecessary but is contraindicated, because any surgery at the weakened aortic wall can lead to bleeding from the suture line and to aneurysm formation later on.

If open repair is not necessary in the stable patient, why should endograft stenting be applied? It has been shown, that the entry of the dissection can be sealed by the stent-grafting, but most often many re-entries can be found. Fortunately enough, though the re-entry perfusion of the organs and the extremities remains possible, the danger of aneurysm formation and rupture remains as well. The indications for open surgery in patients with chronic type B dissection are well defined today and open surgery has proved to be highly successful, if the correct indications are followed.

Consequently, if aortic dilatation progresses to an aneurysm we recommend replacement by the open method including segmental arteries into the proximal and distal anastomosis as has been shown by Connolly *et al.*[29] This strategy allows preservation of collateral circulation to the spinal cord and to the visceral organs. This is not always the case with stent-grafting.[19] The most important complication from open surgery is spinal cord damage, which cannot be avoided by stent-grafting either. On the contrary, stent-grafting has only limited applicability and leaves the patient with great uncertainty for the future.

Endovascular stent-grafting is not a definitive procedure. This is known by its advocates, who subsequently cover up also healthy parts of the aorta and even segmental and visceral arteries by lengthy and multiple grafts. Stent-grafting aneurysm formation and even rupture has been described in the literature.[11,30] Open repair might become a necessary but difficult task.

At the moment of acute aortic dissection we do not know which patient will develop an aneurysm and if this will appear early or late. Therefore, in a stable patient, neither open surgery nor prophylactic stent-grafting is indicated, because this strategy would be a treatment of a radiological image and not of the patient himself. As these patients have to be followed by modern imaging, an aneurysm might be discovered later. Yet we do not know which diameter presents the threshold of rupture, while in the asymptomatic patient treatment below 6 cm transverse diameter is generally felt to be not necessary.

Why are endovascular stent-grafts today inserted in dilated dissected aortas and in dissected aneurysms of a smaller diameter? Where is the justification? The indication for open surgery is always the prevention from rupture and recurrent dissection, but these complications appear only in large aneurysms. Why should stent-grafts be inserted in smaller aneurysms in aortas, which show only a dilatation? If in these particular cases open surgery can be avoided by endovascular stent-grafting with the same efficacy, the latter would be clearly preferable, if durable, but the superiority of stent-grafting has not been proved today. Open surgery can solve the problem definitely; can we really expect the same thing from endovascular stent-grafting?

Old studies on open repair and recent studies on endovascular stent-grafting – where do we go?

As far as the risk of open surgery is concerned, the results of some series should be studied in detail. Crawford *et al.,* as early as 1981, published their results of open surgery for descending thoracic aorta aneurysms in over 100 patients without bypass and shunting and achieved an early mortality rate of below 10%.[7] In comparison, Greenberg reported almost 20 years later a 20% mortality rate (12.5% in elective and 33% in urgent cases) for the endovascular method.[11]

Assessing the results, it is important to take into consideration, that with the exception of one single case no emergencies were included while only patients with good landing zones for stent-grafting were preferred. A mortality rate of 20% for elective treatment is rather high. It is of course not known how many patients were waiting for how many days in order to undergo treatment, because the endograft had to be manufactured and tailored to the size of the individual aorta. It is known already from publications and presentations, that quite a few patients waited too long and died, before the endograft was delivered and could be applied.

Furthermore, Greenberg *et al.* pointed out, that the risk for open surgery was found to be elevated in four patients with contained rupture and in seven with chronic obstructive pulmonary disease (COPD). However, neither contained rupture nor COPD, which is usually present in the majority of those elderly patients, presents a contraindication against open surgery. One particular patient, who had undergone previous TAA resection ruptured from penetration of the stent-graft into the aortic arch and died. Was it realistic to expect, that this type of aneurysm could heal by endografting? Three patients had to undergo emergency conversion to open surgery due to graft migration, which definitely does not appear in open surgery.

Borst *et al.*, in 1994, published results of 123 patients who had undergone, between 1986 and 1992, open surgery with standardized left heart bypass using the biomedicus pump.[8] Ten patients were excluded from the study, because only brief periods of aortic X-clamping were expected. The early mortality rate was only 3% with a late mortality rate of 7% and a permanent spinal complication rate of 2.3%. Migration, bulging of the graft, endoleaks, ruptures, infections, thrombosis, access complications, additional procedures for failure of the primary one, further dissections, thrombosis of the graft, penetrations and even visceral ischaemia and stroke did not occur in Borst's series so where do the supporters of endografting find the justification for stent-grafting?

Is it really justified to expose the patient to this experimental type of treatment for the sake of the development of a new method, which is of course very attractive but does not lead to complete and durable exclusion of the aneurysm. If the aneurysm cannot be prevented from rupture and this is the one and only indication for repairing or excluding an aneurysm, why should such a method be used clinically? And one must add, how is inoperability for open surgery defined? Is it more the inability of the surgeon, the anaesthesiologist or the institution, which we do not want to mention or truly the health condition of the patient? Don't we admit anymore, that differences in expertise and capability exist on the surgical sector and that some institutions can provide much better results than others?

The national audit in Great Britain from 1998 showed, that for TAA surgery procedures the mortality rate was 33% in patients with pump or bypass and 28% without. Does a nation-wide level with such disastrous results reflect the bad health status of the patient or does it demonstrate only the level of experience which might be lacking? Should these results support endovascular grafting, although the new method has not been shown nation-wide to be better than open repair, or at least has similar results?

The future of endovascular stent-grafting

Ten years of learning curve, several generations of stent-grafts with many already withdrawn from the market, is this not enough to restrict this treatment to a small number of experts and institutions and patients instead of widespread use, especially, if mortality and morbidity figures are no better than those being published for open repair? And if it is true that patients demand this type of treatment because they have been informed by the media, then who gave this optimistic and unrealistic information to the media except those who want to push endovascular treatment further? Those who want to perform either open repair or endovascular stent-grafting are obliged, to give the patient the present rates of complication and survival for both methods. However, it is not enough to mention an individual's good or bad results, but also the results of centres probably more experienced in either of the two techniques.

In a much more demanding type of open surgery, the replacement of the thoracoabdominal aorta, experts have reached a mortality rate of only 8% and a very low rate of spinal cord complications[31] while the same is true for the rather limited replacement of the descending thoracic aorta. In endovascular surgery we are lacking guidelines and well-defined indications, about in which circumstances this technique might serve the patient's needs better than open surgery and these should be developed on a scientific basis. Devices can be tested first in animals and the appropriate application can be performed in humans later. Additionally, we have to await mid- and long-term results for those grafts which did maintain their function so far without secondary intervention. We have observed many unexpected complications from endografting for infrarenal aortic aneurysms. Why do we not restrict ourselves to a very limited and clearly defined indication in the thoracic aorta?

Finally it is alarming, that sometimes surgeons and radiologists, who never achieved significant experience with open repair, vigorously promote the insertion of endovascular stent-grafts.

In conclusion, due to the uncertainty of durability and taken into account that mortality and morbidity rates are not significantly lower than those for open repair in experienced hands, endovascular stent-grafts should not be implanted without a strict research protocol and only in small numbers.

The complications after open repair are related to the condition of the patient and the type of the aneurysm, while endografting has additional complications which are related to the device. The success of open repair lasts 10, 20 and even 30 years. Therefore we should reduce the number of stent-grafts and wait for the mid- and long-term results of the grafts which have been implanted so far. We will probably be unexpectedly surprised as was the case in the infrarenal region.

Endovascular stent-grafting is still experimental on human beings. It has not replaced open repair.

Summary

- Endovascular stent-grafting is not durable.

- It does not protect totally from rupture.

- Morbidity and mortality rates are not significantly lower than for open repair.

- Unlike open repair, endovascular stent-grafting has device-related complications.

- The indications for stent-grafting of the descending thoracic aorta are not defined.

- Endovascular stent-grafting is still experimental in human beings.

- It has not replaced open repair.

References

1. Bickerstaff LK, Pairolero PC, Hollier LH *et al*. Thoracic aortic aneurysms: a population based study. *Surgery* 1982; **92**: 1103–1108.
2. Hamerlijnck R, De Geest R, Brutel de la Revière A. Surgical correction of descending thoracic aortic aneurysms with shunt or bypass techniques versus simple aortic cross-clamping. *Eur J Cardiothorac Surg* 1989; **3**: 37–43.
3. Najafi H, Javid H, Hunter JA *et al*. An update of treatment of aneurysms of the descending thoracic aorta. *World J Surg* 1980; **4**: 553–561.
4. DeBakey ME, Cooley DA. Successful resection of aneurysm of the thoracic aorta and replacement by graft. *JAMA* 1953; **152**: 673–636.
5. Volodos NL, Karpovich IP, Troyan VI *et al*. Clinical experience of the use of self-fixing synthetic prostheses for remote endoprosthetics of the thoracic and abdominal aorta and iliac areries through femoral artery and intraoperative endoprosthesis for aortic reconstruction. *Vasa* Suppl 1991; **33**: 93–5.

6. Clouse WD, Hallett JW, Schaff HV *et al*. Improved prognosis of thoracic aortic aneurysms. *JAMA* 1998; **280**: 1926–1929.

7. Crawford ES, Walker HS, Saleh SA, Normann NA. Graft replacement of aneurysm in descending thoracic aorta: results without bypass or shunting. *Surgery* 1981; **89**: 73–85.

8. Borst HG, Jurmann M, Bühner B, Laas J. Risk of replacement of descending aorta with a standardized left heart bypass technique. *J Thorac Cardiovasc Surg* 1994; **107**: 126–133.

9. D'Ayala M. Endovascular grafting for thoracic aortic aneurysms. In: Marin ML, Hollier LH (eds). *Endovascular Grafting: Advanced Treatment for Vascular Disease*. New York: Futura Publishing, 2000; 95–107.

10. Gaines PA, Gerrard DJ, Reidy JF. The endovascular management of thoracic aortic disease – some controversial Issues. *Eur J Vas Endovasc Surg* 2002; **23**: 162–164.

11. Greenberg R, Resch T, Nyman U *et al*. Endovascular repair of descending thoracic aortic aneurysms: an early experience with intermediate-term follow-up. *J Vasc Surg* 2000; **31**: 147–156.

12. Juvonen T, Biancari F, Ylönen K *et al*. Combined surgical and endovascular treatment of pseudoaneurysms of the visceral arteries and of the left iliac arteries after thoracoabdominal aortic surgery. *Eur J Vasc Endovasc Surg* 2001; **22**: 275–277.

13. Kasirajan K, Dolmatch B, Ouriel K, Clair D. Delayed onset of ascending paralysis after thoracic aortic stent graft deployment. *J Vasc Surg* 2000; **31**: 196–199.

14. Kato N, Hirano T, Kawaguchi T *et al*. Aneurysmal degeneration of the aorta after stent-graft repair of acute aortic dissection. *J Vasc Surg* 2001; **34**: 513–518.

15. Kilaru S, Beavers FP, Heller JA *et al*. Endoluminal stent graft repair of traumatic thoracic aortic pseudoaneurysm. *Eur J Vasc Endovasc Surg* 2002; **24**: 456–458.

16. May J, White G, Waugh R *et al*. Comparison of first- and second-generation prostheses for endoluminal repair of abdominal aortic aneurysms: A 6-year study with life table analysis. *J Vasc Surg* 2000; **32**: 124–129,

17. Najibi S, Terramani TT, Weiss VJ *et al*. Endoluminal versus open treatment of descending thoracic aortic aneurysms. *J Vasc Surg* 2002; **36**: 732–737.

18. Palombi M, Berardi F, Sposato S *et al*. Endovascular treatment of a ruptured thoracic aortic aneurysm. *Eur J Vasc Endovasc Surg* 2000; **19**: 101–102 .

19. Pasic M, Bergs P, Knollmann F *et al*. Delayed retrograde aortic dissection after endovascular stenting of the descending thoracic aorta. *J Vasc Surg* 2002; **36**: 184–186.

20. Rehders, T, Nienaber CA. Complications of stent-graft placement in the thoracic aorta. In: A Branchereau, M Jacobs: *Complications in Vascular and Endovascular Surgery*. New York: Futura Publishing, 2001: 185–191.

21. Saccani S, Nicolini F, Beghi *et al*. Thoracic aortic stents: a combined solution for complex cases. *Eur J Vasc Endovasc Surg* 2002; **2**: 423–427.

22. Schoder M, Grabenwöger M, Hölzenbein TH *et al*. Endovascular stent-graft-repair of complicated penetrating atherosclerotic ulcers of the descending thoracic aorta. *J Vasc Surg* 2002; **36**: 720–726.

23. Taylor PR, Gaines PA, McGuinness CL *et al*. Thoracic aortic stent grafts – early experience from two centres using commercially available devices. *Eur J Vasc Endovasc Surg* 2001; **22**: 70–76.

24. White RA, Donayre CE, Walot I *et al*. Endovascular exclusion of descending thoracic aortic aneurysms and chronic dissections: Initial clinical results with the AneuRx device. *J Vasc Surg* 2001; **33**: 927–934.

25. Schepens MAAM, Defauw J, Hamerlijnck R *et al*. Surgical treatment of thoracoabdominal aortic aneurysms by simple crossclamping. *J Thorac Cardiovasc Surg* 1994; **107**: 134–42.

26. Umscheid T, Eckstein HH, Noppeney T, Weber H, Niedermeier HP. Quality management of infrarenal aortic aneurysms of the German Society of Vascular Surgery – Results 2000. *Gefässchirurgie* 2001; **6**: 194–200.

27. Wheat MW, Palmer RF, Bartley TD, Seelman RC. Treatment of dissectin aneurysms of the aorta without surgery. *J Thorac Cardiovasc Surg* 1965; **50**: 364.

28. Borst HG, Heinemann MK, Stone CD. *Surgical Treatment of Aortic Dissection*. Edinburgh: Churchill Livingstone, 1996.

29. Connolly JE. Prevention of paraplegia secondary to operations on the aorta. *J Cardiovasc Surg* 1986; **27**: 410–417.

30. Dake MD, Miller DC, Mitchell RS *et al*. The first generation of endovascular stent grafts for patients with aneurysms of the descending aorta. *J Thorac Cardiovasc Surg* 1999; **116**: 689–704.

31. Safi HJ, Subramaniam MH, Miller CC *et al*. Progress in the management of type I thoraco-abdominal and descending thoracic aortic aneurysms. *Ann Vasc Surg* 1999; **13**: 457–462.

Endografting for thoracic aneurysm has replaced the need for open surgery

Charing Cross Editorial Comments towards Consensus

The endovascular argument is that it can be done and a major operation can be avoided and therefore it should be done. Both sides are aware that there are no satisfactory comparative data but Professor Sandmann argues that endovascular stent-grafting is not durable and it does not protect totally from rupture. He says that the morbidity and mortality rates are not significantly lower than for open repair. The authors describe endovascular stent-grafting as still 'an experiment on the human being'.

These surgical groups are diametrically opposed and a clash can be anticipated on the day.

R M Greenhalgh
Editor

Medicine beats angioplasty and stent for renal artery stenosis

For the motion

George Hamilton

Introduction

Progressive atherosclerotic renal vascular disease is a major cause of end-stage renal failure in the elderly, accounting for about 15% of older patients requiring dialysis.[1,2] The true prevalence of this condition is unknown and varies according to presentation but it occurs most commonly in high risk patients with co-existent vascular disease affecting other systems. It is commonly found in patients with coronary artery disease and a history of stroke[3,4] but is particularly common in patients with peripheral vascular disease or congestive cardiac failure.[5,6]

Decisions to treat renal artery stenosis by revascularization are relatively straightforward in certain groups of patients recognized as most likely to benefit (Table 1). Such clinical decisions are much more difficult to make in the majority of renal artery stenoses where the clinical evidence for intervention is inadequate. Such decisions are made largely on the basis of prevention of progression of renal failure, progression of renal artery stenosis and much less commonly to treat hypertension. There remains great controversy concerning the best treatment, particularly with regard to renal artery stent angioplasty where clinical outcome has not matched the good technical results achieved by this intervention. Patients with progressive atherosclerotic renal vascular disease are a heterogeneous group with different presentations, different spectrum of pathologies and response to treatment. The debate regarding best treatment and particularly the disappointing clinical results of angioplasty, can best be informed by understanding these factors.

Table 1. Patient groups most likely to benefit from renal revascularization

1. Progressive renal failure of short duration (<6 months)
2. Pulmonary oedema and refractory congestive cardiac failure (volume overload)
3. Severe renal failure precipitated by ACE-inhibitor treatment
4. Refractory hypertension
5. Severe stenosis (>90%)
6. Renal length > 8cm

What is atherosclerotic renovascular disease?

Atherosclerotic renovascular disease is a complex condition in which renal artery stenosis of varying severities is frequently present, together with hypertension and varying degrees of renal failure. The combination of hypertension and parenchymal renal disease is commonly known as ischaemic nephropathy. Renovascular hypertension and ischaemic nephropathy are complex pathophysiological conditions. Renal artery stenosis is a localized anatomical condition, which may compromise renal perfusion and be a source for renal atheroembolism, but in many patients progressive atherosclerotic renal vascular disease may play a very minor role in the pathophysiology of their condition. Selection of patients for treatment should logically be made on the basis of the underlying pathophysiology rather than purely on the basis of the anatomical lesion.

Renovascular hypertension is often of mixed origin since many patients will have essential hypertension as the underlying major initiating risk factor for the development of their arteriosclerosis. Indeed this combination of essential and renovascular hypertension is frequently present.[7] Renal revascularization will have no effect on the intrarenal changes of essential hypertension, or on intrarenal arteriosclerosis, factors which help to explain the low cure rates seen in patients having revascularization for hypertension.

Ischaemic nephropathy is an even more complex pathological entity. Histological analysis of kidneys suffering long-standing renal artery stenosis reveals cortical infarcts, nephrosclerosis, small vessel arteriosclerosis, endothelial damage and much cholesterol embolization.[8] This parenchymal disease may be present as a result of hypertension-induced nephrosclerosis, or as a result of aging, or diabetes if present, or secondary to atheroembolism, but most commonly as a result of combinations of these pathologies. All of these factors can be present in progressive atherosclerotic renal vascular disease quite independently of an associated renal artery stenosis, particularly when it is not severe.[9] However, the severity of renal artery stenosis correlates well with clinical outcome. A recent prospective 2-year study found renal survival was 97.5% in patients with unilateral stenosis, 82% with bilateral stenosis, and 45% in patients with unilateral stenosis plus contralateral occlusion.[10]

Atheroembolism

Atheroembolism in the kidney causes occlusion by cholesterol and other particulate matter of the arcuate and interlobular arteries and of the glomerular capillaries. Renal atheroembolism classically occurs after anticoagulation, or after aortic catheterization and less frequently after aortic surgery. It is increasingly being recognized that spontaneous and insidious renal atheroembolism may be more common than previously suspected in the elderly arteriosclerotic.[11] Because this condition can only reliably be diagnosed by renal biopsy, its true incidence is underestimated. Furthermore renal atheroembolism commonly complicates invasive vascular procedures such as arteriography, coronary and renal angiography/angioplasty.[12] Significant atheroembolism was found in a recent pilot study of renal stenting protected with a distal protection device.[13] In 32 renal angioplasties, in all cases visible arteriosclerotic debris was removed with an average of 100 particles of 0.2mm mean diameter, with one particle measuring a staggering 6 mm! As in carotid stent angioplasty, the introduction of protection devices has confirmed that significant embolism complicates every angioplasty procedure.

For the above reasons it becomes clear that treatment based on revascularization will have variable results depending on the degree of underlying parenchymal damage and co-existence of essential hypertension, both of which will not be affected by improved perfusion. Indeed progression to end-stage renal failure will occur in up to 25% of successful revascularizations. This has led to the suggestion that exposure of a diseased renal parenchyma to increased blood pressure after a successful revascularization may actually accelerate intrarenal arteriosclerosis, nephrosclerosis and renal failure. A successful outcome from revascularization will depend critically on the balance between vascular hypoperfusion and the extent of irreversible parenchymal disease. In addition the inevitable atheroembolic showering into the renal parenchyma during stent angioplasty can only adversely affect the outcome.

What is a clinically significant renal artery stenosis?

The widely accepted convention is that an arterial stenosis becomes significant once it becomes greater than 50%. The effect of the stenosis, however, is known to be dependent on its anatomical site and the end organ served. Experimental studies in dogs have shown that a 40% reduction in renal perfusion will result from a 75–90% stenosis of the renal artery.[14] Autoregulation of renal blood flow and the capacity to develop a collateral circulation efficiently are two further factors which will act to mitigate compromised perfusion pressure particularly in the lower grade stenoses.

In man there is little evidence available to accurately define what constitutes significant renal artery stenosis. The most objective evidence available is based on a clinical study correlating activation of the renin-angiotesin system with angiographic grading of renal artery stenosis. This was performed in a group of patients with renovascular hypertension but with good kidney function where the renin-angiotensin system activation was detected by captopril stimulated renal vein renin measurements. Unilateral or bilateral hypersecretion of renin was found only with greater than 80% renal artery stenosis as found on angiography.[15] This clinical study suggests that significant reduction in renal blood flow occurs only when renal arterial stenosis is 80% or greater. Review of the published literature indicates that a very sizable proportion of angioplasties undertaken for renal artery stenosis were performed in non-critical stenosis, less than 80%, where significant reperfusion was unlikely to be achieved and provides a further explanation for the disappointing results achieved with stent angioplasty.

What is the risk of progression of renal artery stenosis?

There is a significant risk for progression of renal artery stenosis in some, but it must be stressed that this does not occur in the majority of patients. The risk of progression appears to be related primarily to the severity of the disease at the time of diagnosis. In a recent prospective study using accurately and reliably performed renal duplex scanning, the cumulative incidence of progression of renal artery stenosis was found to be 35% at 3 years and 51% at 5 years. The 3-year incidence of progression was found to differ according to the degree of stenosis at presentation. When the initial renal artery stenosis was less than 60%, progression occurred in 28% but when the initial stenosis was greater than 60% progression occurred in 49%.[16] Most importantly in this prospectively studied series of 295 kidneys, progression to occlusion was low with only nine or 3% developing occlusion. Predictive risk factors for renal artery progression were found to be high-grade stenosis, hypertension and diabetes mellitus. Half of these patients did not develop any progression of renal artery stenosis, an important clinical fact which has not been sufficiently recognized in management decisions.

Previous estimates of progression and rates of occlusion were found to be higher but unlike the results described above which were in a prospective study using duplex scanning, these original studies were based on serial angiography largely performed for other indications. A review of five reports with a total of 237 patients gave a rate of progression (worsening of existing stenosis of the renal artery or development of contralateral renal artery stenosis) in 49% of these patients over 6–180 months follow-up. Progression to complete occlusion occurred in 98 cases or 14%. This study overestimates the risk of progression and occlusion because these were patients in whom angiography was largely indicated because of worsening vascular disease, a cohort well known to have significantly increased risk of severe renal artery stenosis.[17] In summary it is clear that progression does not occur in all renal artery stenosis, even those which are high grade, and furthermore that complete occlusion develops at a rate much lower than previous angiographic studies had suggested.

Survival of patients with progressive atherosclerotic renal vascular disease

The benefit of any treatment, particularly interventions with significant morbidity and mortality, and cost, must be considered in the context of the patient's likely life expectancy. A recent Swedish study of hypertensive patients with progressive atherosclerotic renal vascular disease showed that cardiovascular events were much more frequent than end-stage renal failure, with 33 of 44 dying from cardiovascular events, nine patients dying from non-cardiac causes and only two progressing to end-stage renal failure.[18]

Patient selection for treatment in progressive atherosclerotic renal vascular disease

Renal artery stenosis is one factor in the complex pathology of progressive atherosclerotic renal vascular disease which anatomically can be treated by stent angioplasty. However, the primary aim of treatment should be to prolong dialysis-free survival and patient survival and should not be primarily focused on abolishing a stenosis. In many patients the renal artery stenosis is clinically silent, and particularly in the older patient, improvement is less likely after revascularization. These patients should not be exposed to the complications and risks of stent angioplasty unless there is refractory hypertension, recurrent heart failure or rapidly developing renal failure in a renal artery stenosis greater than 80%. Medical management in all of these patients is mandatory. In the greater majority this treatment alone will prevent vascular events in patients who are much more likely to die of non-renal causes before developing end-stage renal failure.

Medical management

Best medical therapy is a concept which is central to the management of all patients with vascular disease. The goals of modern medical management are treatment of heart disease and other related conditions such as diabetes, and more specifically, in progressive atherosclerotic renal vascular disease, the aggressive control of hypertension and reversal or delay of developing renal failure. The drugs with documented value in achieving these goals are anti-hypertensives, lipid-lowering agents and anti-platelet agents.

Hypertension

There are two patterns of renovascular hypertension which can develop and are often mixed. In a unilateral renal artery stenosis (one clip, two kidney model) hypertension is mediated by renin release from the affected kidney. In bilateral stenosis or in a stenosis of a solitary kidney, (one kidney, one clip model) there is a mixed picture of renin release and increased volume. These patients have a well recognized tendency to pulmonary oedema and heart failure[19] but will also respond to treatment with angiotensin converting enzyme (ACE)-inhibitors. The advent of ACE-inhibitors has significantly improved control of renovascular hypertension.

Enthusiasm for medical treatment of renovascular hypertension is a relatively recent development. Revascularization had better results in the older series when ACE-inhibitors and other powerful anti-hypertensive agents had not been introduced.[20] Also there were concerns that ACE inhibition might worsen renal function by inhibition of angiotensin II mediated glomerular efferent arteriolar vasoconstriction, which acts to maintain glomerular filtration pressure in the presence of diminished renal arterial pressure. This complication of ACE-inhibitors is well recognized in patients with bilateral renal artery disease but ongoing clinical experience has shown that the potential for acute renal function deterioration has been overstated. In patients with bilateral renal stenosis, acute and significant deterioration in renal function occurred in less than 20% and only 5% needed discontinuation of ACE-inhibitor.[20] Most episodes of renal failure involve minor increases in creatinine and when treatment is stopped, the acute renal failure is reversible. There is experimental evidence that ACE-inhibitors may hasten renal atrophy in the ischaemic kidney but the long-term benefits of treatment far outweigh the theoretical disadvantages. Not only is excellent blood pressure control achieved but improved renal microcirculation results in the majority treated with ACE-inhibitors.[21,22] The current consensus is that excellent blood pressure control can safely be achieved with ACE-inhibitors providing that renal function and renal size (of both kidneys) are frequently monitored.

Other powerful anti-hypertensive agents have recently been introduced and description of these agents is beyond the scope of this paper. As a result of modern powerful anti-hypertensive medications, renovascular hypertension is controlled solely by medical therapy in the great majority of patients. Indeed, blood pressure control is now so good that many patients with renovascular hypertension remain undiagnosed by their primary physicians.

Preservation of renal function

Powerful lipid lowering agents and anti-platelet drugs have been introduced to great effect over this last decade. In particular the statins have been shown to improve survival in patients with coronary artery disease in several controlled trials. These drugs not only reduce cholesterol but have several other actions at the microcirculatory level, including reducing endothelial dysfunction, and have been shown to halt progression of arteriosclerotic lesions in the coronary circulation.

Similar effects would be expected to occur in the arteriosclerotic kidney and on the renal artery stenosis itself. Conclusive evidence is lacking but there have been case reports of documented regression of atherosclerotic renal artery disease with aggressive lipid-lowering therapy.[23] Simvastatin has been shown to halt progressive renal failure in a patient with renal atheroembolism.[24]

There are no large studies assessing the effect of lipid-lowering therapy on renal disease but there is one recently reported meta-analysis which confirms a beneficial effect.[25] This meta-analysis was on 13 small controlled trials of the effects of lipid lowering therapy on glomerular filtration rate, proteinuria or albuminuria. A significantly lower rate of decline in glomerular filtration rate, and improved proteinuria, were found in the treated group compared with controls. The Mayo Clinic recently reported results of a group of patients with significant progressive atherosclerotic renal vascular disease who were given modern conservative treatment without revascularization. Only 10% of patients with renal artery stenosis greater than 70% had resistant hypertension or progressive renal failure.[26] The proven ability of lipid lowering and anti-platelet therapy to prevent life-threatening coronary and cerebrovascular events and the probability that the renal circulation will also benefit, provide compelling arguments for the use of medical therapy in progressive atherosclerotic renal vascular disease as the primary treatment.

Results of renal angioplasty and stent

Because of the common problem of elastic recoil and high restenosis rates with simple angioplasty for osteal lesions, the overwhelming majority of renal artery stenoses are now treated by stent angioplasty.[27] Stent angioplasty gives excellent technical success rates typically 95–100% but restenosis remains a problem with rates between 17 and 29% being reported at 6 months.[27,28] All series report successful treatment of restenosis by re-angioplasty usually within the first 6 months but few have looked at long-term patency.[29,30] These studies reported primary patency rates of 92% and 81.5% at 1 and 2 years respectively, but secondary patency rates achieved in the long term were not clear.

There is a significant complication rate associated with this intervention. A review of the reported series of the last decade (1991–2001) revealed a median major complication rate of 5% (range 0–33%) and a median peri-procedural mortality of 1.2% (range 0–14.2%).[31] A recent large series of 148 renal artery stentings from Australia documented a major procedural complication rate of 7% with cholesterol embolization occurring in 2.8%, an overall complication rate of 13.3% and one procedure-related death.[28] A prospectively studied series of 63 stent angioplasties from Holland reported complications in 44% of patients with puncture wound haemorrhage in 17%, femoral artery aneurysm in 10%, renal artery injury of 6%, cholesterol embolization in 11%, cholesterol embolization with renal dysfunction in 8%, but with no deaths.[32] Two patients (3.2%) developed end-stage renal failure because of stent deployment, probably from atheroembolism.

Hypertension

There are three randomized comparisons of renal angioplasty with medical treatment, all of which found only minimal differences in blood pressure between patients treated by revascularization or by best medical therapy.[33-35] The number of anti-hypertensives required to control blood pressure was lower after angioplasty, thus it will significantly reduce but rarely abolish the need for these agents. The cost of this saving on drugs, however, is the significant morbidity in an elderly group of patients as described above.

There are no reported randomized trials comparing stent angioplasty with best medical therapy, but a randomized trial comparing renal angioplasty with stent angioplasty showed higher patency rates after stenting but no difference in their effects on blood pressure and renal function.[36]

Preservation of renal function

Review of the major studies of renal angioplasty of the last decade indicates improvement in renal function occurring in approximately 25%, with stabilization or no change, occurring in about 50%.[31] Most of these studies were uncontrolled. Data from randomized studies comparing angioplasty, stent angioplasty, and medication alone showed no significant difference in renal function as measured by serum creatinine between the groups (Table 2). Most patients in these studies had unilateral stenosis and therefore renal function could have been maintained by the normal kidney. A study from Guy's Hospital where individual kidney function was measured by

Table 2. Renal function in prospective trials of angioplasty and medical therapy for progressive atherosclerotic renal vascular disease (modified from Ref 38)

Reference	Treatment	Mean follow-up (months)	Mean initial plasma creatinine (µM/litre)	Mean change in plasma creatinine (µM/litre)
Webster et al.[33]				
Unilateral stenosis	Medication (n=13)	3–54	168	0
	Intervention (n=14)		138	8
Bilateral stenosis	Medication (n=12)		148	4
	Intervention (n=16)		182	1
Plouin et al.[34]	Medication (n=26)	6	105	−9
	Intervention (n=23)		96	1
Van Jaarsveld[35]	Medication (n=50)	6.7	115	−9
	Intervention (n=56)		106	0
Van de Ven[36]	Stent (n=42)	6	150	24
	Without stent (n=42)		133	24

synchronous glomerular filtration rate measurement and renal isotope studies, failed to show any improvement in short-term renal function of the treated kidney after angioplasty.[37]

A further shortcoming of these studies is that most of the data are short-term. Revascularization by stent angioplasty may prevent occlusion since no occlusions were reported in stent angioplasty patients in the short-term (6–12 months) while in one study there was a 9% progression to occlusion in the medication only group.[35] Conversely, significant stent restenosis is common up to and after 12 months, and angioplasty without doubt causes atheroembolism with probable infarction and progression of renal failure. The picture is confused but a major benefit from stent angioplasty seems unlikely. All of the available data cannot provide answers to the question of effectiveness of angioplasty with or without stent in preventing progression of renal failure. The ongoing ASTRAL Trial in the UK and the STAR Trial in the Netherlands, will provide much needed clinical evidence to determine whether revascularization by angioplasty carries any true benefit over aggressive best medical therapy.

Summary

- Progressive atherosclerotic renal vascular disease is a complex disease of hypertension and ischaemic nephropathy where hypoperfusion from renal artery stenosis is in most cases of minor significance.

- Essential hypertension forms a major part of renovascular hypertension which will not respond to revascularization.

- Progression of renal artery stenosis and of renal failure is not as common as previously described (even in severe renal artery stenosis).

- Patients with progressive atherosclerotic renal vascular disease mostly die from other vascular causes before developing end-stage renal failure.

- Renal stent angioplasty carries significant peri-procedural risk of morbidity and death.

- Atheroembolism complicates all angioplasties.

- Available data shows no significant benefit from stent angioplasty in preservation of renal function but only reduction of antihypertensive therapy.

- Best medical management is at least as effective in preservation of renal function without the risks of angioplasty and of atheroembolism.

References

1. Scoble JE, Maher AR, Hamilton G. Atherosclerotic renal vascular disease causing renal failure – case for treatment. *Clin Nephrol* 1989; 31: 119–112.
2. Mailloux LU, Napolitano B, Bellucci AG *et al*. Renal vascular disease causing end stage renal disease incidence, clinical correlates and outcomes: a twenty year clinical experience. *Am J Kidney Vis* 1994; 24: 622–629.

3. Uzu T, Inoue T, Fujii T *et al.* Prevalence and predictors of renal artery stenosis in patients with myocardial infarction. *Am J Kidney Vis* 1997; **29**: 733–738.

4. Kuroda S, Nishiea N, Uzu T *et al.* Prevalence of renal artery stenosis in autopsy patients with stroke. *Stroke* 2000; **31**: 61–65.

5. Missouris CG, Buckenham T, Cappucci FP, MacGregor GA. Renal artery stenosis: a common and important problem in patients with peripheral vascular disease. *Am J Med* 1994; **96**: 10–14.

6. MacDowall P, Kalra PA, O'Donoghue DJ *et al.* Risk of morbidity from renovascular disease in elderly patients with congestive cardiac failure. *Lancet* 1998; **352**: 13–16.

7. Pickering TG. Diagnosis and evaluation of renovascular hypertension. *Circulation* 1991: **83**; 1146–1154.

8. Greco BA, Breyer JA. Atherosclerotic ischemic renal disease. *Am J Kidney Vis* 1997; **29**: 167–187.

9. Conlon PJ, O'Riordan E, Kalra PA. New insights into the epidemiologic and clinical manifestations of atherosclerotic renovascular disease. *Am J Kidney Vis* 2000; **35**: 573–587.

10. Connolly JO, Higgins RM, Walters HL *et al.* Presentation, clinical features and outcome in different patterns of atherosclerotic renovascular disease. *QJM* 1994; **87**: 413–421.

11. Smyth JS, Scoble JE. Atheroembolism. *Curr Treat Options Cardiovasc Med* 2002; **4**: 255–265.

12. Modi KS, Venkateswara KR. Atheroembolic renal disease. *J Am Soc Nephrol* 2001; **12**: 1781–1787.

13. Henry M, Klonaris C, Henry I *et al.* Protected renal stenting with the PercuSurge GuardWire device: a pilot study. *J Endovasc Ther* 2001; **8**: 227–237.

14. Imanishi M, Akabane S, Takamiya M *et al.* Critical degree of renal artery stenosis that causes hypertension in dogs. *Angiology* 1992; **43**: 833–842.

15. Simon G. What is critical renal artery stenosis? Implications for treatment. *AJH* 2000; **13**: 1189–1193.

16. Caps MT, Periassinoto C, Zierler RE. *Circulation* 1998; **98**: 2866–2872.

17. Rimmer JM, Gennari FG. Atherosclerotic renovascular disease and progressive renal failure. *Ann Intern Med* 1993; **118**: 712–719.

18. Johansson M, Herlitz H, Jensen G *et al.* Increased cardiovascular mortality in hypertensive patients with renal artery stenosis. Relation to sympathetic activation, renal function and treatment regimens. *J Hypertens* 1999; **17**: 1743–1750.

19. Bloch MJ, Trost DW, Pickering TG *et al.* Prevention of recurrent pulmonary edema in patients with bilateral renovascular disease through renal artery stent placement. *Am J Hypertens* 1998; **12**: 1–7.

20. Bloch MJ, Pickering T. Renal vascular disease: medical management, angioplasty and stenting. *Semin Nephrol* 2000; **20**: 474–488.

21. Zuchelli P, Zuccala A, Borghi M *et al.* Long term comparison between captopril and nifedipine in the progression of renal insufficiency. *Kidney Int* 1992; **42**: 452–458.

22. Inman SR, Stowe NT, Vidt DG. Role of the microcirculation in antihypertensive therapy. *Cleve Clin J Med* 1994; **61**: 356–361.

23. Khong TK, Missouris CG, Belli A-M, MacGregor GA. Case report: Regression of atherosclerotic renal artery stenosis with aggressive lipid lowering therapy. *J Human Hypertens* 2001; **15**: 431–433.

24. Yonemura K, Ikegaya N, Fujigaki Y *et al.* Potential therapeutic effect of simvastatin on progressive renal failure and nephrotic range proteinuria caused by renal cholesterol embolism. *Am J Med Sci* 2001; **322**: 50–52.

25. Fried LF, Orchard TJ, Kasiske BL for the Lipids and Renal Disease Progression Meta-Analysis Study Group. *Kidney Int* 2001; **59**: 260–269.

26. Chabova V, Schirger A, Stanson AW *et al.* Outcomes of atherosclerotic renal artery stenosis managed without revascularisation. *Mayo Clin Proc* 2000; **75**: 437–444.

27. Leertouwer TC, Gussenhoven EJ, Bosch JL *et al.* Stent placement for renal artery stenosis: where do we stand? A meta-analysis. *Radiology* 2000; **78**: 78–85.

28. Perkovic V, Thomson KR, Mitchell PJ *et al.* Treatment of renovascular disease with percutaneous stent insertion: long term outcomes. *Austral Radiol* 2001; **45**: 438–443.

29 Henry M, Amor M, Henry I *et al.* Stent placement in the renal artery: Three year experience with the Palmaz stent. *J Vasc Interv Radiol* 1996; **7**: 343–350.

30. Blum U, Krumme B, Flugel P *et al.* Treatment of ostial renal artery stenosis with vascular endoprostheses after successful balloon angioplasty. *N Engl J Med* 1997; **336**: 459–465.

31. Hamilton G. Early and late failure of endovascular renal artery repair. In: Branchereau A, Jacobs M (eds). *Complications in Vascular and Endovascular Surgery* Part II. Armonk, NY: Futura Publishing Company Inc. 2002: 195–217.

32. Beutler JJ, van Ampting JMA, van de Ven PJG *et al.* Long term effects of arterial stenting on kidney function for patients with ostial atherosclerotic renal artery stenosis and renal insufficiency. *J Am Soc Nephrol* 2001; **12**: 1475–1481.

33. Webster J, Marshall F, Abdalla M *et al.* Randomised comparison of percutaneous angioplasty vs continued medical therapy for hypertensive patients with atheromatous renal artery stenosis. Scottish and Newcastle Renal Artery Stenosis Collaborative Group. *J Hum Hypertens* 1998; **12**: 329–335.

34. Ploiun PF, Chatellier G, Darne B, Raynaud A. Blood pressure outcome of angioplasty in atherosclerotic renal artery stenosis: a randomised trial. Essai Multicentrique Medicaments vs Angioplastie (EMMA) Study Group. *Hypertension* 1998; **31**: 823–829.

35. van Jaarsveld BC, Krijnen P, Pieterman H *et al.* The effect of balloon angioplasty on hypertension in atherosclerotic renal artery stenosis. Dutch Renal Artery Stenosis Intervention Cooperative Group. *N Engl J Med* 2000; **342**: 1007–1014.

36. van de Ven PJ, Kaatee R, Beutler JJ *et al.* Arterial stenting and balloon angioplasty in ostial atherosclerotic renovascular disease: a randomised trial. *Lancet* 1999; **353**: 282–286.

37. Farmer CKT, Reidy J, Kalra PA *et al.* Individual kidney function before and after angioplasty. *Lancet* 1998; **352**: 288–289.

38. Plouin PF, Rossignol P, Bobrie G. Atherosclerotic renal artery stenosis: to treat conservatively, to dilate, to stent, or to operate? *J Am Soc Nephrol* 2001; **12**: 2190–2196.

Medicine beats angioplasty and stent for renal artery stenosis

Against the motion

Jon G Moss

Introduction

Atherosclerotic renal artery stenosis is a common condition affecting up to 53% of unselected patients at postmortem.[1] It is particularly prevalent in patients with other co-morbid vascular disease (coronary, cerebrovascular and peripheral vascular disease). In this population it is frequently overlooked or simply ignored. This cynicism has developed over the last 20 years and has been reinforced by the poor results achieved in three recent randomized controlled trials comparing angioplasty with best medical treatment in patients with hypertension.[2–4]

However, all three trials showed a trend in favour of angioplasty (albeit with wide confidence limits) and were underpowered to detect a small but clinically important benefit from angioplasty. In addition these trials predated the stenting era. Furthermore, the high crossover rate from the medical arm to the angioplasty arm made analysis by the intention to treat principle unreliable. A recent meta-analysis of these trials showed a small but significant improvement in systolic blood pressure (Fig. 1) but

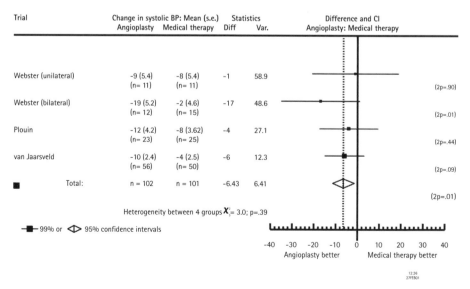

Figure 1. Change in systolic blood pressure (between baseline and 6 months): angioplasty versus medical treatment. Reproduced with permission from Ref. 5.

217

only a trend supporting angioplasty for diastolic blood pressure.[5] A larger trial is needed to confirm any perceived blood pressure benefit from angioplasty and these small studies should not be overinterpreted.

Atherosclerotic renal artery stenosis has more recently been linked with progressive renal failure. It has been estimated that atherosclerotic renal artery stenosis accounts for at least 15% of patients entering a renal dialysis programme. In patients aged over 60 years it is the commonest cause responsible for 25% of renal replacement treatment.[6] The potential to modify or halt this process by angioplasty and or stenting has become a major focus of clinical research (ASTRAL and STAR trials).

Although there are many uncontrolled studies showing atherosclerotic renal artery stenosis to be a progressive disease it was not until the landmark work from Strandness`s group in Seattle using ultrasound that this was fully accepted. Using Doppler ultrasound in a prospective series of patients they showed that <60% stenoses had a 42% of progressing to >60%, and >60% lesions had a 11% chance of progressing to occlusion over a 2-year follow-up period (Fig. 2).[7]

Scoble and the group at Guys hospital (London) using a dual radioisotope technique to measure individual glomerular filtration rate in a group of patients showed that once a renal artery occludes renal function is all but lost – being reduced to a paltry 2.6 ml/min (mean).[8]

It is worth assembling these separate pieces of vital information to get the message across. Atherosclerotic renal artery stenosis is a prevalent progressive disease, which can lead to occlusion of the renal artery with likely loss of any useful function from that kidney. The argument to prevent this process by angioplasty or stenting is strong.

Previous research has shown that approximately 70% of patients have stable or improved renal function 1 month after renal stent placement.[9,10] Examination of reciprocal serum creatinine plots in a small uncontrolled series indicated that renal artery stenting was associated with a four-fold reduction in the rate of progression of renal failure after stent placement (Fig. 3).[10]

Much of the published literature has focused on the results of angioplasty without stenting. Of the 210 patients in the three randomized controlled blood pressure trials only two received a stent in addition to angioplasty.[2-4] The Dutch randomized trial compared the technical and patency outcomes of angioplasty and stenting and showed a clear and significant superiority in favour of stents (Table 1); indeed the trial was stopped prematurely.[11] Unfortunately this trial was not powered to look at any clinical outcomes. However, it is reasonable to postulate that the clinical benefit from stenting may be superior to angioplasty alone.

On occasion a patient will present with acute renal failure due to occlusion of the renal artery where the presence of collaterals maintains tissue viability but not function (Fig. 4a–b). Restoring blood flow with a stent can sometimes dramatically restore

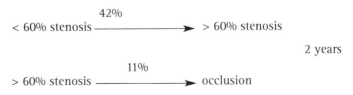

Figure 2. The probability of a < 60% stenosis and a > 60% stenosis progressing over a 2-year period.[7]

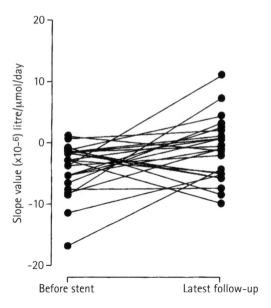

Figure 3. Reciprocal serum creatinine plots for 23 patients with atherosclerotic renal artery stenosis before and after renal stenting. Zero denotes stable renal function, negative values deteriorating and positive improving renal function. The mean (SE) of the slopes of reciprocal serum creatinine values was −4.34 (0.85) litre/μmol/day before stent placement and −0.55(1.0) litre /μmol /day after stent placement (p<0.01). Reproduced with permission from Ref.10.

Table 1. Random controlled trials comparing stents with angioplasty in 85 patients[11]

	Stents	Angioplasty
Technical success	88%	57%
Primary 6-month patency	75%	29%

renal function in this situation (Fig. 4c). It is difficult to envisage a role for medical treatment in this scenario.

Flash pulmonary oedema is an ill understood condition where atherosclerotic renal artery stenosis impedes the ability of the kidneys to excrete sodium and water causing fluid overload. Often there is diastolic cardiac dysfunction but normal systolic function. Angioplasty or stenting has been shown to reverse this process by revascularization in some but not all patients and again few would argue to withhold stenting in this situation.

The use of ACE inhibitors and angiotensin II receptor antagonists has increased as trials have demonstrated clear benefits in clinical conditions such as cardiac failure. The presence of atherosclerotic renal artery stenosis may precipitate acute renal failure with these drugs as the angiotensin effect on the efferent arteriole is blocked reducing perfusion pressure to a critical level. Correcting the stenosis by angioplasty or stenting can allow these important drugs to be reinstated. Once again there is no medical alternative in this situation.

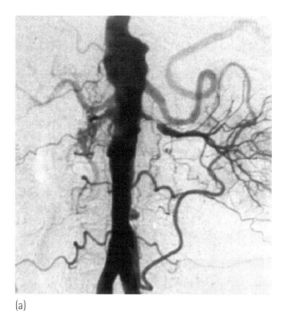

(a)

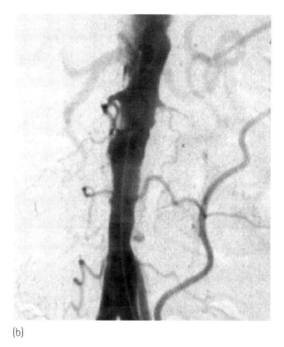

(b)

Figure 4a,b. Initial aortogram (a) shows an occluded right renal artery and a severely stenosed left renal artery. The patient presented 2 months later with acute renal failure requiring dialysis (b).

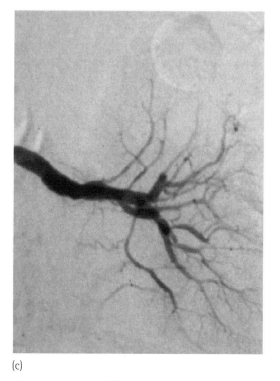

(c)

Figure 4c. The left renal artery was stented (c) and the patient's renal function recovered.

Technique

The technique is fairly standardized and has been described elsewhere.[12] Most operators will require some preoperative imaging (usually a magnetic resonance angiogram), which will help decide upon the access route (usually femoral). Patients should be kept well hydrated before and after the procedure.

Critics of endovascular renal revascularization often quote high complication rates from the literature. However, the technique has developed over the years due to technological advances borrowed from the carotid stent experience and indeed is still evolving. Examples of recent advances and their potential benefits are shown below.

1. Small platform stents – less traumatic probably less atheroembolism
   – smaller, fewer groin complications.
2. Carbon dioxide contrast – eradicates risk of contrast nephropathy.
3. Renoprotective drugs – reduces incidence of contrast nephropathy.
4. Protection devices – under evaluation, but likely to reduce atheroembolism.
5. Covered stents – permit endovascular treatment of vessel rupture.

Atheroembolism undoubtedly occurs during any form of revascularization. Largely anecdotal work in the carotid territory using small platform stents and particularly protection systems suggests these reduce the risk of atheroembolic stroke. It seems reasonable to assume that these measures will also reduce atheroembolism in the kidney. Although protection devices have been used for renal stenting a dedicated device is still not available.[13]

When serious complications do occur such as renal artery perforation covered stents allow an endovascular solution avoiding surgery in this high-risk population.

Medical treatment

The argument for using drug treatment alone is weak. No drug has been shown to improve renal function in atherosclerotic renal artery stenosis and once the artery has occluded a mechanical solution is the only option that offers some potential to recover renal function. Although the hypertension trials suggested no overall gain from angioplasty the studies were too small. In addition up to 50% of those randomized to drug treatment subsequently 'crossed over' and underwent angioplasty making the interpretation of the data from an intention to treat principle difficult. Small underpowered trials always have the potential to fail to detect important clinical differences between two treatments.

Summary

- Atherosclerotic renal artery stenosis is a progressive disease which can lead to vessel occlusion with loss of renal function.

- Atherosclerotic renal artery stenosis is the commonest aetiology for patients aged over 60 requiring dialysis.

- Atherosclerotic renal artery stenosis causes flash pulmonary oedema and can prevent use of ACE inhibitors.

- Stenting has a high technical success and patency rate.

- Complications have reduced with technological and other advances.

- Meta-analysis has shown trends in favour of revascularization over drugs alone.

- ASTRAL trial is randomizing 1000 to further investigate the effect of stenting on renal function.

References

1. Holley KE, Hunt JC, Brown AL et al. Renal artery stenosis: a clinical-pathological study in normotensive and hypertensive patients. Am J Med 1964; 37: 14–22.
2. Plouin P-F, Chatellier G, Darne B et al. Blood pressure outcome of angioplasty in atherosclerotic renal artery stenosis. Hypertension 1998; 31: 823–829.
3. Webster J, Marshall F, Abdalla M et al. Randomised comparison of percutaneous angioplasty vs continued medical therapy for hypertensive patients with atheromatous renal artery stenosis. J Hum Hypertens 1998; 12: 329–335.
4. Van Jaarsveld BC, Krijnen P, Pieterman H et al. The effects of balloon angioplasty on hypertension in atherosclerotic renal artery stenosis. N Engl J Med 2000; 342: 1007–1014.

5. Ives N, Wheatley K, Gray R. Continuing uncertainty about the value of revascularisation in atherosclerotic renovascular disease: a meta-analysis of previous trials. *Nephrol Dial Transplant* 2003; 18: 298–304.
6. Mailloux LU, Napolitano B, Belluci AG *et al*. Renal vascular disease causing end-stage renal disease, incidence, clinical correlates and outcomes: a 20 year clinical experience. *Am J Kidney Dis* 1994; 24: 622–629.
7. Zierler RE, Bergelin RO, Isaacson JA *et al*. Natural history of atherosclerotic renal artery stenosis: A prospective study with duplex ultrasonography. *J Vasc Surg* 1994; 19: 250–258.
8. Scoble JE, Mikhail A, Reidy J, Cook GJR. Individual kidney function in atherosclerotic renal artery disease. *Nephrol Dial Transplant* 1998; 13: 1048–1049.
9. Rees CR, Palmaz JC, Becker GJ. Palmaz stent in atherosclerotic stenoses involving the ostia of the renal arteries: preliminary report of a multicentre study. *Radiology* 1991; 181: 507–514.
10. Harden PN, Macleod MJ, Rodger RS *et al*. Effect of renal-artery stenting on progression of renovascular renal failure. *Lancet* 1997; 349: 1133–1136.
11. Van de ven PJG, Kaatee R, Beutler JJ *et al*. Arterial stenting and balloon angioplasty in ostial atherosclerotic renovascular disease: a randomised trial. *Lancet* 1999; 353: 282–286.
12. Moss JG. Renal artery lesions should be treated by angioplasty and stent. *The Evidence for Vascular or Endovascular Reconstruction*. London: Saunders, 2002; 215–221.
13. Henry M, Klonaris C, Henry I *et al*. Protective renal artery stenting with the PercuSurge GuideWire device: a pilot study. *J Endovasc Ther* 2001; 8: 227–237.

Medicine beats angioplasty and stent for renal artery stenosis

Charing Cross Editorial Comments towards Consensus

The authors refer mainly to atherosclerotic renal artery stenosis and George Hamilton argues that essential hypertension forms a major part of renal vascular hypertension and does not respond to renal revascularization. He also argues that progression from renal artery stenosis to renal failure is not as common as previously described and in any case the patients mostly die of other vascular causes ahead of renal failure. He stresses the high procedural morbidity for renal stent angioplasty and says that available data show no significant benefit for stent angioplasty in preservation of renal function. Mr Hamilton concludes that the best medical treatment is at least as effective in preservation of renal function without the risks of angioplasty and embolism.

John Moss refers to the important Astral Trial in which a thousand patients are being randomized in order to investigate the effect of stenting on renal function. He comments also on the Star Trial and states that meta-analysis has shown trends in favour of revascularization over drugs alone. He draws attention to the high technical success and patency rate following renal artery stenting.

This will be an ideal debate to remind and inform on the latest renal artery stenosis thinking.

Roger M Greenhalgh
Editor

Renal angioplasty needs protection

For the motion

M Henry, I Henry, PC Rath, G Lakshmi, R Shiram, C Klonaris, M Hugel

Introduction

A renal artery stenosis can result in renovascular hypertension. It accounts for 1–2% of all cases of hypertension[1] and it is one of the important causes of correctable hypertension. A renal artery stenosis can also lead to renal insufficiency, cardiac failure with pulmonary oedema, and unstable angina.

Endovascular treatment is now a well accepted alternative for revascularization[2-3] and the first treatment to be proposed.

This method has been proposed as the standard for care for non-ostial renal artery stenosis and although initial studies concerning the treatment of ostial lesions yielded varying results,[4-5] recent series suggest that vascular endoprostheses are highly effective in the ostial segment with an excellent procedural success rate (98–100%), a good long-term angiographic stent patency rate of 86–92% and a low complication rate.[6-12] The benefit of angioplasty for renal artery stenosis includes complete cure or at least easier management of hypertension in addition to preservation or improvement of renal function.[13]

However, post-procedural deterioration of the renal function occurs in a subset of patients after percutaneous renal angioplasty.[14-16] Atheroembolism during the procedure has been implicated as a precipitating factor for this complication.[17-19]

In order to eliminate or reduce the risk of atheroembolic material being carried into the renal parenchyma, we applied a novel technique consisting of balloon angioplasty and stenting under protection with distal balloon protection or filters, a concept currently being evaluated in carotid artery angioplasty.

Material and methods

Patients characteristics

From January 1999 to October 2002, 61 renal artery stenoses were treated in 52 patients with hypertension (32 males, 20 females), mean age 67.7±11.5 years (22–87) who were diagnosed with atherosclerotic renal artery stenosis by renal duplex scanning and digital subtraction angiography; they were treated with percutaneous angioplasty and stenting under distal embolic protection. Because of the currently available dimensions of the device, patients with renal artery diameter > 6 mm were excluded for occlusion balloon and patients with renal artery diameter > 5.5 mm excluded for filters, as were patients with bifurcated or trifurcated renal arteries in which the lesion was positioned < 2 cm from the division. Written informed consents were obtained from all patients in this study.

One bilateral procedure was performed in eight patients, and we treated two renal arteries on the same side in one patient.

Five patients had a solitary or single functioning kidney; 34 patients had normal baseline renal function (serum creatinine ≥1.4 mg/dl), 13 had moderate renal insufficiency (serum creatinine 1.5–1.9 mg/dl) and five had severe renal dysfunction (serum creatinine ≥2.0 mg/dl). The renal artery stenosis was located at the ostiums in 56 cases. Mean diameter stenosis was 84.0±8.5% (70–95%). Mean lesion length was 11.6±3.1 mm (8–29). The diameter of the artery was estimated at 6 mm 38 arteries and 5 mm in 23 arteries; 35 patients had diffuse severe atherosclerosis of the abdominal aorta; 11 patients had diabetes mellitus; 36 were current smokers; 32 had hyperlipidaemia; 33 associated coronary diseases. Cerebrovascular diseases were found in 12 and peripheral artery diseases in 22.

Protected renal angioplasty/stenting techniques

Placement of a guiding catheter at the renal ostium

All procedures were performed under local anaesthesia and intravenous sedation. A 7 or 8 F guiding catheter was placed at the ostium of the renal artery via a percutaneous femoral approach in all patients except one presenting with total occlusion of both iliac arteries, necessitating a humeral approach. In case of high grade lesions or those with acute angles between the aorta and the renal artery, a coaxial technique with a 5F Simmons type selective catheter placed inside the guiding catheter was used to catheterize the renal artery. The lesions were then crossed with a coronary 0.014 inch wire. The guiding catheter was slowly advanced at the renal ostium over the Simmons catheter and then the coronary wire and the Simmons catheter were both removed.

Placement of the protection devices

Two types of protection devices were used:

Occlusion balloon

The Guardwire system (Medtronic Minneapolis, MN, USA) is the same as that used for carotid protection. The technique has been previously described.[20] The Guardwire consists of three components:

1. The Guardwire temporary occlusion catheter is a 0.014 or 0.018 inch hollow tube angioplasty wire made of nitinol. Incorporated into its distal segment is an inflatable, compliant elastometric balloon with a radiopaque marker. The diameter of the balloon (5–6 mm) is chosen depending on the diameter of the artery. The distal 3.5 cm of the wire is floppy and shapable. The wire is available in lengths of 190 and 300 cm, allowing monorail or over-the-wire techniques for angioplasty and stenting.
2. The proximal end of the hypotube wire incorporates a Microseal device that keeps the elastometric balloon inflated to protect the kidney from

atheroembolism during intraluminal manoeuvres and at the same time allows catheter exchange at the proximal end, similar to commonly used guidewires.
3. The 5.2F export aspiration catheter is placed over the shaft of the Guardwire prior to distal balloon deflation to aspirate the debris through a 1 mm sidehole. This catheter is tapered to the guidewire to avoid the risk of debris generation or stent dislodgment during its advancement into the renal artery.

The Percusurge technique was used in 38 procedures (Figs 1, 2).

Filters
Two types of filters were used in our series :

1. EPI Filter wires (Boston Scientific, Natick Mass, USA) in 22 patients (Figs 3, 4).
2. Angioguard Filters (Cordis Corporation, Warren NJ, USA) in one patient.

The filters have pores of 80–120 microns (µ) allowing a permanent flow during the procedure. They are highly flexible with good steerability and trackability. The radiopaque loop (EPI) and the radiopaque markers (EPI, Angioguard) allow an easy placement into the renal arteries. EPI filter is a monorail system facilitating the procedure as for a coronary procedure.

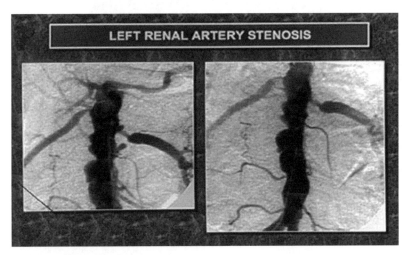

Figure 1. Left renal artery stenosis.

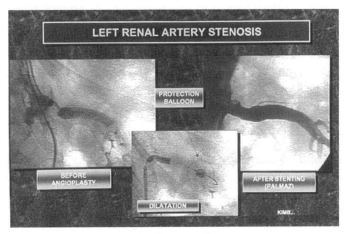

Figure 2. Renal angioplasty under protection (Percusurge).

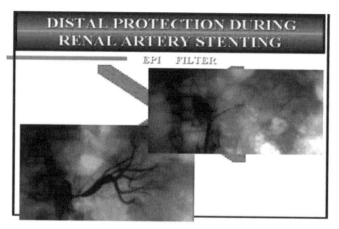

Figure 3. Left renal artery stenosis. EPI filter.

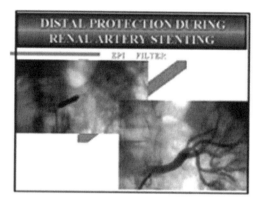

Figure 4. Renal angioplasty under protection (EPI filter).

With the guiding catheter appropriately positioned, the protection device is carefully advanced across the lesions and positioned 2 or 3 cm beyond the target site. With a Percusurge device, the Microseal adapter is attached and the occlusion balloon inflated to occlude the renal artery. On detaching the adapter, the occlusion balloon remains inflated. With a filter, it is deployed by removing carefully the sheath delivery. Contrast injection checks the good positioning of the protection device.

Stenting

A predilatation of the stenosis under protection was done for 17 tight calcified ostial stenoses and for the five non-ostial lesions. A direct stenting was done for 39 ostial lesions. The non-ostial lesions were stented because of the significant residual stenosis post-dilatation. For ostial lesions, care was taken to position the stent so that it would protrude slightly into the aortic lumen ~1–2 mm. The proximal part is flared. Different stents models were used. Because we were familiar with each of those stent types, no specific selection criteria were applied.

Protection device retrieval

Percusurge device

After stent deployment, the aspiration catheter was advanced over the wire to the level of the lesion and positioned adjacent to the protection balloon. Any debris was removed using a 20 ml syringe connected to the proximal end of this catheter. Two aspirations were performed. After removing the aspiration catheter, the Microseal adapter was reattached to the Guardwire and the occlusion balloon deflated allowing normal vessel flow. If the angiographic result was satisfactory, the device was removed.

Filters

Angiographic control was performed after stent deployment. If the result was satisfactory, the filter was withdrawn with the removal sheath. To facilitate protection, device withdrawal, and prevent it from getting caught on the stent, the guiding catheter was routinely advanced into the stent up its distal end. The aspirated blood or the filters were sent to the laboratory for analysis.

Medications – patients surveillance

Before the procedure, patients were given ticlopidine (500 mg) or clopidogrel (75 mg/day) and aspirin (100 mg/day). During the procedure, an intravenous bolus of 5000 units of unfractioned heparin and 3 mg of cefamandole nitrate were routinely administrated at the beginning of the procedure.

The post-procedural drug regimen included aspirin (100 mg/day) indefinitely and ticlopidine (250 mg/day) or clopidogrel (75 mg/day) for 1 month. Patients remained in the hospital for 48 hours to monitor serum creatinine levels and adjust blood pressure medications. Renal duplex scanning was scheduled the day after the procedure, at 6 and 12 months and then annually. Angiography was performed when a restenosis was suspected on the basis of positive clinical and duplex scan findings. Serum creatinine values were measured before and after the procedure (day 1) and at 1 and 6 months, with bi-annual measurements thereafter.

Definitions and statistical analyses

Ostial lesions were defined as stenoses >50% occurring within 5 mm of the aortic lumen as assessed by arteriography.[10]

Immediate technical success was defined as residual stenosis < 30% of the reference diameter (measured by quantitative angiographic analysis) without significant periprocedural complications.

Inability to successfully place the Guardwire at the correct position to protect the kidney throughout the procedure was considered to be a failure of the device.

Duplex criteria for restenosis were a loss of the early systolic notch and a systolic velocity > 1.5m/s. The angiographic criterion for restenosis was the development of luminal narrowing >50% of the reference diameter.

Reversal of hypertension was defined as diastolic blood pressure <90 mmHg and no need for any medication. Improvement corresponded to a diastolic pressure of 91–109 mmHg with at least 15% decrease from the preprocedural level or a diastolic pressure of 91–109 mmHg with decline of at least 10% from the preprocedural level and withdrawal of at least one drug from the treatment regimen.[21]

Moderate renal insufficiency was defined as baseline serum creatinine from 1.5 to 1.9 mg/dl, a value ≥2.0 mg/dl was categorized as severe insufficiency.[10,22] A decrease >0.2 mg/dl from the preprocedural creatinine values represented an improvement, whereas values within ±0.2 mg/dl of baseline were considered unchanged. An increase >0.2 mg/dl was considered as deterioration in renal function.[22]

Determination of vessel diameter was made by sizing the guiding catheter against the normal vessel distal to the lesion using quantitative analysis.

Continuous data are presented as mean ±SD and categorical data as percentages.

Statistical differences between groups were determined by the Student's *t* test.

Statistical significance was taken at p < 0.05

All calculations were performed with the SPSS Program (SPSS Version 7.5, Chicago, IL, USA).

Results

All stenoses were easily crossed with the protection devices either Guardwire or filters thanks to their low profile and good flexibility. We had no difficulty deflating the occlusion balloon and removing the protection devices.

Different stent models were used: Cordis P154 (n=6), Corinthian (n=11), Genesis (n=10), M3 (n=2), Medtronic Ave (n=15), Nir (n=15), Herculink (n=13), Biotronik (n=1).

Some patients required two stents in the same artery to treat a long lesion. Technical success was obtained for all arteries (100%) with good stent deployment, no significant residual stenosis, and complete covering of the lesion.

Mean renal artery occlusion time with the Percusurge technique was 6.46±2.42 min.

When stents were deployed primarily, mean occlusion time was 5.02±1.53 min. In cases of predilatation and subsequent stenting (necessiting aspiration, deflation of the balloon, angiographic control and reinflation of the balloon), the mean occlusion time was 7.57±2.48 min.

The mean time *in situ* for filters was 4.20±1.10 min, shorter than with occlusion balloon.

Two patients developed an arterial spasm (one with the Percusurge device, one with an EPI filter) at the site of the protection device, which immediately responded to local vasodilatation therapy.

We have never seen a dissection of the vessel artery due to a protection device.

Particulate analysis

With the Percusurge technique and the aspiration catheter, we aspirated visible debris in all patients (the same as for the carotid procedures).

The aspirated blood samples were analysed and studied by microscopy and scanning electron microscopy. Different particles were isolated and identified. Their number varied from 13 to 208 per procedure (mean 98.1±60.0), and diameter ranged from 38 to 6206 μm (mean 201.2±76.2 μm). Excluding one 6.2 mm fragment, the mean particle diameter was 188.0±49.8 μm. In cases of direct stenting, the average number of extracted particles per procedure was 112.0±73.5. When predilatation of the lesion was performed, the mean particle number was 86.0±47.0 (p=0.36). Also, we did not notice a significant statistical difference between the mean diameters of the particles after direct stenting or after predilatation (190±44.5 mm vs 210.0±96.0 mm, respectively, p=0.56).

For the three non-ostial lesions, aspiration was performed both after angioplasty and after stenting, and more particles were collected with the second aspiration (64 vs 80). The particles were atheromatous plaques, cholesterol crystals, necrotic cores, fibrin, thrombi, platelets, and macrophage foam cells. With filters we removed visible debris in 70% of the cases. Two filters were totally blocked by large particles, with a flow totally interrupted. The flow was restored after removal of the filter. One patient was 26 years old.

Follow-up

The mean follow-up period was 23.8±15.6 months (2–46 months). In all cases, follow-up was beyond the period for development of clinical manifestations of atheroembolism.

Three patients died from myocardial infarction, one at day 3 (a patient who underwent coronary angioplasty before renal stenting) one at 6 months and one at 1 year follow-up.

Two patients were lost to follow-up after one year. Table 1 shows the mean value for urea and creatinine preprocedurally (J-1) and after the procedure (J+1), at 1 month, 6 months, 1 year and 3 years. There is no statistically significant difference during the follow-up.

Table 1. Effects on renal function

	No. of patients	Urea mean value g/litre	Creatinine mean value mg/litre	p Value
J – 1	52	0.43±0.17	13.43±4.34	
J + 1	52	0.39±0.15	12.42±4.26	
J + 30	51	0.42±0.13	13.29±4.00	NS
J + 180	41	0.44±0.12	11.62±2.89	
2 years	28	0.40±0.12	11.06±2.43	
3 years	19	0.52±0.23	12.65±4.42	

Table 2 shows the effects on the renal function at 6 months, 2 and 3 years in patients with normal renal function and in patients with moderate and severe renal insufficiency.

Table 2. Effects on renal function

	6 Months				2 Years				3 Years			
	No. of patients	Stabilization	I	D	No. of patients	Stabilization	I	D	No. of patients	Stabilization	I	D
Normal renal function	31	31			19	18		1*	12	11		1*
Moderate renal insufficiency	11	6		5	7	2	4	1	6	1	4	1
Severe renal insufficiency	3			3	2		2		1		1	
Total	45	37	8	0	28	20	6	2	19	12	5	2

I: Improvement of renal function; D: Deterioration of renal function.   * Patient with bilateral angioplasty (one without protection)

At 6 months (41 patients), we observed no deterioration of the renal function and seven improvements in patients with renal insufficiency.

At 2 years (28 patients), and 3 years (19 patients), we observed only two deteriorations of the renal function.

1. One in a patient with normal renal function before the procedure, normal renal function at 6 months follow-up and who developed a renal insufficiency at 2 years. This patient was treated for bilateral stenosis, one side without protection.
2. One in a patient with moderate renal insufficiency.

Six patients remained improved at 2 years, and five at 3 years.

Table 3 shows the effects of the procedure on hypertension. Systolic and diastolic blood pressure dropped significantly. The number of medications also declined significantly. Nine patients were cured, 31 improved, and 12 remained unchanged.

Table 3. Effects on blood pressure

	Before procedure mmHg	After procedure mmHg	Mean reduction mmHg	p Value
Systolic blood pressure	169±15.1	149.8±12.3	19.2±9.4	p<0.01
Diastolic blood pressure	104±13	92.8±6.7	11.2±8.7	p<0.01
Number of medications	2.31±0.7	1.19±0.8	1.12±0.7	p<0.01

Discussion

Renal artery stenosis is more and more diagnosed in patients suffering from hypertension and renal insufficiency thanks to non-invasive diagnostic techniques (duplex-scan, CT scan, MRI) but also to systematic renal angiography performed during cardiac catheterization, coronary procedures and particularly in hypertensive, or multivascular diseased patients. The prevalence of renal artery stenosis is high. Rihal[23] found a renal artery stenosis >50% in 19.2% of patients during cardiac catheterization of 297 hypertensive patients (bilateral in 3.7%; stenosis >70% in 7% of patients). The natural history of renal artery stenosis is to progress over time resulting in renal artery occlusion, loss of renal mass, and subsequent decrease in kidney function. Vessels with the most severe stenoses result in total occlusion in 16% of patients.[24-26] So some authors advocate early stenting for significant renal artery stenosis.[22-27]

The treatment of a renal artery stenosis includes medical therapy, balloon angioplasty and surgery. Surgery remains at high-risk with a 2–7% perioperative mortality rate, a 17–31% morbidity and deterioration in renal function in 11–31% of patients, with reocclusion or restenosis in 3–4%.[28-30]

Percutaneous transluminal renal angioplasty (PTRA) technique has become the corner-stone for the therapeutic strategy for addressing renal artery stenosis and is now the first treatment to be proposed. Several series reported the successful use of endovascular stents for treating suboptimal angioplasty results and as a primary intervention for atherosclerotic lesions and particularly ostial lesions with better immediate and long-term results than with PTA alone.[7-11,14,31-33]

The procedural success in these studies is excellent (98–100%) with a low complications rate[8,9,32] and a long-term patency rate of 85–98%. The benefits of PTRA are complete cure (7–19%) or at least easier management of hypertension (52–74%), stabilization or improvement of renal function.

Recent studies regarding the effects of PTRA or stenting on renal function show that a large percentage of patients seem to benefit from the procedure, with a stabilization or improvement in renal function.[8–12,22,34–36] Renal stenting in selected patients could slow the progression of renovascular renal failure and may delay the need for renal replacement therapy.[37] Nevertheless, there is a high mortality rate in patients with severe impairment of renal function despite successful treatment of renal artery stenoses.[38–39] An earlier diagnosis and treatment of renal artery stenosis may lead to better outcome.

In many of the published series, a decline in renal function was noted in a subset of patients even after successful initial technical results. Harden,[37] in a series of 32 patients with chronic renal insufficiency, found improvement or stabilization of renal function in 69% of patients but deterioration in 31%. Dorros et al.[14] used primary stent placement for atherosclerotic renal artery stenosis in 76 patients. The 6-month follow-up showed that serum creatinine values improved in 30%, were unchanged in 48% and deteriorated in 22% of the patients. A deterioration of the renal function was observed in only 5% of patients with normal renal function, but in 42% of patients with a creatinine between 1.5 and 1.9 mg/dl and 47% in patients with a creatinine >2 mg/dl.

In a later study[22] of 141 patients, with 6-month follow-up, they reported that renal function stabilized or improved in the two-thirds of unilateral stenosis patients, whereas one-third had an increase in creatinine by >0.2 mg/dl above baseline. Lack of complete angiographic follow-up limited their understanding of the worsening renal function in patients with normal baseline creatinine after successful revascularization.

Isles et al.[40] published a series of ten studies examining 416 stent placement procedures in 379 patients treated for renal artery stenosis. The technical success was high in all studies (96–100%), renal function improved in 26%, stabilized in 48%, but deteriorated in 26% of the patients. Subramanian et al.[41] observed a worsening in renal function in 24% of non-diabetic patients and 27% of diabetic patients with renal insufficiency at 47.4±31.2 months post-renal stenting.

Recently, Guerrero[42] in a retrospective series of 72 consecutive patients reported a deterioration of the renal function in 7% of the patients with normal creatinine, and in 31% of patients with renal insufficiency.

Many factors may account for this functional deterioration: contrast media-induced nephrotoxicity progression of concomitant nephrosclerosis, lesion recurrence, exposure of the diseased glomeruli to high arterial pressure after the procedure with disease acceleration. Atheroembolism during the procedure could also play an important role. Cholesterol atheromatous embolism is an increasingly recognized cause of acute renal failure.[43] These embolisms are caused by the release of microscopic plaque fragments and cholesterol crystals from the renal artery lesion or the atherosclerotic aorta into parenchymal renal vasculature during the procedure.[43–46] Instrument manipulation in the aorta and renal arteries can result in detachment and embolism of atheromatous debris from ulcerated plaques. The large size of the devices used, increased length or specific difficulties of the procedure may be contributory. Walker[47] recently demonstrated the great potential for embolic debris during the placement of the guiding catheter, sheath or diagnostic catheter. He performed an aggressive aspiration of the guiding catheter or sheath before any contrast injection. Large particles of atherosclerotic debris (1–3 mm) were discovered in 41.7% of the patients.

Patients with severe atheromatous disease of the aorta and its branches, ulcerated plaques, associated lesions such as aneurysm, dissection, are candidates or these complications. Oral and intravenous anticoagulants and thrombolytic drugs can also induce atheroembolism.[48-49]

The true incidence of atheroembolism is uncertain because many patients can have a silent course because of the large functional kidney reserve, which allows normal serum creatinine values despite a significant decline in total glomerular filtration. Therefore only the most severe cases may be detected, especially in patients with pre-procedural renal dysfunction and limited functional reserve. If in a normal kidney 50% of the nephrons are destroyed, we observe only little or no change in renal function.

Few studies have addressed the problem of atheroembolism after renal artery interventions, but, interestingly, it was the predominant complication in all of them. Boisclair *et al.*[16] published their results of successful stent placement in 33 patients either for immediate angioplasty failure or recurrent stenosis. Seven patients developed complications, including four with renal artery emboli. In another study, Van de Ven *et al.*[17] reported that after successful stenting in 24 patients with an atherosclerotic ostial renal artery stenosis, two developed renal insufficiency due to cholesterol embolism. Wilms *et al.*[19] observed two cases of renal deterioration, including a case of massive cholesterol embolism, among 11 patients with stent-supported renal angioplasty.

Commeau[50] reported recently an acute deterioration of renal function due to cholesterol embolism and necessitating hemodialysis. Morice[51] also published two cases of partial renal infarctions in a series of 80 patients.

Clinical manifestations of the disease are also non-specific. Thadhani *et al.*[52] retrospectively evaluated 52 patients with both renal failure and histologically proven atheroembolism after angiography or cardiovascular surgery over a 10-year period. Within 30 days of their procedure, 50% of the patients had cutaneous signs of atheroembolism and 14% had documented blood eosinophilia. Most patients reach a peak serum creatinine level over 3–8 weeks[53] but onset is usually sooner.[16] Although proteinuria and nephrotic syndrome are uncommon, Haqqie *et al.*[53] reported four patients with histopathologically documented atheroembolism who developed nephrotic-range proteinuria. They suggested that atheroembolism should be considered in the differential diagnosis of nephrotic syndrome in elderly patients with serious vascular disease. Similar conclusions were made by Greenberg *et al.*[54] after reviewing the clinical features and histological findings of 24 patients found to have cholesterol atheroembolism at renal biopsy; 19 had recently undergone an invasive vascular procedure.

Atheroembolism can give rise to different degrees of renal impairment:

1. Only a moderate loss of renal function.
2. Severe renal failure requiring dialysis.
3. Acute sceneries with abrupt and sudden onset of renal failure.
4. More frequently a progressive loss of renal function over weeks (3–8 weeks).
5. Chronic stable and asymptomatic renal insufficiency.

Even in cases with high clinical suspicion, the diagnosis of atheroembolism is difficult to establish using routine laboratory tests. Renal biopsy is the only definitive diagnostic tool; although it is valuable to exclude other potentially treatable disease processes, its routine application for confirmation of a disease amenable only to supportive treatment is problematic. For these reasons, it is not surprising that atheroembolism after renal artery interventions is often misdiagnosed as drug-induced nephrotoxicity or the progression of nephrosclerosis.

Renal atheroembolism definitely poses a risk of renal function deterioration and decreased survival in patients undergoing endovascular procedures for renal artery stenosis. Due to the increasing number of such patients, the cost of renal function deterioration and subsequent end-stage renal disease requiring dialysis represents a significant long-term problem. Its importance is clearly demonstrated in a recent work by Krishnamurthi et al.,[55] who evaluated its impact on survival in 44 patients who had surgery for atherosclerotic renal artery stenosis and concomitant intraoperative renal biopsy for detection of atheroemboli. Atheroembolic disease was identified in the biopsy specimens in 16 (36%) patients and correlated significantly with decreased survival (54% 5-year survival in this group versus 85% in patients without atheroembolism, p=0.011).

Boero[56] recently pointed out the bad prognosis of renal atheroembolism. In a series of 22 patients with an onset of symptoms from few hours to 60 days, 11 patients (50%) were on dialysis with a partial functional recovery in four; 11 patients (50%) died.

So we can say that cholesterol embolism is involved in a high incidence of renal failure and a high mortality rate.

No specific treatment can be proposed for renal atheroembolism. Corticosteroid therapy in conjunction with plasma exchange was suggested by Hasegawa,[57] renal transplantation for end-stage renal disease by Kammerl.[58]

So the main problem is to avoid atheroembolic events during renal interventions. The selection of the patients may limit the risk but we have to treat more and more elderly high-risk patients, with advanced atheromatous diseases and it is difficult to contraindicate these patients. Technical points are very important to mention.

The procedures should be as atraumatic as possible with use of small devices and adaptation of coronary angioplasty techniques. Direct stenting is not sufficient to avoid embolism. If we compare with carotid procedures, we know that stent dilatation is the most embolic step. Recently, Feldman et al.[59] recognizing the risk of atheroembolism, reported their 'no-touch' technique, which consists of placing a second 0.035-inch J-wire within the guiding catheter during cannulation of the renal artery to prevent the tip of the catheter from rubbing the aortic wall in an effort to minimize the contact with atherosclerotic plaques and reduce the potential for embolization.

Walker[47] proposed that a careful aspiration of catheter before injections or interventions should routinely be performed during renal interventions.

Beyond these technical considerations to circumvent atheroembolisms, we applied the concept of protected renal angioplasty and stenting.

The rationale for distal embolic protection is similar to that of brain protection during angioplasty and stenting of the carotid arteries. Several studies have shown that protection devices with occlusion balloon or filter are efficient to reduce the risk of embolization to the brain[60,61] and that these techniques are mandatory in this field and the standard of care.[62] We postulated that the same technique could be suitable in the management of renal artery stenosis mitigating the risk of atheroembolism.

Our results show stabilization or improvement of renal function and no deterioration at 6-month follow-up. Only two deteriorations appeared at 2-year follow-up, but one in a patient with bilateral stenosis, one side treated without protection. These results seem favourable if we compare with literature data and may well be attributed to the use of a protection device during the procedure. It is noteworthy that visible atherosclerotic debris was extracted in all cases with balloon occlusion techniques and in 70% of the cases with filters. In one instance, we removed a fragment measuring 6.2 mm in its maximum diameter, large enough to produce macroembolism or new renal artery occlusion. Two filters were totally blocked by debris showing the role of protection devices.

In our experience, protected renal angioplasty and stenting seems to have the same effects on hypertension as performing the procedures without protection:[8] significant decreases in systolic and diastolic blood pressure, easier blood pressure control, and reduced antihypertensive medications. Larger randomized studies are needed to confirm this observation. Moreover, if we can reduce the renal function deterioration rate after protected renal angioplasty and stenting, this could influence the long-term prognosis of hypertension, and further studies are needed to appreciate the impact of unchanged renal function on hypertension.

Although no device-related complications occurred in this small series of patients, adding another instrument to the procedure while trying to prevent complications could create new problems. The potential for renal artery thrombosis during protection is negligible, even with occlusion balloon, because the patients are receiving heparin and antiplatelet therapy; moreover, the duration of occlusion is usually short, less than the time required to perform the distal anastomosis of a conventional aortorenal bypass. The risk of dissection with a protection device is negligeable, but we have to mention the possibility of spasm (two cases in our series) although this is easily treated medically. Also the interventionist should remember that this technique doe not protect the kidney from atheroembolism during attempts to initially catheterize the renal artery and cross the lesion. The technique proposed by Walker[47] could reduce the risk of embolization during these steps.

The indications for this technique of renal protection may be discussed. Is the technique indicated for all patients undergoing endovascular treatment for renal artery stenosis, as protection devices seem indicated for all carotid angioplasties? Or should it be limited to some patients? Selective indications should at least be pointed out:

1. Elderly patients.
2. Patients with renal insufficiency and a creatinine > 1.4 mg/dl.
3. Bilateral renal stenosis.
4. Solitary or single functioning kidney.
5. Patients with diseased aorta and renal ostia.
6. Maybe diabetes.

Conclusion

Renal artery angioplasty and stenting is largely performed with very good technical success, good anatomical results, a low complications rate and a good long-term patency rate. The effects on blood pressure are encouraging. However, the deterioration of renal function after the procedure may limit the immediate benefits of this technique. Atheroembolism seems to play an important role. Physicians dedicated to this field should be aware of the risks of atheroembolism and deterioration of renal function after renal interventional procedures.

Renal protection is a new approach to improve the results of PTRA and stenting.

Safety, feasibility, efficiency of protected renal angioplasty is demonstrated. Distal protection is not merely particulate retrieval. It may be the standard of care in the near future.

The absence of randomization and the small number of patients in our series is a clear limitation. Larger or randomized studies are awaited and will be needed to definitely address the utility of this approach and better document its beneficial effects on renal function and perhaps on hypertension and its long-term prognosis.

Some problems remain:

1. The cost of this technique.
2. The best protection devices have to be determined.
3. Improvements in protection devices are needed for this renal protection.
4. Indications have to be specified.

Summary

- Renal artery angioplasty and stenting is a safe and efficient procedure.

- Good anatomical results and long-term patency.

- But a concern: post-procedural deterioration of the renal function in 20-45 % of the patients.

- Atheroembolism seems to play an important role.

- Role of protection devices to avoid embolism during procedure.

- Distal protection is not merely particulate retrieved.

- May be the standard of care in the near future.

References

1. Berglund G, Anderson O, Wilhelmsen T. Prevalence of primary and secondary hypertension studies in a random population sample. *Br Med J* 1976; 2: 554–556.
2. Novick AC. Options for therapy of ischemic nephropathy: role of angioplasty and surgery. *Semin Nephrol* 1996; 16: 53–60.
3. Zuccala A, Zucchelli P. Ischemic nephropathy: diagnosis and treatment. *J Nephrol* 1998; 11: 318–324.
4. Klinge J, Mali PTM, Puijlaert CBA *et al.* Percutaneous transluminal renal angioplasty: initial and long-term results. *Radiology* 1989; 171: 501–506.
5. Canzanello VJ, Millan VG, Spiegel JE *et al.* Percutaneous transluminal renal angioplasty in management of atherosclerotic renovascular hypertension: results in 100 patients. *Hypertension* 1989; 13: 163–172.
6. Sos TA, Pickering TG, Sniderman K *et al.* Percutaneous transluminal renal angioplasty in renovascular hypertension due to atheroma or fibromuscular dysplasia. *N Engl J Med* 1983; 309: 274–279.
7. Van de Ven PJ, Kaatee R, Beutler JJ *et al.* Arterial stenting and balloon angioplasty in ostial atherosclerotic renovascular disease: a randomised trial. *Lancet* 1999; 353: 282–286.
8. Henry M, Amor M, Henry I *et al.* Stents in the treatment of renal artery stenosis: long-term follow-up. *J Endovasc Surg* 1999; 6: 42–51.
9. Henry M, Amor M, Henry I *et al.* Stent placement in the renal artery: three-year experience with the Palmaz stent. *J Vasc Interv Radiol* 1996; 7: 343–350.
10. Blum U, Krumme B, Flugel P *et al.* Treatment of ostial renal artery stenosis with vascular endoprostheses after unsuccessful balloon angioplasty. *N Engl J Med* 1997; 336: 459–465.
11. Iannone LA, Underwood P, Nath A *et al.* Effect of primary balloon expandable renal artery stents on long-term patency, renal function and balloon pressure in hypertension and renal insufficient patients with renal artery stenosis. *Cathet Cardiovasc Diagn* 1996; 37: 243–250.
12. Von Knorring J, Edgren J, Lepantalo M. Long-term results of percutaneous transluminal angioplasty in renovascular hypertension. *Acta Radiol* 1996; 37: 36–40.
13. Kuhlmann U, Greminger A *et al.* Long-term experience in percutaneous transluminal dilatation of renal artery stenosis. *Am J Med* 1985; 79: 692–698.
14. Dorros G, Jaff M, Jain A *et al.* Follow-up of primary Palmaz-Schatz stent placement for atherosclerotic renal artery stenosis. *Am J Cardiol* 1995; 75: 1051–1055.

15. Isles CG, Robertson S, Hill D. Management of renovascular disease: a review of renal artery stenting in ten studies. *Q J Med* 1999; **92**: 159–167.

16. Boisclair C, Therasse E, Olivia VL *et al.* Treatment of renal angioplasty failure by perculaneous renal artery stenting with Palmaz stents: midterm technical and clinical results. *Am J Roentgenol* 1997; **168**: 245–251.

17. Van de Ven PJ, Beutler JJ, Kaatee R *et al.* Transluminal vascular stent for ostial atheosclerotic renal artery stenosis. *Lancet* 1995; **346**: 672–674.

18. Wilms G, Staessen J, Baert AL *et al.* Percutaneous transluminal renal angioplasty and renal function. *Radiology* 1989; **29**: 195–200.

19. Wilms GE, Peene PT, Baert AL *et al.* Renal artery stent placement with use of the Wallstent endoprosthesis. *Radiology* 1991; **179**: 457–462.

20. Henry M, Kconaris C, Henry I. Renal stenting with its percusing guardwire device: a pilot study. *J Endovasc Ther* 2001; **8**: 227–237

21. Standards of Practice Committee of the Society of Cardiovascular and Interventional Radiology, Guidelines for percutaneous transluminal angiology. *Radiology* 1990; **177**: 619–626.

22. Dorros G, Jaff M, Mathiak L *et al.* Four year follow-up of Palmaz-Schatz stent revascularization as treatment for atherosclerotic renal artery stenosis. *Circulation* 1998; **98**: 642–647.

23. Rihal CS, Textor SC, Breen JF *et al.* Incidental renal artery stenosis among a prospective cohort of hypertensive patients undergoing coronary angiography. *Mayo Clin Proc* 2002; **77**: 309–316.

24. Schreiber MJ, Pohl MA, Novick AC. The natural history of atherosclerotic and fibrous renal artery disease. *Urol Clin North Am* 1984; **11**: 383–392.

25. Srandness DE Jr. Natural history of renal artery stenosis. *Am J Kidney Dis* 1994; **24**: 630–635.

26. Zierler RE. Screening for renal artery stenosis: is it justified. *Mayo Clin Proc* 2002; **77**: 307–308.

27. White CJ. Open renal arteries are better than closed renal arteries. *Cathet Cardiovasc Diagn* 1998; **45**: 9–10.

28. Novick AC, Ziegelbaum M, Vidt DG *et al.* Trends in surgical revascularization for renal artery disease: Ten years' experience. *JAMA* 1987; **257**: 498–501.

29. Weibull H, Bergqvist D, Bergentz SE *et al.* PTRA versus surgical reconstruction of atherosclerotic renal stenosis: a prospective randomized study. *J Vasc Surg* 1993; **18**: 841–852.

30. Cambria RP. Surgery: Indications and variables that affect procedural outcome, as well as morbidity and mortality. *J Invas Cardiol* 1998; **10**: 55–58.

31. Dorros G, Prince C, Mathia KL *et al.* Stenting of a renal artery stenosis achieves better relief of the obstructive lesion than baloon angioplasty. *Cathet Cardiovasc Diagn* 1993; **29**: 191–198.

32. Zeller TH. Endovascular treatment of renal artery stenosis: technical aspects. Long term clinical results and restenosis rate in Paris. *Course Revascularization Book* 2000: 333–364.

33. Rocha Sing KJ, Miskkel GJ, Kathodi RE *et al.* Clinical predictors of improved long-term blood pressure control after successful stenting of hypertensive patients with obstructive renal artery atherosclerosis. *Cathet Cardiovasc Interv* 1999; **47**: 167–172.

34. Taylor A, Sheppard D, Macleod MJ *et al.* Renal artery stent placement in renal artery stenosis: technical and early clinical results. *Clin Radiol* 1997; **52**: 451–457.

35. Paulsen D, Klow NE, Rogstad B *et al.* Preservation of renal function by percutaneous transluminal angioplasty in ischaemic renal disease. *Nephrol Dial Transplant* 1999; **14**: 1454–14561.

36. Rodriguez-Lopez JA, Werner A, Ray LI *et al.* Renal artery stenosis treated with stent deployment : indications, technique, and outcome in 108 patients. *J Vasc Surg* 1999; **29**: 617–624.

37. Harden PN, MacLeaod MJ, Rodger *RSC et al.* Effect on renal-artery stenting on progression of renovascular renal failure. *Lancet* 1997; **349**: 1133–1136.

38. Mailloux LU, Napolitano B, Bellucci AG *et al.* Renal vascular disease causing end-stage renal disease, incidence, clinical correlates, and outcomes: A 20-year clinical experience. *Am J Kidney Dis* 1994; **4**: 622–629.

39. Durros G. Long-term effects of stent revascularization upon blood pressure management renal function and patient survival. *J Invasive Cardiol* 1998; **10**: 51–53.

40. Isles CG, Robertson S, Hill D. Management of renovascular disease: a review of renal artery stenting in ten studies. *Q J Med* 1999; **92**: 159–167.

41. Subramanian R, Silva JA, Ramee SR *et al.* Beneficial effects of chronic renal insufficiency. *Eur Heart J* 2002; **97**: 577.

42. Guerrero M, Kunjmmen B, Khaleel R *et al.* Stabilization of renal function after renal artery stenting. *Am J Cardiol* 2002; **90**: 63H.

43. Scolari F, Bracchi M, Valzorio B *et al.* Cholesterol atheromatus embolism: an increasingly recognized cause of acute renal failure. *Nephrol Dial Trasplant* 1996; **11**: 1607–1612.

44. Meyrier A. Renal vascular lesions in the elderly: nephrosclerosis or atheromatous renal disease? *Nephrol Dial Transplant* 1996; **11** (Suppl 9): 45–52.

45. Saleem S, Lakkis FG, Martinez-Maldonado M. Atheroembolic renal disease. *Semin Nephrol* 1996; **16**: 309–318.

46. Mayo RR, Swartz RD. Redefining the incidence of clinically detectable atheroembolism. *Am J Med* 1996; **100**: 524–529.

47. Walker C, Kowalski J, Knan M *et al*. Proximal protection before distal protection: preventing large atheroemboly during renal intervention. *Am J Cardiol* 2002; **90**: 28H.

48. Rauh G, Spengel FA. Blue toe syndrome after initiation of low-dose anticoagulation. *Eur J Med Res* 1998; **3**: 278–280.

49. Belenfant X, d'Auzac C, Bariety J *et al*. Cholesterol crystal embolism during treatment with low-molecular-weight heparin [in French]. *Presse Med* 1997; **26**: 1236–1237.

50. Commeau P, Barragan P, Huret B *et al*. Direct stenting in the treatment of renal artery stenosis: immediate and in-hospital results. *Am J Cardiol* 2001; TCT 74.

51. Morice MC, Marcoj, Laborde JC *et al*. The French registry on renal stenting. *Am J Cardiol* 2002; **90**: 67H.

52. Thadani RI, Camargo CA Jr, Xavier RJ *et al*. Atheroembolic renal failure after invasive procedures. Natural history based on 52 histologically proven cases. *Medicine (Baltimore)* 1995; **74**: 350–358.

53. Haqqie SS, Urizar RE, Singh J. Nephrotic-range proteinuria in renal atheroembolic disease: report of four cases. *Am J Kidney Dis* 1996; **28**: 493–501.

54. Greenberg A, Bastacky SI, Iqbal A *et al*. Focal segmental glomerulosclerosis associated with nephrotic syndrome in cholesterol atheroembolism: clinicopathological correlations. *Am J Kidney Dis* 1997; **29**: 334–344.

55. Krishnamurthi V, Novick AC, Myles JL. Atheroembolic renal disease: effect on morbidity and survival after renovascularization for atherosclerotic renal artery stenting. *Catheter Cardiovasc Interv* 1999; **46**: 245–248.

56. Boero R, Borcam M, Ladarola GM *et al*. Acute kidney failure caused by cholesterol embolism. *Minerva Urol Nefrol* 2000; **52**: 119–122.

57. Hasegawa M, Kawashima S, Shikanom *et al*. The evolution of corticosteroral therapy in conjunction with plasma exchange in the treatment of cholesterol embolic disease. A report of 5 cases. *Am J Nephrol* 2000; **20**: 263–267.

58. Kammerl MC, Fishereder M, Zulke C *et al*. Renal transplantation in a patient and stage renal disease due to cholesterol embolism. *Transplantation* 2001; **71**: 149–151.

59. Feldman RL, Wargovich TJ, Bittl JA. No-touch technique for reducing aortic wall trauma during renal artery stenting. *Catheter Cardiovasc Interv* 1999; **46**: 245–248.

60. Henry M, Henry I, Klonaris C *et al*. Benefits of cerebral protection during carotid stenting with the percusurge guardwire system: midterm results. *J Endovasc Ther* 2002; **9**: 1–13.

61. Reimers B, Corvaja N, Moshiris *et al*. Cerebral protection with filter devices during carotid artery stenting. *Circulation* 2001; **104**: 12–15.

62. Roubin GS. Carotid angioplasty and stenting under cerebral protection: the standard of care. *Int Congress XV Scottsdole* 11–14 February 2002.

Renal angioplasty needs protection

Against the motion
Tony Nicholson

Introduction

Protection is defined as 'the act of defending from trouble, harm or attack'.[1] There are many things that can go wrong during any endovascular intervention and for the most part these can be kept to a minimum by training, experience and clinical judgement. However, despite these safeguards there are some complications in renal intervention that happen due to the pathophysiology of the disease or the chemical agents used to define it. These are usually due to atherosclerotic embolization and renal infarction or contrast nephrotoxicity and can cause either insignificant temporary, or devastating permanent renal failure. In the last 2 years various mechanical devices[2] and pharmacological agents[3] have been developed that might protect the kidney from such insults during endovascular interventions. Do they work and are they necessary in all cases?

The two most common causes of renovascular disease are atherosclerosis and fibromuscular dysplasia. Others such as neurofibromatosis and aortic dissection are rarer though Takayasu's disease is very common in the Far East and South America. Endovascular treatment of such symptomatic diseases in the renal arteries is now widely accepted as being relatively safe and efficacious in the right clinical setting. However, renal failure following intervention, due to atheroembolism or contrast toxicity, is only described in atherosclerotic renovascular disease, usually (though not exclusively) where there is a degree of pre-existing renal failure. It would seem therefore that protection is unnecessary in all cases but that we should examine its potential in the atherosclerotic patient.

The incidence of renal insufficiency post-endovascular renal intervention

An analysis of the literature from 24 published series in the 1990s citing 1187 patients who had undergone percutaneous transluminal renal angioplasty (PTRA) +/- stenting for atheromatous renovascular disease, reveals a 1% incidence of permanent renal insufficiency and a 3.3% incidence of temporary renal insufficiency.[4] Segmental infarction occurs in 1.3% but is significant in less than 1%.

Two more recent papers from Henry *et al.*[5,6] described follow-up in 269 patients who had renal stent implantation for mainly ostial atherosclerotic renovascular disease. Most of these patients had undergone suboptimal PTRA suggesting that the degree of manipulation was maximal and that not insignificant amounts of contrast were used. Though the papers do describe a small number of mechanical complications, neither paper describes any incidence of clinically significant atheroembolism or contrast nephrotoxicity. It is not surprising, therefore, that the same group later found no evidence of renal insufficiency after using an atheroembolic renal protection device, in a different cohort of patients undergoing renal stenting for ostial atheromatous.[2] What is surprising is that they should recommend the routine use of a protection device in all renal interventions.

Cholesterol embolization or contrast nephrotoxicity?

None of the above papers mention the role of contrast as a nephrotoxic agent or the use of pharmacological protection. Indeed when discussing post-interventional renal failure few authors consider both atheroembolization and contrast nephrotoxicity together though there is literature evidence that the latter is the more important factor prognostically.[7] Unless the patient has livido reticularis with a raised erythrocyte sedimentation rate (ESR), C-reactive protein (CRP) and an eosinophillia it is impossible to know in the early phase whether a rise in creatinine is due to cholesterol or contrast. The more insidious late rise in creatinine occasionally seen is often blamed on embolization but can equally be due to poor patient selection for intervention or progressive atherosclerotic disease. Even renal biopsies are unhelpful at this stage as cholesterol clefts can be seen in many of these patients where no intervention has taken place.[8]

Atheroembolization and the need for protection

There is a considerable literature on renal atheroembolic disease. An early paper of Thurlbeck and Castleman[8] showed that in post mortem analysis of aortic aneurysm repair followed by death there was an incidence of renal atheroembolic disease of greater than 70%. It also showed, however, that there is a greater than 20% incidence of atheroembolic disease in individuals with no intervention but severe aortic atherosclerotic disease. Flory[9] showed that the pathophysiology of this condition is related to cholesterol crystal embolization to the renal vascular bed. He also showed that it could be a multisystem disease involving many organs characterized by livido reticularis, raised ESR, CRP and an eosinophillia. Such clinical scenarios are highly unusual following renal intervention and are still the subject of case reports.

What is the data available on embolization during endovascular interventions?

Muscle biopsies in patients undergoing angiography alone have shown subclinical cholesterol embolization in 25% of patients.[10] This, and the fact that cholesterol can be found in renal biopsies where there is no intervention, would suggest that ostial plaque is inherently unstable. Rapp *et al.*[11] using an *ex vivo* preparation of carotid arteries with intervention and analysis of effluent showed that emboli were produced at all stages of an intervention from the passing of an initial fine guidewire, through PTA to stent insertion (Fig.1).

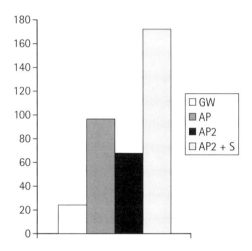

Figure 1. Rapp *et al.*[11] *In vitro* manipulations of carotid artery segments. GW: guidewire insertion. AP: first angioplasty. AP2: second angioplasty. AP2+S: angioplasty plus stent insertion.

If embolization is the usual case during intervention, why is it not more often a clinical problem?

Kimura *et al.*[12] using microspheres to mimic atheroembolic disease suggested that cholesterol crystals occlude arteries between 55 and 900 microns (μ) in diameter. In the kidney these would correspond to renal arteries of interlobular and arcuate size down to glomerular capillaries. Two further important points emerged from this paper. The first was that the outcomes in terms of proteinuria and renal dysfunction were dose-dependent. Only with larger doses of microspheres did proteinuria occur and only at the largest dose was there a decline in renal function. With low doses of microspheres there was no proteinuria or renal dysfunction. Second, this effect took 12 weeks to occur. This is in keeping with the insidiously progressive form of atheroembolic disease rather than the acute catastrophic form described following renal intervention. So the clinical effect of cholesterol embolization appears to be dose-dependant.

What is the cholesterol load to the kidney during intervention?

This is difficult to determine. There has been Doppler analysis of cerebral blood flow during carotid intervention.[13] It is not clear what the signals represent but it is probable that they do reflect debris in the carotid circulation. There are no data on renal artery Doppler recognition of emboli and intervention. However, there is an interesting paper on iliac angioplasty. The authors recorded Doppler signals over the femoral arteries after iliac angioplasty.[14] Their control group consisted of patients undergoing renal angioplasty. Although the signal was low compared with iliac angioplasty there were embolic events recorded for 2 hours after renal angioplasty in the femoral arteries. Does this suggest that the embolic load during PTRA would be even greater to the target organ or could it be that shear stress due to flow in an artery at right angles to the aorta is actually partly renoprotective?

Can we prevent embolization during intervention?

There are three types of atheroembolic protective device from a number of manufacturers. One developed for carotid angioplasty and stent placement involves reversal of blood flow through the carotid during the angioplasty procedure and is not applicable to the renal artery. The second type of device is the occlusion balloon and is the type used in the study by Henry *et al.*[2] It has a crossing profile of 2.7 Fr, which is just under 1mm. This would be about the size of the channel in a critically stenosed 6mm diameter renal artery. One could easily see how the manipulation of such a device across a tight stenosis could dislodge unstable plaque as previously demonstrated.[11] In addition its deployment position might be difficult with early branch vessel division (Fig. 2). It also relies on aspiration of effluent after stent deployment. There is no evidence that aspiration can be completely performed. The third type of device is a filter

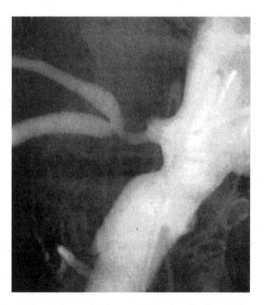

Figure 2. Early division of the main renal artery would make effective deployment of a protection device impossible.

that is deployed distal to the angioplasty site to catch some of the fragments that may be dislodged. The crossing profile of these devices is from 3.1–3.9 Fr. They are therefore even more likely to dislodge plaque during manipulation. The pore sizes of the available filters vary from 80–150 µ. Kimura's work[10] has demonstrated that smaller cholesterol crystals can still obstruct glomerular capillaries. In addition the deployment problems cited for the balloon occlusion device also apply to these filters.

What evidence is there that filters might be effective during renal intervention?

Baim *et al.*[15] randomized 800 patients to stent placement with or without a protective device during coronary intervention and showed a significant difference in terms of the defined endpoints. The device used in this study was the occlusive balloon device. There was a significant reduction in death, myocardial infarction and emergency bypass, from 16.5% to 9.6% when a protection device was used. These represent very short-term events and there does not appear to be a similar scenario to the progressive dysfunction seen with renal atheroembolic disease. The only paper on the use of protection devices in the renal arteries is the previously cited preliminary report by Henry *et al.*[2] Here a balloon occlusion device was also used. The patients had excellent initial renal function and were undergoing intervention for hypertension control. The authors noticed no change in renal function on follow-up but found debris with all the patients of a size that would fit the vessel size affected in the Flory paper.

It is clear that atheroemboli are the rule in any intervention in atherosclerotic disease. However, it is also clear that important clinical sequelae are uncommon. Renal angioplasty and stent placement will release atheroemboli to the renal circulation but this is mainly in low dose and the effect is not overwhelming as angioplasty/stent placement are associated with an improvement in renal function. It is unlikely that any protection device will preclude any cholesterol embolization: experimental data shows that even the guidewire will produce this. However, it is also possible that the heterogeneous response of kidneys to angioplasty with atherosclerotic disease compared with the beneficial response to angioplasty in fibromuscular dysplasia may depend on the dose of cholesterol crystals released by the procedure. At present neither of the two randomized trials underway in Europe (STAR and ASTRAL) have addressed the issue of protection devices. It may be possible that smaller trials, which include those most at risk with single kidney function measurements, can be performed to address this issue. Until that is done the costs and extra manipulations involved with renal protection devices cannot be justified.

Contrast nephrotoxicity and the need for protection

Contrast-associated nephropathy is a potentially serious sequelae of contrast media that manifests as symptoms ranging from acute, irreversible renal failure to minor changes in tubular function. Indeed in diabetics with pre-existing renal failure who have been dehydrated prior to pyelography with ionic contrast media the incidence of significant creatinine rise is greater than 90%.[16] However, the use of non-ionic media and pre-procedural hydration reduces this to between 0 and 3%.[17] Nevertheless, the incidence of acute renal failure due to contrast agents surpasses that due to aminoglycoside antibiotics.[18] Those at highest risk remain those with diabetes and pre-existing renal failure where the incidence of contrast nephropathy remains high at 10–35% despite non-ionic media and hydration.[3] Where there are no risk factors nephrotoxicity is not a problem[19] though if patients are studied carefully a 'creatinine bump' consisting of a transient increase in serum creatinine of 0.5 µg/dl over base-line at 48 hours can be seen.[7]

The exact mechanism is poorly understood but it is believed to be vascoconstrictive, affecting the outer medulla where most of the metabolic effort involving ion exchange occurs. This causes ischaemia to the tubular cells in the ascending limb and cellular damage ensues. Like ischaemia elsewhere this is mediated by free radicals. N-acetylcysteine, a free radical scavenger has been shown to be effective at preventing renal deterioration due to contrast toxicity.[3] More recently feneldopam mesylate, a dopamine type 1 receptor agonist, has been shown to be a potent vasodilator of the medullary tubular arteries and to completely eliminate the contrast-induced 'creatinine bump' in all patients and to reduce significant increases to less than 4% in the high risk population.[20]

Summary

- Clinically significant renal failure due to atheroembolism and/or contrast toxicity during endovascular renal interventions has an incidence of 1%–3%.

- Only patients with symptomatic atheromatous renovascular disease are at risk of atheroembolism during endovascular procedures.

- Clinically apparent renal failure depends on the atheroembolic load and only occurs with a high dose of embolized cholesterol.

- The group at highest risk is diabetics with pre-existing renal failure.

- Atheroembolization occurs during the deployment of protection devices and their effective deployment is dependant on renal artery anatomy.

- There is no evidence at the present time for the use of balloon occlusion or filtration protection devices during renal intervention.

- There is good evidence for the use of pharmacological protection against contrast nephropathy in high risk groups during endovascular renal interventions.

References

1. *Collins English Dictionary* London: Harper Collins, 1995.
2. Henry M, Klonaris C, Henry I *et al*. Protected renal stenting with the PercuSurge Guard Wire device: a pilot study. *J Endovasc Ther* 2001; **8**: 227–237.
3. Tepel M, van der Giet M, Schwarzfeld C *et al*. Prevention of radiographic contrast agent induced reductions in renal function by acetylcysteine. *N Engl J Med* 2000; **343**: 180–184.
4. Moss JG. Renal and visceral artery intervention. In: Dyet, Ettles and Nicholson (eds). *Textbook of Endovascular Procedures*. London: Edinburgh: Churchill Livingstone, 2000.
5. Henry M, Amor M, Henry I *et al*. Stents in the treatment of renal artery stenosis: long-term follow-up. *J Endovasc Surg* 1999; **6**: 42–51.
6. Henry M, Amor M, Henry I *et al*. Stent placement in the renal artery: three year experience with the Palmatz stent. *JVIR* 1996; **7**: 343–350.

7. Gruberg L, Mintz GS, Mehran R *et al.* The prognostic implications of further renal function deterioration within 48 hours of interventional coronary procedures in patients with pre-existing chronic renal insufficviency. *JACC* 2000; **36**: 1542–1548.

8. Thurlbeck WM, Castleman B. Atheromatous emboli to the kidneys after aortic surgery. *N Engl J Med* 1957; **257**: 442–447.

9. Flory CM. Arterial occlusions produced by emboli from eroded aortic atheromatous plaques. *Am J Pathol* 1945; **21**: 549–565.

10. Ramirez G, O'Neill WM, Lambert R *et al.* Cholesterol embolization: a complication of angiography. *Arch Intern Med* 1978; **138**: 1430.

11. Rapp JH, Pan XM, Sharp FR *et al.* Atheroemboli to the brain: size threshold for causing acute neuronal cell death. *J Vasc Surg* 2000; **32**: 68–76.

12. Kimura M, Suzuki T, Hishida A. A rat model of progressive chronic renal failure produced by microembolism. *Am J Pathol* 1999; **155**: 1371–1380.

13. Jordan WD, Voellinger DC, Doblar DD *et al.* Microemboli detected by transcranial Doppler monitoring in patients during carotid angioplasty versus carotid endarterectomy. *Cardiovasc Surg* 1999; **7**: 33–38.

14. Al-Hamali S, Baskervile P, Fraser S *et al.* Detection of distal emboli in patients with peripheral arterial stenosis before and after iliac angioplasty. *J Vasc Surg* 1999; **29**: 345–351.

15. Baim DS, Wahr D, George B *et al.* Randomized trial of a distal embolic protection device during percutaneous intervention of saphenous vein aorto-coronary bypass grafts. *Circulation* 2002; **105**: 1285–1290.

16. Harkonan S, Kjellstrand CM. Exacerbation of diabetic renal failure following intravenous pyelography. *Am J Med* 1977; **63**: 939–946.

17. Cruz C, Hricak H, Samhouri F *et al.* Contrast media for angiography: effect on renal function. *Radiology* 1986; **158**: 109–112.

18. Hou SH, Bushinsky DA, Wish JB *et al.* Hospital acquired renal insufficiency: a prospective study. *Am J Med* 1983; **74**: 243–248.

19. Barrett BJ. Contrast nephrotoxicity. *J Am Assoc Nephrol* 1994; **5**: 125–137.

20. Chamsuddin AA, Kowalik KJ, Bjarnson H *et al.* Using a dopamine 1A receptor agonist in high risk patients to ameliorate contrast associated nephropathy. *Am J Roentgenol* 2002; **179**: 591–596.

Renal angioplasty needs protection

Charing Cross Editorial Comments towards Consensus

The starting point is the experience from carotid angioplasty. Initially angioplasty was performed without cerebral protection and although the pioneers spoke well of the procedure, later the same pioneers were heard to state that carotid angioplasty should only be performed with cerebral protection! It has now become accepted that cerebral protection is mandatory for the cerebral circulation. I have almost heard the case made that it is legally actionable not to have cerebral protection. We will not go into the argument that it was deemed correct to do angioplasty before cerebral protection but the history of this matter is surely relevant. The kidney has a single artery and in some respects even more than the brain, the kidney is very unforgiving if embolization occurs. Using the cerebral and carotid experience, it would surely follow that protection is logical. Nevertheless renal artery stenosis, with or without stent, is frequently performed without protection.

Tony Nicholson argues that clinically significant renal failure in angioplasty procedure has an incidence rate as low as 1–3%. He argues that the embolism occurs during deployment and the renal artery anatomy is a main determinant. He stresses that there is no evidence at the present time for the use of balloon occlusion or filtration protection devices during renal intervention. However, he argues that there is good evidence for the use of pharmacological protection against contrast nephropathy in high risk groups during endovascular renal interventions.

So once again we have the logical expectation that protection should be valuable but the lack of evidence that it is. Time will tell.

Roger M Greenhalgh
Editor

Patients with intermittent claudication should have supervised exercise and medical treatment ahead of any intervention

For the motion

Clifford P Shearman, Stephen Baxter

Introduction

Atherosclerotic peripheral arterial disease is a surprisingly common problem. The Edinburgh Artery Study examined 1592 male and female subjects aged 55–74 years from the general population. Intermittent claudication was experienced by 4% of this group and a further 25% had evidence of asymptomatic arterial disease.[1] However, after 5 years only 28.8% of those with claudication still experienced symptoms and only 8.2% had reached a point where they had been thought to require intervention. There is considerable evidence to support this finding.[2] Peripheral arterial disease is a very common problem in the population, but it will rarely deteriorate to the point that the limb is threatened. The symptoms of the majority of patients will, if anything, improve without any specific intervention.

The real problem lies with the excess cardiovascular mortality experienced by patients with peripheral arterial disease; 60% of claudicants will die from myocardial infarction (MI) and 10% will die from stroke.[3] Patients presenting with claudication are as likely to die a cardiovascular death as a patient who has already had an MI.[4] This is a mortality rate 3.8 times greater than the normal population and it is hard to find a patient group at greater risk of cardiovascular death than patients with claudication.[5] Despite this problem having been recognized for nearly a century there seems to have been little enthusiasm to tackle it. Patients with peripheral arterial disease are much less likely to receive advice or intervention to reduce their risk of cardiovascular death compared with patients who have coronary artery disease.[6] It is a sobering thought to realise, even for the enthusiasts of interventional treatment of claudication, that by 5 years the death rate from cardiovascular disease exceeds that of bypass failure.[7]

There can be little doubt then that irrespective of how the patient is advised regarding treatment of their walking disability a concerted effort must be made to reduce their chances of dying a cardiovascular death. Failure to do so is a missed opportunity.

Evidence for risk factor modification

Medical treatment involves identification of modifiable factors such as smoking, hyperlipidaemia and hypertension or therapy such as antiplatelet agents or exercise.

The most obvious aim of risk factor modification is to reduce the patient's chance of cardiovascular death. There are, however, other potential benefits. It has become apparent that the atherosclerotic plaque is a highly biologically active lesion. Complex inflammatory processes result in changes in plaque cellular content and behaviour that can result in plaque instability and rupture (Fig. 1). Most clinical episodes appear to be related to these events and the possibility of pharmacologically inducing plaque stability seems a real possibility.[8] A secondary benefit of risk factor modification may also be improved walking ability and a more positive approach to their disease. This appears to be particularly true for exercise.

The evidence for this approach is examined below (Table 1).

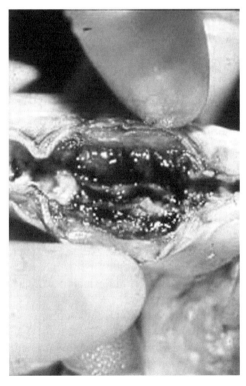

Figure 1. Ruptured atherosclerotic plaque in a coronary artery covered with fresh thrombus. Post-mortem appearances in male who suffered a fatal myocardial infarction. Courtesy of Dr P Gallagher, Department of Pathology, Southampton General Hospital, UK.

Table 1. Risk factors

Fixed	Modifiable	Therapeutic
Age	Smoking	Antiplatelet agents
Sex	Hypertension	Exercise
Genotype	Lipids	ACE inhibitors
	Diabetes	Oestrogen*
	Diet*	
	Hyperhomocysteinaemia*	

* Unproven

Smoking

Smoking is the single most important risk factor for the development of peripheral arterial disease and contributes to 40 300 cardiovascular deaths per year in the UK.[9] Smoking cessation is associated with a significant cardiovascular benefit resulting in a reduction of MI and stroke. Smoking cessation also has positive rheological effects which in theory may improve walking. The direct effects on peripheral arterial disease of stopping smoking are less clear as there have been no large high quality studies to rely upon. A systematic review found only weak evidence (non-randomized studies) of a non-significant improvement of walking in claudicants who successfully stopped.[10] Patients who are motivated to stop smoking are probably more able to make life style changes generally and so this may of course contribute to any benefit seen.

Over the longer term, however, patients who cease are less likely to develop critical limb ischaemia or die from MI than those who continue to smoke.[11] These results mirror the benefits of smoking cessation seen in the very large Coronary Artery Surgical Study (CASS) study where patients who continued to smoke after coronary re-vascularization fared much worse than those who stopped.[12]

There can be no doubt there is much to gain and nothing to lose in helping a claudicant stop smoking. The real challenge remains of how to achieve this. Simply telling patients to stop is of limited benefit and only around 2% will succeed whereas an organized approach from an experienced team using techniques such as nicotine replacement therapy can result in 30% cessation rates and is highly cost-effective.[13] It is surprising that currently relatively few claudicants receive this help.

Lipid lowering therapy

The benefits of lipid lowering therapy in patients with coronary artery disease have been clearly established and it appears that those at highest cardiovascular risk gain the greatest benefit from therapy.[5] Patients with peripheral arterial disease have considerable cardiovascular risk, far in excess of many of the groups in the large studies that showed benefit from treatment. Despite this logical extrapolation of the results there still remains some hesitancy to treat patients with peripheral arterial disease and elevated cholesterol.

In a systematic review of the available evidence Leng concluded that lipid therapy in peripheral arterial disease resulted in a non-significant reduction in mortality, but showed no apparent effect on non-fatal events. There was, however, a suggestion that therapy may slow progression of the disease.[14] Subsequent studies support this and statins appear to have a beneficial effect on the plaque biology independent of their lipid lowering, properties which may reduce clinical episodes.[15] The side-effects of treatment of hyperlipidaemia appear relatively minor and screening for it is simple and economical.

Recent evidence has confirmed the role of lipid lowering therapy in peripheral arterial disease. The Heart Protection Study randomized 20 536 patients with total cholesterol levels of >3.5mmol/litre who were considered to be at increased cardiovascular risk to simvastatin or placebo. In the 2701 subjects with peripheral arterial disease alone the major cardiovascular event rate for the simvastatin group was 247/1000 and for the placebo group 305/1000. This was a statistically significant reduction.[16]

On the evidence above the case for treating any claudicant with elevated cholesterol seems overwhelming. There may even be a case for treating all patients with peripheral arterial disease, irrespective of their cholesterol level.

Hypertension is associated with a two- to three-fold increase in cardiovascular events and is a major risk factor for peripheral arterial disease.[4] Treatment will reduce the cardiovascular risk. Angiotensin-converting enzyme inhibitors (ACE) may be of direct benefit. In the Heart Outcomes Prevention Evaluation Study patients with peripheral arterial disease given ramipril had a significant reduction in cardiovascular events compared with placebo.[17]

Diabetes mellitus

Good glycaemic control will reduce microvascular complications, but does not affect cardiovascular risk.[18] Type 2 diabetes forms part of the metabolic syndrome (syndrome X).[19] This is a cluster of abnormalities including hypertension, dyslipidaemia, insulin resistance and a procoagulant state that accelerate the progress of atherosclerosis. Patients with type 2 diabetes have a markedly increased risk of cardiovascular death and treatment of associated risk factors is likely to be of major benefit.[20]

Antiplatelet therapy

Aspirin is the most widely used antiplatelet drug and there is evidence to suggest it is very powerful at reducing cardiovascular events (27% relative risk reduction) in patients with established atheromatous disease.[21] This, however, was associated with an increase in non-fatal bleeding complications although on balance the risk of bleeding was outweighed by the benefits. Further analysis confirmed that this advantage was apparent in patients with peripheral arterial disease.[22] The CAPRIE Study, a large randomized trial of 19 185 patients comparing clopidogrel with aspirin, showed a significant reduction in expected cardiovascular events, with clopidogrel achieving a slight advantage (relative risk reduction of 8.7%). The subgroup with peripheral arterial disease gained the greatest benefit overall.[23] Currently clopidogrel is indicated in patients with peripheral arterial disease who are unable to take aspirin.

At a local level antiplatelet agents may be of benefit in preventing arterial occlusion, restenosis after angioplasty and bypass graft failure. Some evidence also suggests that aspirin may reduce the need for subsequent intervention in claudicants.[24]

There are very few reasons why a patient with claudication should not be taking an antiplatelet agent. Disappointingly a large number of patients with peripheral arterial disease seen in specialist clinics fail to do so.[25]

Exercise

Although there is no single study that demonstrates the benefits of exercise, two systematic reviews suggested significant improvements of approximately 150% in walking distances of patients included in exercise programmes.[10,26] Theoretical concerns over the risk associated with exercise seem unfounded and biological disease markers of inflammation tend to improve.[27] It does seem that exercise must be continued indefinitely to maintain the gain which raises problems of compliance. As with smoking cessation attitudes to exercise programmes need to be managed carefully to gain maximum benefit.[28] Although walking seems to be the best form of exercise for a claudicant, upper limb exercises also seem to be of benefit, presumably improving general cardiovascular fitness.[29] This allows patients who have difficulty with conventional exercise programmes the opportunity to benefit.

Although there is limited evidence, the only two randomized studies comparing exercise with angioplasty found that patients fared better in the long term after exercise.[30] Exercise programmes are cost-effective and safe.[31] Taking all this into account it seems hard to ever justify interventional treatment unless exercise has been tried and failed.

Vasoactive drugs

A number of agents have been used to improve walking ability in claudicants. However, the effect of treatment is often small and the cost-effectiveness difficult to determine.[10] Recent evidence from four randomized controlled studies suggests that the phosphodiesterase III inhibitor cilostazol may improve pain free and maximum walking distance by 38–80m and 28–84 m respectively.[4] It also improves quality of life above placebo. The role of this drug although promising is yet to be determined.

Evidence for intervention

Given that many patients with claudication will symptomatically improve or lose their symptoms spontaneously and that the limb is rarely at risk, the only justification for intervention can be short-term improvement of quality of life.

Angioplasty may seem appealing as short-term benefit is more easily achieved than with exercise. However, the treatment is more costly both in the long and short term and is associated with a 3% risk of major complication and a small risk of limb loss.[32] Many patients with claudication are unsuitable for angioplasty and acceptable results can only be obtained in relatively minor lesions. In a large randomized controlled study, although surgical bypass improved walking and quality of life more than either angioplasty or exercise, the treatment effects were small and no attempt was made to address cost-effectiveness.[33]

It is apparent that in carefully selected patients in whom the risk is low it is possible to achieve good results with re-vascularization procedures. It has yet to be established how to select these patients or if there is any advantage for any of these patients compared with medical treatment. Certainly it follows that their medical treatment must first be optimized and cardiovascular risk minimized to achieve the best results from intervention.

Evidence for primary intervention

Can primary intervention ever be justified in a patient with claudication without modification of risk factors? With regards to blood pressure, diabetes, cholesterol, smoking and aspirin the answer must be no. Neglect of these aspects of care will expose the patient to an unnecessarily high risk of cardiovascular mortality and morbidity and may reduce the chance of success of any intervention. The longer a patient survives after a successful intervention the more cost-effective will be the treatment.

Exercise programmes have not been enthusiastically adopted and many patients are not offered exercise treatment. The risks of intervention and recurrence are often not appreciated by the patient. Who, given the choice between an expensive, relatively dangerous treatment that has not been shown to be any better than a safe economic therapy, if properly counselled, would not opt for exercise first?

Medical treatment of peripheral arterial disease can have a major impact on survival of the patient and reduction of their symptoms. Delivering this care to the vascular patient is difficult and new strategies to do this are needed. It may not be as challenging or interesting to the clinician as angioplasty or surgery, but this is no excuse to neglect medical treatment in favour of intervention.

Summary

- Claudication is a very common problem.

- The majority of patients remain stable or improve spontaneously.

- The cardiovascular mortality and morbidity is very high.

- Modification of risk factors will significantly reduce mortality.

- Exercise is currently as good as any intervention over the long term and is safe and economic.

- Intervention will benefit a few selected patients and carries risk as well as being expensive.

- Medical therapy is difficult to deliver and will only work with an enthusiastic multidisciplinary team.

- High quality studies of medical treatment and exercise versus intervention are needed.

References

1. Leng GC, Lee AJ, Fowkes FG *et al.* Incidence, natural history and cardiovascular events in symptomatic and asymptomatic peripheral arterial disease in the general population. *Int J Epidemiol* 1996; 25: 1172–1181.
2. TransAtlantic Inter-Society Consensus (TASC). Management of peripheral arterial disease. *J Vasc Surg* 2000; 1(suppl): 1–296.
3. Smith GD, Shipley MJ, Rose G. Intermittent claudication, heart disease risk factors and mortality; the Whitehall study. *Circulation* 1990; 82: 1925–1931.
4. Hiatt WR. Medical treatment of peripheral arterial disease and claudication. *N Engl J Med* 2001; 344: 1608–1621.
5. Haq IU, Yeo WW, Jackson PR, Ramsay LE *et al.* The case for cholesterol reduction in peripheral arterial disease. *Critical Ischaemia* 1997; 7: 15–22.
6. Hirsch AT, Criqui MH, Treat-Jacobenson *et al.* Peripheral arterial disease detection, awareness, and treatment in primary care. *JAMA* 2001; 286: 1317–1324.
7. Szilagyi DE, Hageman JH, Smith RF *et al.* Autogenous vein grafting in femoropopliteal atherosclerosis: the limits of its effectiveness. *Surgery* 1979; 86: 836–851.
8. Libby P. Changing concepts of atherogenesis. *J Int Med* 2000; 247: 349–358.
9. Coronary Heart Disease National Service Framework. London: Dept of Health, March 2000.
10. Girolami B, Bernardi E, Prins MH *et al.* Treatment of intermittent claudication with physical training, smoking cessation, pentoxyifylline, or nafronyl. *Arch Intern Med* 1999; 159: 337–345.

11. Smith I, Franks PJ, Greenhalgh RM *et al*. The influence of smoking cessation and hypertriglyceridaemia on the progression of peripheral vascular disease and the onset of critical ischaemia. *Eur J Vasc Endovasc Surg* 1996; 11: 402–408.

12. Cavender JB, Rogers WJ, Fisher LD *et al*. Effects of smoking on survival and morbidity in patients randomised to medical or surgical therapy in the Coronary Artery Surgery Study (CASS): 10 year follow up. *J Am Coll Cardiol* 1992; 20: 287–294.

13. Jackson C, White D. Smoking cessation in the 21st century. In: Beard JD, Murray S (eds). *Pathways of Care in Vascular Surgery*. Shrewsbury: TFM Publishing Limited. 2002: 31–38.

14. Leng GC, Price JF, Jepson RG. Lipid-lowering for lower limb atherosclerosis (Cochrane Review). In: *The Cochrane Library,* Issue 3, 2001. Oxford: Update Software.

15. Palinsky W. New evidence for beneficial effects of statins unrelated to lipid lowering. *Arterioscler Thromb Vasc Biol* 2001; 21: 3–5.

16. Heart Projection Study Collaborative Group. MRC/BHF Heart protection study of cholesterol lowering with simvastatin in 20536 high-risk individuals: a randomised placebo-controlled trial. *Lancet* 2002; 360: 7–22.

17. The Heart Outcome Prevention Evaluation Study Investigators. Effects of an angiotensin-converting enzyme inhibitor, ramapril, on cardiovascular events in high risk patients. *N Engl* J *Med* 2000; 342: 145–153.

18. UK Prospective Diabetes Study (UKPDS) Group. Intensive blood glucose control with sulphonlyureas or insulin compared with conventional treatment and risk of complications in patients with type 2 diabetes (UKPDS 33). *Lancet* 1998; 352: 837–853.

19. Reaven GM. Mulitple CHD risk factors in type 2 diabetes: beyond glycaemic control. *Diabetes Obes Metabol* 2002; Supp 1: S13.

20. Byrne CD, Wild SH. Diabetes care needs evidence based intervention to reduce risk of vascular disease. *Br Med J* 2000; 320: 1554–1555.

21. Antiplatelet Trialists' Collaboration. Collaborative overview of randomised trials of antiplatelet therapy- I: prevention of death, myocardial infarction, and stroke by prolonged antiplatelet therapy in various categories of patient. *Br Med J* 1994; 308: 81–106.

22. Antiplatelet Trialists' Collaboration.Collaborative meta-analysis of randomised trials of antiplatelet therapy for prevention of death, myocardial infarction, and stroke in high risk patients. *Br Med J* 2002; 324: 71–86.

23. CAPRIE Steering Committee. A randomised, blinded, trial of clopidogrel versus aspirin in patients at risk of ischaemic events (CAPRIE) *Lancet* 1996; 348: 1329–1339.

24. Girolami B, Bernardi E, Prins MH *et al*. Antithrombotic drugs in the primary medical management of intermittent claudication: a meta analysis. *Thromb Haemost* 1999; 81: 715–722.

25. Davies A. The practical management of claudication. *Br Med J* 2000; 321: 911–912.

26. Leng GC, Fowler B, Ernst E. Exercise for intermittent claudication. In: *The Cochrane Library*, Issue 3, 2002. Oxford: Update Software.

27. Tisi PV, Hulse M, Chulakadabba A *et al*. Exercise training for intermittent claudication: does it adversely affect biochemical markers of the exercise-induced inflammatory response? *Eur J Vasc Endovasc Surg* 1997; 14: 344–50.

28. Morris-Vincent P, Theophilus T. Exercise programmes for claudicants. In: Beard JD, Murray S (eds). *Pathways of Care in Vascular Surgery*. Shrewsbury: TFM Publishing Limited, 2002: 19–30.

29. Walker RD, Nawaz S, Wilkinson CH *et al*. Influence of upper- and lower-limb exercise training on cardiovascular function and walking distance in patients with intermittent claudication. *J Vasc Surg* 2000; 31: 662–669.

30. Fowkes FG, Gillespie IN. Angioplasty (versus non-surgical management) for intermittent claudication. In: *The Cochrane Library*, Issue 3, 2000. Oxford: Update Software.

31. Tan KH, de Crossart L, Edwards PR. Exercise training and peripheral vascular disease. *Br J Surg* 2000; 87: 553–562.

32. Shearman CP. Management of intermittent claudication. *Br J Surg* 2002; 89: 529–531.

33. Taft C, Karlsson J, Gelin J *et al*. Treatment efficacy of intermittent claudication by invasive therapy, supervised physical exercise training compared to no treatment in unselected randomised patients II: one year results of health-related quality of life. *Eur J Vasc Endovasc Surg* 2001; 22: 114–23.

Patients with intermittent claudication should have supervised exercise and medical treatment ahead of any intervention

Against the motion
C Vaughan Ruckley

Introduction

Intermittent claudication is a benign condition in the majority of cases and early intervention is unnecessary. It is therefore all the more important to recognize the special group of patients for whom early intervention is appropriate. Let us first identify the areas of agreement.

The commonest cause of claudication is peripheral atherosclerotic occlusive disease In this disease the crucial importance of claudication as a presenting symptom, is as a warning flag that the patient is at high risk of life-threatening cardiovascular events, notably myocardial infarction and stroke.[1-3] Therefore a high priority is that the patient should be assessed for risk factors. Diabetes, dyslipidaemia and thrombophilia may all need medical treatment. The patient should be encouraged to stop smoking and to take exercise. Another high priority is the investigation for evidence of arterial disease affecting other systems. Hypertension and ischaemic heart disease may need medical therapy. Few would demur with this general approach.

Where Primary Care is functioning effectively we would expect that, for most patients with claudication, risk factor control and the investigation and treatment of co-existing cardiovascular disease would have been initiated in Primary Care before referral to a vascular specialist. Indeed many patients do not need to be referred at all. The patient referred with claudication to a vascular specialist is therefore likely to be unusual in some way; perhaps an uncertain diagnosis, perhaps symptoms which are unusually severe or of acute onset, perhaps a failure to control risk factors, perhaps a perceived need for urgent intervention.

The unqualified statement that 'patients with intermittent claudication should have supervised exercise and medical treatment ahead of any intervention' is potentially dangerous dogma. Like all dogma it defies rational thought and stultifies initiative. It implies that all patient with claudication have the same pathology, the same distribution of disease, the same co-morbidity and the same social circumstances. Claudication may be caused by obstruction to arterial blood flow affecting arteries anywhere between the heart and the small vessels in the calf. It may be caused by obstruction to venous return. Vascular claudication is mimicked by several non-vascular conditions. The list of vascular and non-vascular causes is a long one (Table 1).

Table 1. Intermittent claudication – differential diagnosis

Vascular causes
Atherosclerosis
Arterial embolism
Adventitial cyst of the popliteal artery
Popliteal artery entrapment syndrome
Chronic compartment syndrome
Thromboangiitis obliterans
Coarctation
Takayasu's disease
Arterial fibrodysplasia
Iliac syndrome of the cyclist
Persistent sciatic artery
Primary vascular tumours
Iliofemoral venous obstruction

Non-vascular causes
Neurogenic claudication
Lumbar disc disease
Arthropathy
Baker's cyst

Even within the peripheral atherosclerotic occlusive disease category the timescale of the disease may vary from acute onset and rapid progression to symptoms essentially stable for many years. Importantly, patients also differ widely in the impact that claudication has upon their lives. This is not a condition meriting standardized management. It demands a holistic approach adjusted to the pathology and the needs of the individual. The role and value of supervised exercise therapy is a different issue and will be discussed separately.

In assessing the patient with claudication the first step is to diagnose the cause. Second, we need to identify the location of the lesion and third, we consider the severity of the symptoms and their social and economic impact on the patient's life. Finally, the appropriateness and timing of any intervention is considered.

The cause

The clinical diagnosis of 'claudication' (muscle pain during exercise and relieved by rest) is on a par with 'headache' or 'lumbago', it tells us nothing about the underlying pathology. If the motion in this debate had stated 'Patients with intermittent claudication *due to atherosclerotic obliterative arterial disease* should have .... Etc' the proposal in this debate on behalf of supervised exercise and medical treatment would have applied to a high proportion of presenting patients. A possible danger of blanket recommendations or guidelines for the management of claudication is that unusual causes of the symptoms may be overlooked.

A frequently overlooked cause of claudication is embolism, whether originating from a central source or locally from a lesion such as an aneurysm. Claudication occurring under the age of 50 should always raise the possibility of popliteal entrapment or cystic adventitial disease, conditions which are also notoriously overlooked.

Conditions such as these may require prompt intervention independent of or concurrent with the medical management of risk factors. Even within the peripheral atherosclerotic occlusive disease category thrombolytic therapy (which, with local infusion techniques, can reasonably be described as an intervention) has a role in some new claudicants and also in previously stable claudicants whose symptoms worsen because of thrombosis superimposed on atherosclerotic stenosis (particularly those with thrombus-dominant rather than plaque-dominant occlusions).[4] In venous claudication the patient will have a history of iliofemoral venous thrombosis and there will be associated swelling. In none of these circumstances, nor any of the non-vascular conditions listed in Table 1, is there evidence that exercise, supervised or otherwise, has anything to offer.

Table 2. Weighted-average primary patency rates following endoluminal intervention in patients with intermittent claudication, including technical failures *(Adapted from TASC 2000 [4])*

	Technical success (%)	Primary patency rate (%)		
		1 year	3 years	5 years
PTA iliac stenosis	95	78	66	61
Stents iliac stenosis	99	90	74	72
PTA femoropopliteal	90	61	51	48
Stents femoropopliteal	90	67	–	–

The location of the lesion

The more proximal the lesion the more likely is it that early intervention will be appropriate. There is a strong argument for treating critical, localized short segment iliac stenoses (TASC type A lesions) before they progress to occlusions. Such lesions of the iliac arteries respond favourably to percutaneous transluminal angioplasty (PTA) +/- stenting, Literature review shows that the 5-year patency rates for stenting iliac stenoses is 72%[4] and is likely to be better when strictly limited to type A lesions. (Table 2). A similar case cannot be made for femoropopliteal PTA +/- stenting in which the results and the complication rates are less favourable.[4] Although in the short term transluminal angioplasty of femoropopliteal lesions may relieve symptoms of claudication, the clinical trial evidence does not suggest long-term benefit.[5,6] In summary, on present evidence, a strong case can be made for early intervention in selected patients with claudication due to peripheral atherosclerotic occlusive disease, the most favourable lesion being iliac short segment stenosis.

Symptom severity and impact on life

Many elderly patients with claudication caused by peripheral atherosclerotic occlusive disease are not seriously impeded in their life style and the only therapy required is modification of risk factors, combined where practical with regular exercise. For the younger patient who is in employment, especially in an occupation that involves a significant amount of walking, claudication can be a serious impediment which threatens the livelihood. It is important that symptoms are relieved quickly. This is unlikely to be achieved by medical therapy.

The effective control of risk factors requires prolonged monitoring and the adjustment of choice and dosage of drug therapy. The evaluation of the outcome of medical management may take years. Supervised exercise therapy may be geographically impractical for some patients and regular sessions may not be compatible with employment. Furthermore the best that can be said of exercise therapy is that over a period of time it diminishes the leg symptoms. The complete relief of leg symptoms restores the capacity to resume normal activities including exercise programmes with potential cardiorespiratory benefits. Early intervention, before or concurrent with medical therapy, is the treatment of choice for selected patients.

Exercise therapy

The taking of regular exercise is common sense advice for all patients, whether or not it can be proven by randomized trial to impact favourably on claudication. The published evidence on exercise in claudication has been subjected to meta-analysis;[7] it has been the subject of a Cochrane Collaboration review[8] and has also been reviewed in the Transatlantic Inter-Society Consensus on the Management of Peripheral Arterial Disease.[4]

The evidence shows that exercise improves walking distance. This applies to unsupervised exercise[9] although the balance of evidence favours supervised exercise.[8] Thrice-weekly sessions of 1 hour's duration are recommended. The exercise needs to be supervised by a trained physiotherapist. Although some trials have reported improvements in haemodynamic parameters the correlation with walking distance is poor.[4] No improvement in major cardiovascular events has been shown. The case that supervised exercise programmes should be resourced by a state funded healthcare system has not yet been made. It can be challenged by considering the following aspects: trial size, patient compliance and selection, timescales, end-points and cost-benefit.

The size of clinical trials

In Leng's Cochrane analysis ten trials met the required quality criteria. The number of randomized patients ranged from 12 to 67 (mean 30).[8] The total number of patients in the 10 trials was 305. In eight trials the exercise was supervised. The small size of these trials contrasts with the thousands of patients on whom the evidence for secondary prevention agents such as aspirin and statins is based. Consequently it has required meta-analysis to provide a sufficient body of evidence to demonstrate that exercise confers significant benefit.

Compliance and selection

Patient acceptance of, and compliance with, exercise programmes is very variable. There are a number of reasons including geography, co-morbidity and social circumstances which affect both initial recruitment and drop-out rates. For example, in a German study of 201 patients recommended for exercise, it was found that 34% had contraindications, and 36% refused to participate for a variety of reasons. In contrast an American study showed that only 9% of patients referred for exercise training were excluded on screening for the programme. Selection, however, may take place at various stages. Claudication is a very common condition in vascular practice. Logically therefore the small size of published trials implies a high degree of patient selection. Published data on the benefits of exercise must be viewed in the light of the fact that they do not apply to the whole claudication population.

Timescales

Any long-term benefit for exercise programmes is unproven. The longest reported exercise regimen in 11 randomized controlled trials of exercise rehabilitation was 6 months and the longest follow-up 15 months.[4] Claudication is a chronic disease with a timescale of many years in most sufferers. Until trials are conducted on more realistic timescales the evidence must be viewed with caution.

Endpoints

As noted earlier, claudication is a warning flag of major vascular risk. The endpoints adopted in secondary prevention trials of pharmacological prophylaxis with antithrombotic agents and statins have been deaths from heart attack or stroke. There is no information as to whether exercise therapy in the patient with claudication has an impact on deaths from major vascular events. Improvement in walking distance, while unquestionably of value to the patient, is by comparison a relatively 'soft' endpoint, which may not be sustained in the long term.

Cost-benefit

The major component of health service costs is staff salaries. Supervised exercise therapy is therefore expensive. In a cash-limited healthcare system priorities have to be considered. Given the indifferent quality of the evidence for exercise therapy itemized above, the question has to be asked whether the salaries of a physiotherapists can be justified to provide supervised exercise sessions throughout the health service for the limited proportion of patients with claudication who are likely to benefit? Competing for funds are preventative measures (population screening and risk factor control) whose proven impact on cardiovascular death rates carry far greater cost benefits than supervised exercise programmes.

Summary

- An individual and holistic approach to the patient with claudication is essential.

- Claudication has a variety of vascular and non-vascular causes, many of which require early intervention and in which exercise therapy has no role.

- The patient with localized atherosclerotic iliac stenosis should be treated by stenting, before, or concurrent with, medical therapy.

- The trials upon which recommendations on exercise therapy are based have been relatively small and short term.

- Supervised exercise therapy improves walking distance but has not been shown to be cost-effective either in terms of long-lasting symptom relief or the prevention of major cardiovascular events.

- There are many higher priorities for health service funding than supervised exercise therapy.

References

1. Davey Smith S, Shipley MJ. Prognosis of intermittent claudication. In: *Epidemiology of Peripheral Vascular Disease.* Fowkes GFR (ed). London: Springer-Verlag, 1991: 315-322.
2. Dormandy J A. Factors affecting clinical progression and mortality. In: *Epidemiology of Peripheral Vascular Disease.* Fowkes GFR (ed). London: Springer-Verlag, 1991: 325-330.
3. Janzon LUC. Prevention of vascular events in claudicants. In: *Epidemiology of Peripheral Vascular Disease.* Fowkes GFR (ed). London: Springer-Verlag, 1991: 343-346.
4. TransAtlantic Inter-Society Consensus (TASC). Management of peripheral arterial disease (PAD) *Eur J Vasc Endovasc Dis* (suppl) 2000; **19**: S47-114.
5. Perkins JMT, Collin JC, Creasy TF *et al.* Exercise training versus angioplasty for stable claudication: long and medium term results of a randomised controlled trial. *Eur J Vasc Endovasc Surg* 1996; **11**: 409-413.
6. Whyman MR, Fowkes FGR, Kerracher EMG *et al.* Is intermittent claudication improved by percutaneous angioplasty? A randomised controlled trial. *J Vasc Surg* 1997; **26**: 551-557.
7. Gardner AW, Poehlman ET. Exercise rehabilitation for the treatment of claudication pain. *JAMA* 995; **274**: 975-980.
8. Leng GC. Exercise for intermittent claudication. *The Cochrane Library,* Issue 2. 2002.
9. Greenhalgh RM, Powell JT. Screening men for aortic aneurysms. *Br Med J* 2002; **325**: 1123-1124.

Patients with intermittent claudication should have supervised exercise and medical treatment ahead of intervention

Charing Cross Editorial Comments towards Consensus

I feel a pang of conscience for having asked my friend Vaughan Ruckley to oppose this motion and he had little time to prepare this excellent chapter.

Cliff Shearman made a very strong case to establish the logic for supervised exercise and medical treatment for intermittent claudication.

Vaughan Ruckley has latched onto the expected benefit from iliac angioplasty and stenting. He has pre-empted the potential findings of the Mild to Moderate Intermittent Claudication (MIMIC) Trial which will test whether angioplasty is superior to best medical treatment and supervised exercise in patients with aortoiliac lesions.

Roger M Greenhalgh
Editor

Angioplasty is the first-line treatment in critical limb ischaemia

For the motion
Cristian Salas, Amman Bolia

Introduction

Critical limb ischaemia is becoming an increasingly common condition in our aging population. An estimated prevalence of 400–1000 patients per million population per year will be seeking treatment throughout UK.[1,2]

The optimal modern management of these patients demands a team approach combining the skills of non-invasive vascular imaging, interventional radiology and vascular surgery in order to offer the best treatment with few complications.

The recommendation from the Second European Consensus Document on critical limb ischaemia that all patients should be considered for reconstructive surgery[3] has been followed in most of the vascular units, shifting dramatically the management from primary amputation to limb salvage procedures.

A national survey in 1993 showed that nearly 70% of patients presenting with critical limb ischaemia were offered some form of revascularization as primary treatment, with a 75% chance of successful limb salvage. Compared with amputation, it has a significantly lower mortality rate, shorter duration of stay, lower cost and lower proportion of patients requiring long-term institutional support.[2]

Patients with critical limb ischaemia often present acutely in the vascular units, and the provision of beds, radiological investigation (or treatment) and theatre space has to be provided in addition to the elective work of the hospital. As a consequence many vascular units are feeling the strain of an exhausting workload, with a real threat of collapse of units with critical limb ischaemia patients.[1]

There is a real perception among vascular surgeons in Great Britain and Ireland that the total workload relating to critical limb ischaemia is very high, with enormous pressure imposed upon National Health Service (NHS) resources. As this condition has its peak in the 70–79 year age group, it must be anticipated that this burden will grow progressively as the life expectancy of our population increases.[2]

Modalities of treatment

Although it is generally accepted that revascularization should be attempted whenever possible, the role of percutaneous transluminal angioplasty (PTA) or surgery achieving this goal has become a source of controversy.[4] Doubts about technical success rate and long-term patency of PTA have been raised, leading to calls for randomized controlled trials.

To date there is no evidence-based data to support either modality as a first-line treatment. Most of the studies that do not support PTA as a treatment for critical limb ischaemia were done in late 1980s and early 1990s, collecting series of patients unsuitable for surgical repair and the only endovascular technique used was transluminal angioplasty.

Nowadays, with technological advances such as small, high pressure, low profile balloons, steerable hydrophilic guidewires, better quality images, road mapping facilities, use of different vasodilators as well as the introduction of percutaneous subintimal angioplasty (PSA), the scope of practice of angioplasty has increased a great deal.

Evidence: Endovascular vs surgical treatment

As noted before, there are no studies with a high level of evidence comparing the endovascular treatment with surgical treatment for critical limb ischaemia. However, we will present the data available so far.

Critical limb ischaemia with aortoiliac disease

Although the majority of patients with critical limb ischaemia have multi-level disease, a small group of patients present with iliac disease either isolated or in concomitance with infrainguinal lesions. Raising the issue about which therapeutic option has to be considered in treating these patients, there is general consensus that endovascular techniques such as PTA and/or stent have the advantage of lower morbidity and mortality compared with open revascularization. However, endovascular procedures are generally performed on patients with less severe disease than those undergoing surgical treatment. Regarding patency, the results of endovascular procedures are inferior, with 4 years primary patency rates of 53% for PTA and 67% for stent placement, compared with the 90% patency at 5 years of aorto-bifemoral bypass.[5]

Since the outcome of each procedure depends mainly on the severity and extent of the lesion, The TransAtlantic Inter-Society Consensus (TASC) document recommends angioplasty as the treatment of choice for TASC type A lesions and surgery in type D lesions. More evidence is needed to make any firm recommendation about the best treatment for TASC types B and C lesions, although currently endovascular treatment is more commonly used for these lesions.[5]

High-risk patients with aortoiliac disease, who are not suitable for aorto-bifemoral repair, are a subset of patients who need special attention. The surgical treatment offered to this group is the so-called extra-anatomic bypass, which, although having low morbidity and mortality, its patency rates compared with the standard aortofemoral bypass are much lower (5-year patency between 33% and 85% in axillo-bifemoral and 60–90% in femorofemoral).[5] This subset of patients can undoubtedly benefit from endovascular therapeutic procedures.

In summary the majority of patients with critical limb ischaemia and aortoiliac disease can be treated with endovascular procedures as a first-line treatment, with the probable exception of type D lesions.

Critical limb ischaemia with infrainguinal disease

Most of the patients presenting with critical limb ischaemia have infrainguinal atherosclerotic disease. To get a better idea of the results of endovascular procedures we have divided the available data according to the technique used (transluminal or subintimal) and the vascular territory treated (suprapopliteal or infrapopliteal), and comparison with surgical treatment.

The section is divided as follows:

a) Transluminal angioplasty technique
 i) Femoropopliteal lesions
 ii) Infrapopliteal lesions
b) Subintimal angioplasty technique
 i) Femoropopliteal lesions
 ii) Infrapopliteal lesions
c) Bypass surgery in infrainguinal disease

(a) Transluminal angioplasty technique

i) Femoropopliteal lesions

Stressing the importance of patient selection, Lofberg et al.[6] reported the results of PTA in 92 patients undergoing 121 procedures; 68 of them were performed in the superficial femoral artery, 13 in the popliteal artery and 40 in both arteries. Technical success rate was 88%. Primary patency rates of the whole series at 1 and 5 years were 40% and 27%. However, in limbs with superficial femoral artery occlusions longer than 5cm the patency was only 12% after 5 years, compared with 32% if the occlusion were equal or less than 5cm long. Also, a 53% primary patency at 5 years was found in limbs with single stenosis in contrast with 42% in those with multiple stenoses. The authors concluded that PTA in femoropopliteal arteries in critical limb ischaemia can be an alternative to bypass surgery in limbs with stenotic lesions and could be a good procedure in high-risk patients, with low life expectancy, who have short occlusive lesions.

Currie et al.[7] reported their failure in treating long occlusions after reporting the results of 51 PTA of the femoropopliteal segment for severe limb ischaemia. Bypass surgery was considered to pose a major risk to all patients in this series; therefore they were selected to undergo PTA. At 2 years, the limb salvage was only 42% and patient survival was 60%. Of the 23 occlusions longer than 5cm successfully treated, 22 procedures failed within 6 months.

Marzelle et al.,[8] in contrast, reported excellent results in 186 cases of endovascular treatment in patients with critical limb ischaemia, mostly in the femoropoliteal vessels. Technical success was achieved in 81%. The cumulative patency rate was 61% at 1 year and 52% at 4 years. The limb salvage rate was 87% at 1 year and 82% at 4 years. The only predictive factors affecting patency were occlusion versus stenosis.

O'Donohue et al.[9] also reported good results in an initial series of 100 infrainguinal angioplasties during a period of 42 months; 56 procedures were performed in patients with critical limb ischaemia. They were followed prospectively with clinical, ankle-brachial pressure index (ABPI) and duplex assessment. Cumulative patency for the entire group at 12 and 18 months was 53% and 43%, including initial failures. The angioplasties done during the initial 21 months had a 1-year patency of 42%, while those performed in the final 21 months had a 74% patency. The 2-year limb salvage rate was 91% in patients with critical limb ischaemia.

In summary, although the results are very variable there seems to be general consensus that transluminal angioplasty in the femoropopliteal region is an accepted and successful method of treating chronic arteriosclerotic stenoses and short occlusions. However, for the treatment of long occlusions the results are poor both in the ability to recanalize and subsequent vessel patency. Therefore, patients with critical limb ischaemia who present with stenoses or short occlusions in the femoropopliteal vessels must be considered for transluminal angioplasty as first-line treatment.

ii) Infrapopliteal lesions

Parsons[10] reported 66 cases of tibial PTA for critical limb ischaemia. With a 1-year cumulative patency and limb salvage rates of 13% and 25%. Treinman[11] reported 25 cases with localized stenosis of below-knee popliteal artery or tibioperoneal trunk, with clinical and haemodynamic success at 1, 2 and 3 years of 59%, 32% and 20%. Both studies agreed that PTA was associated with a high rate of recurrence, needing subsequent intervention and therefore do not support its use.

However, other studies show excellent results. Criado et al.[12] reported 26 cases of PTA of stenosis or short occlusions (< 3cm) of crural arteries with a technical success of 77% and long-term limb salvage of 80%.

Varty et al.[13] showed that infrapopliteal PTA was a safe and successful procedure after reporting the outcome of 40 consecutive limbs performed over a 65-month period (50% of patients presenting with critical limb ischaemia). Primary symptomatic and haemodynamic patency at 2 years was 59% and 68%. The 1-year cumulative limb salvage in the patients with critical limb ischaemia was 77%. There were two major complications (5%), both distal embolizations that were successfully retrieved by percutaneous aspiration with no adverse sequelae. The 30-day mortality was zero.[8]

Sivananthan et al.[14] also reported good results in 50 procedures performed in patients with critical limb ischaemia.. A total of 73 tibial vessels were treated, with a technical success of 96% and a cumulative patency at 1 and 2 years of 73% and 60%.

Finally, studies published in the last 2 years support the use of PTA in carefully selected patients with critical limb ischaemia, with long-term limb salvage rates of 60-80%.[15-18]

These results challenge the general consensus that angioplasty should not be performed in calf vessels.

b) Subintimal angioplasty technique

i) Femoropopliteal lesions

The technique of recanalization using the subintimal approach is well described elsewhere.[19] Although reported about 15 years ago, few other centres outside Leicester have embraced this technique and have published data. The reason may be the need for a long and exhausting learning curve, which may discourage many operators, or there may be a desire to avoid reporting results that may be inferior to the Leicester group.

Recently McCarthy[20] published the results of femoropopliteal subintimal angioplasty of 69 procedures done in patients considered unfit for bypass surgery due to either co-morbidity or unfavourable disease pattern; 62% of the patients presented with critical limb ischaemia and the median length of occlusion was 10 (range 2–50) cm. The initial technical success was 74%. Symptomatic and haemodynamic primary patency at 6 months, including failures, were 60% and 51%. Major complications requiring surgical intervention occurred in 3%.[2]

Reekers[21] reported the results of PSA in 40 patients, 72.5% presenting with critical limb ischaemia. The median length of occlusion in the superficial femoral artery was 17cm and in the popliteal was 12cm. Five patients had occlusions involving both segments with a median length of 28cm. Primary technical success was 85%. Primary and secondary patencies at 1 year were 59% and 60% – and at 2 years were 59% and 55% respectively, including failures. The option for bypass was not endangered in any of the patients with failed PSA.

A study from Leicester[22] involving 200 attempted PSA in femoropopliteal occlusions (11% of patients with critical limb ischaemia) showed a technical success of 81% in occlusion <10cm, 83% in occlusion 11–20cm and 68% in >20cm. There was a 1% rate of major complications and the haemodynamic and symptomatic patency at 1 year on an intention-to-treat basis were 56% and 58% and at 3 years were 46% and 48%.

Another study from the same Centre[23] reported the outcome of patients presenting 54 limbs with critical limb ischaemia in which the primary reason for choosing angioplasty was a high anaesthetic risk (55% of the patients); 65% of the procedures were done in the femoropopliteal vessels. A technical success of 91% was achieved. The symptomatic patency, homodynamic patency, limb salvage and patient survival at 2 years were 77%, 78%, 89% and 76% respectively. The seven patients who failed to improve were not disadvantaged by the attempted angioplasty.

Although only a few reports are available from the literature, the results in treating long occlusions of the femoropopliteal vessels are very good; therefore, when patients with critical limb ischaemia present with long occlusions, our therapeutic option must include subintimal angioplasty.

ii) Infrapopliteal lesions
Subintimal angioplasty in infrapopliteal artery occlusions was first reported in 1994.[24] Subsequently a study in 1997[25] was published of subintimal angioplasty of infrapopliteal arteries in 27 patients with 28 critically ischaemic legs. In 68% of them an adjunctive angioplasty of the superficial femoral artery or popliteal arteries was performed. The median length of occlusion was 7 (range 2–30)cm. Technical success was achieved in 82% of limbs. The cumulative haemodynamic and symptomatic patency at 1 year was 53% and 56%. The limb salvage and patient survival in the same period was 85% and 81%.[11]

Vraux[26] reported their experience with PSA of calf vessels in 36 patients and 40 limbs. All patients were considered unsuitable for surgery (poor general status, swelling, extended ulceration, lack of autogenous conduit). 68% of patients had occlusions more than 10 cm long. The technical and clinical success rates were 78% and 68%. Primary patency (assessed with duplex scan) at 1 year was 56%, including the technical failures. Limb salvage and survival at 6 months were 81% and 78%. An important feature pointed out is that even after late re-occlusions, five out of eight patients healed their ulcers or gangrene.

Ingle[27] recently published a study treating 70 ischaemic limbs with subintimal technique in infrapopliteal vessels. The median length of occlusion was 6 cm. The technical and clinical success was 86% and 80%, with symptomatic patency (freedom from critical limb ischaemia), limb salvage and mortality rate at 3 years of 84%, 94% and 51% respectively.

Based on these results, patients with critical limb ischaemia presenting with long occlusion of the calf vessels can successfully be treated with PSA.

c) Bypass surgery in infrainguinal lesions

Bypass surgery has been considered the 'gold standard' therapeutic modality in patients with critical limb ischaemia. The Second European Consensus Document on chronic leg ischaemia[3] quoted 1-year patency rates for patients with critical limb ischaemia of 75% for above-knee femoropopliteal, 70% for below-knee femoropopliteal and 70% for infrapopliteal grafts using autologous vein. With prosthetic graft the patency decreases, with respective figures reported to be 65%, 60% and 40% at 1 year.

The mortality of this procedure, on the other hand, is reported to be around 7% according to the 2001 National Outcome Audit Report.[28]

Angioplasty vs surgery

Although in the literature we can find studies comparing results of vascular surgery and percutaneous angioplasty, most of them have been done in claudicants or have pitfalls that make them unreliable. Holm et al.[29] reported the results of a prospective, randomized study performed over a 6-year period in 102 patients with critical limb ischaemia, with similar immediate and 1-year success rates for both modalities, but due to a strict inclusion criteria only 5% of the total number of patients treated during this period were accepted in the study.

Another study from Blair et al.[30] comparing transluminal PTA with surgery showed a high 1-month failure rate of 59% for PTA. Therefore, not surprisingly, the authors concluded that surgery was a more durable option.

The Veteran Administration (VA) cooperative study No 199[31] showed that PTA was as successful as surgery if the immediate PTA failures were excluded. The analysis of the PTA failures showed that patients with severely stenotic or occluded arteries were poor candidates for PTA.

Varty[32] published the results of surgery and angioplasty for the treatment of critical limb ischaemia during a 12-month period. The study was not randomized since the policy of the unit was to offer intervention with PTA whenever possible. Revascularization was attempted initially in 75% of patients, with PTA as a treatment in 46% of patients and surgery in 29% of them. The survival rates at 1 year were 91% for surgery and 78% for PTA, whereas the overall 12-month limb salvage rate in both modalities was 76%

A very interesting study by Laurila et al.[33] analysed the cost and cost-effectiveness of femoropopliteal PTA compared with femoropopliteal bypass surgery in patients with critical limb ischaemia. Surgery patients were found to have more severe disease as indicated by lower distal pressures and longer occlusions. Surgery had a slightly better clinical outcome; although the differences were not statistically significant. PTA costs were half of those of vascular surgery. The cost-effectiveness rates were significantly better for the PTA patients. They conclude that PTA should be the treatment of choice in the subset of patients where both procedures are possible.

In summary if we compare the patency of both procedures, bypass procedure has better results than endovascular modalities, but only when it is performed with autologous graft.[3] Since vein is absent or of insufficient quality in up to one-third of patients,[34] by using an alternative conduit a large number of bypasses will experience a significant decrease in patency, matching the results of endovascular procedures.

Regarding the mortality rates of both procedures, many series of angioplasty include patients not suitable for bypass surgery. However, the mortality rate for angioplasty is still very low (around 1%) compared with surgical reconstruction.

The impact of PTA in critical limb ischaemia (the Leicester and Bath experience)

The national average use of angioplasty as a therapeutic modality in patients with critical limb ischaemia is 22%.[2] However, in some units there are changing trends in management of critical limb ischaemia. Nasr et al.[35] from Royal United Hospital in Bath reported their results of patients admitted with ischaemic legs between 1994 and 1999. Patients were divided into three groups according to the date of presentation. Primary PTA rates increased from 44% (1994–1995) to 69% (1998–1999), without compromising patient survival or limb salvage rates.

In Leicester Royal infirmary,[23] during the period 1988–1991 only 23% of patients with critical limb ischaemia were treated with PTA whereas 64% were treated with surgery. A few years later (1994), when intervention with PTA was considered the first line of treatment, of the 75% of patients offered some form of revascularization, PTA became the main therapeutic modality, accounting for 46% of the patients; surgery on the other hand was only used in 27% of patients.[32] The most recent study, as yet unpublished, has shown that in critical limb ischaemia, angioplasty was the first-line therapeutic modality in 64% of patients.

Conclusion and recommendations

As a result of great differences in patient selection and characteristic of lesions, it is impossible to make comparisons between the results of surgery, subintimal or transluminal angioplasties reported thus far.

According to TASC only 5–35% of patients with critical limb ischaemia would be candidates for angioplasty if we selected them by 'favourable anatomy'[5] which in general terms means only stenotic lesions or short occlusions. Since we know from experience that the majority of patients with critical limb ischaemia have occlusions longer than 10 cm, then the only way to increase the scope of treatment by endovascular means is to incorporate in our skills the subintimal angioplasty technique which, based on the reports mentioned, works very well in long occlusions.

If we compare endovascular revascularization with bypass surgery, the results regarding long-term patency are better in the surgical arm, but only when autologous conduit is used. We have to take into consideration, however, that endovascular procedures are simple, with low risk, require a short hospitalization and most of the time are successful regarding healing of ulcers and/or relief of pain (based on limb salvage and freedom from limb ischaemia rates). Furthermore, in the context of the general health characteristic of our patients, with 3-year survival of only 50–60%, a long-term solution is not what many of these elderly frail patients require.

Surgery is often limited by swelling, spreading infection, lack of venous conduit and co-morbidities, which can lead to undertreatment of an important number of patients if PTA is not available.

Another point to be stressed is the amount of work required for bypass reconstruction compared with endovascular procedures. An angioplasty takes an average of 60–90 minutes to be performed and the majority of our patients are discharged the same day or next morning. In one morning session it is possible to treat up to four patients. This is remarkably different from a surgical reconstruction, which is exhausting for patients and surgeons. Besides the average hospital stay of 16 days,[36] a couple of femorodistal bypasses are rarely scheduled in a full day theatre list due to practical difficulties (not enough theatre time or exhaustion of the operator).

Failure after an attempted endovascular revascularization rarely compromises a subsequent surgical bypass option.

As a therapeutic modality PTA continues to evolve and advance in conjunction with the manufacturing of new devices as well as refining technical expertise. Criteria once thought to limit the technical success and long-term results of endovascular procedure have been challenged with the introduction of subintimal angioplasty.

Patient selection is critical, as it is for reconstructive surgery, but with appropriate selection in order to choose the appropriate technique, according to the characteristics of the lesions to be treated, angioplasty as a whole must be considered the first-line treatment in critical limb ischaemia.

Finally we are all waiting for a prospective, randomized study that could compare bypass surgery versus transluminal angioplasty when patients present with short occlusions or stenosis and bypass versus subintimal angioplasty when they face long occlusion, as do the majority of patients with critical limb ischaemia. Meanwhile, angioplasty, transluminal or subintimal, remains an attractive first-line option in the treatment of stenotic and occlusive disease of the iliac and infrainguinal arteries in critical limb ischaemia.

Summary

- There is no high level evidence in the literature supporting surgery or angioplasty as first-line treatment for patients with critical limb ischaemia.

- Angioplasty does not require specialized equipment or materials, and is an inexpensive procedure.

- Subintimal angioplasty has increased the scope of treatment in more patients with critical limb ischaemia than would have been possible by conventional PTA.

- The rates of major complications and mortality are lower with endovascular procedures than bypass surgery.

- While the patency of bypass surgery is better than angioplasty (only when vein conduit is used), the limb salvage rates are very similar in both procedures.

- Failure after an attempted endovascular revascularization rarely compromises a subsequent surgical bypass option.

References

1. Holdsworth RJ, McCollum PT. Results and resource implications of treating end-stage limb ischaemia. *Eur J Vasc Endovasc Surg* 1997; 13: 164–173.
2. The Vascular Surgical Society of Great Britain and Ireland. Critical ischaemia: management and outcome. Report of a national survey. *Eur J Vasc Endovasc Surg* 1995; 17: 108–113.
3. Second European Consensus Document on chronic critical lower limb ischemia. *Eur J Vasc Surg* 1992; 6(Suppl. A): 1–32.

4. Bradbury AW, Ruckley CV. Angioplasty for lower-limb ischaemia: time for randomised controlled trials. *Lancet* 1996; **347** (8997): 277–278.

5. Management of peripheral arterial disease (PAD). TransAtlantic Inter-Society Consensus (TASC). Section D: chronic critical limb ischaemia. *Eur J Vasc Endovasc Surg* 2000; **19**(Suppl A): S144–S243.

6. Lofberg AM, Karacagil S, Ljungman C *et al.* Percutaneous transluminal angioplasty of the femoropopliteal arteries in limbs with chronic critical lower limb ischemia. *J Vasc Surg* 2001; **34**: 114–121.

7. Currie IC, Wakeley CJ, Cole SE *et al.* Femoropopliteal angioplasty for severe limb ischaemia. *Br J Surg* 1994; **81**: 191–193.

8. Marzelle J, Raffoul R, Mekouar T *et al.* Long-term outcome of infra-inguinal endovascular surgery for critical ischemia. *Chirurgie* 1998; **123**: 162–167.

9. O'Donohoe MK, Sultan S, Colgan MP *et al.* Outcome of the first 100 femoropopliteal angioplasties performed in the operating theatre. *Eur J Vasc Endovasc Surg* 1999; **17**: 6–71.

10. Parsons RE, Suggs WD, Lee JJ *et al.* Percutaneous transluminal angioplasty for the treatment of limb threatening ischemia: do the results justify an attempt before bypass grafting? *J Vasc Surg* 1998; **28**: 1066–1071.

11. Treinman GS, Treiman RL, Ichikawa L, Van Allan R. Should percutaneous transluminal angioplasty be recommended for treatment of infrageniculate popliteal artery or tibioperoneal trunk stenosis? *J Vasc Surg* 1995; **22**: 457–463.

12. Criado FJ, Twena M, Abdul-Khoudoud O, Al-Soufi B. Below-knee angioplasty: misguided aggressiveness or reasonable opportunity? *J Invasive Cardiol* 1998; **10**: 415–424.

13. Varty K, Bolia A, Naylor AR *et al.* Infrapopliteal percutaneous transluminal angioplasty: a safe and successful procedure. *Eur J Endovasc Surg* 1995; **9**: 341–345.

14. Sivananthan UM, Browne TF, Thorley PJ, Rees MR. Percutaneous transluminal angioplasty of the tibial arteries. *Br J Surg* 1994; **81**: 1282–1285.

15. Brillu C, Picquet J, Villapadierna F *et al.* Percutaneous transluminal angioplasty for management of critical ischemia in arteries below the knee. *Ann Vasc Surg* 2001; **15**: 175–181.

16. Boyer L, Therre T, Garcier JM *et al.* Infrapopliteal percutaneous transluminal angioplasty for limb salvage. *Acta Radiol* 2000; **41**: 73–77.

17. Jamsen T, Manninen H, Tulla H, Matsi P. The final outcome of primary infrainguinal percutaneous transluminal angioplasty in 100 consecutive patients with chronic critical limb ischemia. *J Vasc Interv Radiol* 2002; **13**: 455–463.

18. Soder HK, Manninen HI, Jaakkola *et al.* Prospective trial of infrapopliteal artery balloon angioplasty for critical limb ischemia: angiographic and clinical results. *J Vasc Interv Radiol* 2000; **11**: 1021–1031.

19. Bolia A, Bell PRF. Femoropopliteal and crural artery recanalization using subintimal angioplasty. *Semin Vasc Surg* 1995; **8**: 253–264.

20. McCarthy RJ, Neary W, Roobottom C *et al.* Short-term results of femoropopliteal subintimal angioplasty. *Br J Surg* 2000; **87**: 1361–1365.

21. Reekers JA, Kromhout JG, Jacobs MJ. Percutaneous intentional extraluminal recanalisation of the femoropopliteal artery. *Eur J Vasc Surg* 1994; **8**: 723–728.

22. London NJ, Srinivasan R, Naylor AR *et al.* Subintimal angioplasty of femoropopliteal artery occlusions: the long-term results. *Eur J Vasc Surg* 1994; **8**: 148–155.

23. London NJ, Varty K, Sayers RD *et al.* Percutaneous transluminal angioplasty for lower-limb critical ischaemia. *Br J Surg* 1995; **82**: 1232–1235.

24. Bolia A, Sayers RD, Thomson MM, Bell PRF. Subintimal and intraluminal recanalization of occluded crural arteries by percutaneous baloon angioplasty. *Eur J Vasc Surg* 1994; **8**: 214–219.

25. Nydahl S, Hartshorne T, Bell PR *et al.* Subintimal angioplasty of infrapopliteal occlusions in critically ischaemic limbs. *Eur J Vasc Endovasc Surg* 1997; **14**: 212–216.

26. Vraux H, Hammer F, Verhelst R *et al.* Subintimal angioplasty of tibial vessel occlusions in the treatment of critical limb ischaemia: mid-term results. *Eur J Vasc Endovasc Surg* 2000; **20**: 441–446.

27. Ingle H, Nasim A, Bolia A *et al.* Subintimal angioplasty of isolated infragenicular vessels in lower limb ischemia: long-term results. *J Endovasc Ther* 2002; **9**: 411–416.

28. The Vascular Surgical Society of Great Britain and Ireland. *National Outcome Audit Report* 2001

29. Holm J, Arfvidsson B, Jivegard L *et al.* Chronic lower limb ischaemia. A prospective randomised controlled study comparing the 1-year results of vascular surgery and percutaneous transluminal angioplasty (PTA). *Eur J Vasc Surg* 1991; **5**: 517–522.

30. Blair JM, Gewertz BL, Moosa H *et al.* Percutaneous transluminal angioplasty versus surgery for limb-threatening ischemia. *J Vasc Surg* 1989; **9**: 698–703.

31. Wolf GL, Wilson SE, Cross AP *et al.* Surgery or balloon angioplasty for peripheral vascular disease:

a randomized clinical trial. Principal investigators and their Associates of Veterans Administration Cooperative Study Number 199. *J Vasc Interv Radiol* 1993; **4**: 639–648.

32. Varty K, Nydahl S, Nasim A *et al. Results* of surgery and angioplasty for the treatment of chronic severe lower limb ischaemia. *Eur J Vasc Endovasc Surg* 1998; **16**: 159–163.

33. Laurila J, Brommels M, Standertskjold-Nordenstam CG *et al.* Cost-effectiveness of percutaneous transluminal angioplasty (PTA) versus vascular surgery in limb-threatening ischaemia. *Int J Angiol* 2000; **9**: 214–219.

34. Tilanus HW, Obertop H, Van Urk H. Saphenous vein or PTFE for femoropopliteal bypass. A prospective randomized trial. *Ann Surg* 1985; **202**: 780–782.

35. Nasr MK, McCarthy RJ, Hardman J *et al.* The increasing role of percutaneous transluminal angioplasty in the primary management of critical limb ischaemia. *Eur J Vasc Endovasc Surg* 2002; **23**: 398–403.

36. Varty K, Nydahl S, Butterworth P *et al.* Changes in the management of critical limb ischaemia. *Eur J Vasc Endovasc Surg* 1996; **83**: 953–956.

Angioplasty is the first-line treatment for critical limb ischaemia

Against the motion
Martin Duddy, Asif Mahmood,
Malcolm Simms

Introduction

Critical ischaemia of a limb occurs when its blood supply becomes inadequate to meet the resting metabolic demands of its constituent tissues. The resulting compromise to functions such as sensation, movement, thermoregulation and most importantly tissue regeneration leads to the development of trophic changes at a rate determined by the severity of the ischaemia and by the degree of environmental stress to which the limb is exposed. Persistence of critical ischaemia leads inevitably to tissue necrosis and limb loss.[1]

Limb ischaemia presents in different guises and degrees of severity but the variable contribution of factors such as trauma (mechanical or thermal), sepsis, neuropathy and concomitant venous disease complicates any ranking, such as the Fontaine Classification, based on symptoms and physical signs.[2] Haemodynamic parameters such as cuff-derived systolic blood pressure at ankle or toe level or ankle-brachial systolic ratio (ABPI) are used to specify a cohort of patients with severe peripheral arterial occlusive disease (PAOD).[3] However, this excludes an important group of critical limb ischaemia patients whose reduced peripheral arterial perfusion pressure is concealed by arterial wall stiffness, usually attributable to mural calcification, including many diabetics, patients aged over 80 years, or those suffering from chronic renal failure.[4] Such patients account for 30–40% of the study group in most clinical series addressing critical limb ischaemia therapy.

The known limitations of sphygmomanometer-based classifications of ischaemic severity have persuaded many clinicians to rely on clinical criteria alone. Unfortunately this can lead to a heterogeneity of case mix that invalidates comparison of data from different centres.

Management options in critical limb ischaemia include first efforts to improve limb blood supply by direct interventions such as percutaneous angioplasty (PTA) or arterial surgery, second amputation procedures and third conservative treatments. The latter include measures to improve nutritional, metabolic, respiratory and cardiovascular status, management of wound infection and indirect circulatory enhancements such as sympathectomy, spinal cord stimulation and vasodilator pharmacotherapy. Personal experience and literature review supports the conclusion that conservative treatments have a largely adjunctive role. Claims for their success in reversing critical limb ischaemia raise the suspicion that the patients studied may not have been suffering from critical ischaemia as defined in our opening sentence.

As though the task of comparing different arterial interventions was not made sufficiently difficult by the problems of defining critical ischaemia, many series continue to mingle the results of treatments in claudicants with those obtained in critical limb ischaemia patients.

The comparing of apples with oranges is a metaphor for the exercise of comparing the outcomes of arterial bypass with percutaneous interventions in critical limb ischaemia. Prior to 1990 few centres suggested that these approaches had similar indications. Bypass was seen as most effective when traversing long and multi-segmental occlusions associated with significant reductions in distal perfusion pressure, these being exactly the conditions associated with most cases of critical limb ischaemia. In contrast, PTA in the infrainguinal segment was traditionally preferred for short occlusions, usually associated with symptoms of claudication.[5] It has only been with the recent introduction of subintimal angioplasty (SAP), with its potential for achieving durable recanalization of long segment infrapopliteal occlusions, that claims have been made for the effectiveness of percutaneous therapy in critical limb ischaemia.[6-9]

Critical limb ischaemia and extent of arterial occlusion

A chronically painful limb exhibiting trophic changes or vasomotor paralysis in conjunction with an ankle systolic pressure below 60mmHg fulfils the classic definition of critical limb ischaemia but many papers describing interventions for purported critical limb ischaemia omit details of ankle systolic pressure or of the anatomic extent of arterial occlusion in their patients.

Occlusion of a single level of the infrainguinal arterial tree usually produces intermittent claudication at worst, whilst classical critical limb ischaemia develops as a result of long multisegment occlusions. However, tissue necrosis, ulceration or gangrene may develop in limbs with short segment arterial occlusion and modest reduction in ankle systolic pressure because of trauma, neuropathy, venous disease or other contributory factors. Most of these limbs are not at risk of developing progressive ischaemic gangrene but tissue regeneration is impaired by relative hypoxia. In such patients successful normalization of ankle systolic pressure, combined with appropriate adjunctive treatment, usually achieves healing. This condition could be referred to as subcritical limb ischaemia, in order to distinguish it from critical limb ischaemia, when a true ankle systolic pressure below 60mmHg associated with long-segment arterial occlusion predicts ultimate loss of the limb in the absence of revascularization.

Because of the difficulty of obtaining valid ankle systolic pressure measurements in a proportion of critical limb ischaemia patients, particularly diabetics, we felt it might be complementary to derive a simple index of the anatomic extent of arterial occlusion in the leg based upon either arteriograms or duplex vascular ultrasound scans.

The system we have devised uses anatomic landmarks to define a series of levels in the lower limb. Levels are defined by the major bifurcations, the adductor hiatus, the peroneal bifurcation/supramalleolar anastomosis and the pedal arch (Fig. 1).

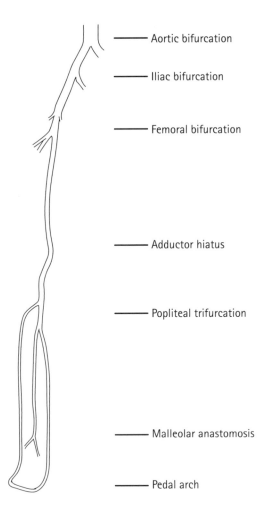

- Aortic bifurcation
- Iliac bifurcation
- Femoral bifurcation
- Adductor hiatus
- Popliteal trifurcation
- Malleolar anastomosis
- Pedal arch

Figure 1. Arterial tree showing levels used to derive occlusion scoring system.

Complete occlusion at or distal to each level scores 1; any stenosis greater than 50% scores 0.5. At the femoral bifurcation, occlusion of the common femoral trunk scores 1, while occlusion of the superficial femoral or profunda femoris scores 0.5 for each vessel. At the adductor hiatus and beyond, an occlusion scores 1 and at the trifurcation and into the calf the score is derived from the least diseased of the three tibial arteries. Figure 2 illustrates examples of this method of scoring applied to typical patterns of infrainguinal occlusion.

Limitations of angioplasty

Certain presentations of critical limb ischaemia are unsuitable for endovascular therapy. Acute on chronic ischaemia developing as a complication of pre-existing occlusive or aneurysmal disease of the leg can be treated with a combination of thrombolysis and angioplasty but recent audit has found this approach to be too slow and unreliable and surgery is preferred.[10–12]

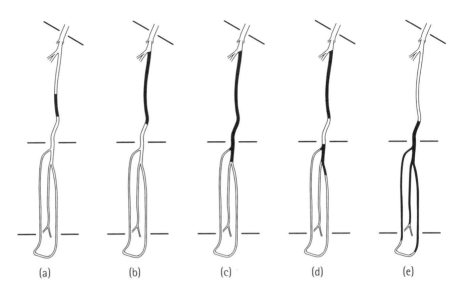

Figure 2. (a) Localized occlusion at adductor hiatus: Score 1; (b) Superficial femoral artery block from groin to adductor hiatus: Score 1.5; (c) Superficial femoral artery block from groin to trifurcation: Score 2.5; (d) Long superficial femoral artery block and tight trifurcation stenosis: Score 2; (e) Complete trifurcation and malleolar block with pedal reconstitution: Score-2.

Extensive atheromatous occlusion of the common femoral artery, either localized or in continuity with iliac occlusion, tends to be inaccessible or resistant to catheter remodelling and is usually best treated surgically.

After failure of an infrainguinal bypass graft it is unusual for the vascular anatomy to favour angioplasty.

Finally, there are few reports of successful endovascular treatment of long tibial artery occlusions traversing the ankle joint. Figure 3 illustrates a successful graft from the above-knee popliteal to the medial plantar artery in a patient with advanced critical limb ischaemia and a plantar Doppler signal that was detectable only in dependency.

Reporting conventions

Clinical series of angioplasty or bypass place variable emphasis on the amount of anatomical, physiological and pathological information supplied on their patient populations. With respect to outcome reporting, the two techniques observe dissimilar conventions.

Surgical outcomes centre on definable endpoints; the graft (patency), the limb (amputation) and the patient (survival). In the case of angioplasty, initial outcome rests on a subjective operator-dependent assessment of immediate angiographic improvement, which can mean any dilatation of a stenosis or any recanalization of an occlusion, irrespective of calibre. Evidence of long-term patency may be based on repeat arteriography, on the maintenance of improved ankle pressure (ABPI) or on continued remission of symptoms.[13]

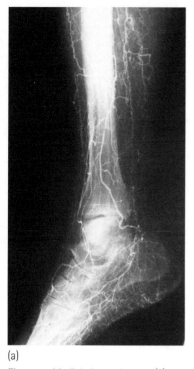 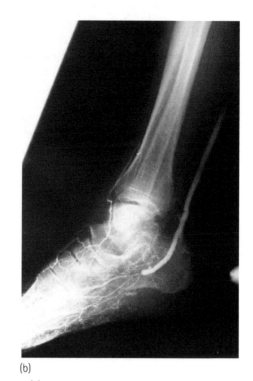

(a)   (b)

Figure 3. Medial plantar bypass: (a) preoperative and (b) postoperative angiograms.

The graft

The patency or otherwise of bypass grafts is easily confirmed; clinical criteria such as observation of tissue perfusion and healing together with pulse palpation are reliable and repeatable. Doubts are easily resolved by duplex ultrasound scanning so that angiography is almost never required solely for the purpose of establishing graft patency.

The limb

Amputation is the commonly accepted endpoint. In critical limb ischaemia, early failure of bypass grafts usually leads to limb loss, whilst occlusion after 6 months is better tolerated.[14,15] Angioplasty failure carries a low morbidity.[16]

Although simple means of assessing limb perfusion exist, in the form of ankle systolic pressure measurement and clinical recording (i.e. measures of pain relief, mobility and wound healing), such outcome data is seldom supplied, either in angioplasty or in bypass series.

The patient

Most series record major morbidity and mortality. Reporting of functional outcome (analgesic requirements, walking distance, functional and social rehabilitation) is usually deficient following treatments for critical limb ischaemia, although improvements in walking distance at 1, 2 and 3 years are usually supplied in papers dealing with angioplasty for claudication.[17]

The angioplasty

There are no absolute criteria for quantifying success in angioplasty. The observation of complete distension of an angioplasty balloon within an arterial stenosis is the usual endpoint, in combination with some evidence of angiographic improvement. Recanalization of infrainguinal occlusions may be complete or partial and a standardized or reproducible system for rating the length or calibre of residual or recurrent stenoses is not in general use. Serial ABPI ankle pressure measurement is a practical means of evaluating both initial success and long term durability of interventional procedures but it is non-specific, is seldom quoted and in fact can improve with conservative management alone. Therefore long-term success or failure following angioplasty may depend largely on subjective clinical judgement and the necessity or otherwise for re-intervention.

Local experience

These data comprise an audit of the recent practice of one surgeon and one radiologist working at one vascular centre over the same time period and simply represent an observation of our contemporary practice. During this time no formal selection protocols for the management of PAOD were in use but the majority of cases were discussed at a multidisciplinary meeting and the management plan was by consensus.

Surgical reconstruction involving infrainguinal bypass

A consecutive inclusive series of 100 infrainguinal bypass graft operations undertaken by one of the four vascular surgeons at this centre between 2000 and 2002 was reviewed by reference to the medical records. There were 27 females and 73 males, aged 42–92 years (mean 74 years) and 29 of the grafts were in diabetics. Presentation was acute on chronic in three cases and due to thrombotic complications of femoral or popliteal aneurysms in five. Failure of a previous graft precipitated recurrent critical ischaemia in 23, and in the remaining 69, ischaemia was attributable to severe PAOD.

Obligatory surgery

In this series of 100 infrainguinal reconstructions the option of angioplasty was not considered to be technically feasible in 64 cases for the following reasons.

In eight cases angioplasty had been undertaken recently without success; in eight there was complete occlusion of all crural arteries extending across the ankle joint necessitating popliteal to pedal bypass; in five the ischaemia was associated with thrombotic complications of femoral and popliteal aneurysms; and in three the degree of acute ischaemia (judged by neurosensory loss) in conjunction with a prior history of chronic ischaemia prompted immediate reconstruction.

Regrafting following failure of a previous infrainguinal bypass accounted for 23 of the cases but the most common reason for not attempting angioplasty was extensive iliofemoral occlusion above an infrainguinal block: there were 13 iliofemoral bypass grafts and in 17 other cases an extended common femoral/external iliac endarterectomy was undertaken. Thus there were a total of 77 reasons for not attempting angio-plasty in 64 cases.

In the remaining 36 cases the decision to undertake bypass reconstruction rather than angioplasty was based on a clinical appraisal of the limb and of its vascular images, whether angiogram, duplex scan or MRA (magnetic resonance arteriogram). This deci-sion was usually taken at a departmental vascular radiology/surgery meeting.

Presentation

Four clinical categories were defined. **Claudication** and **acute on chronic** ischaemia were clinical categories. Chronic ischaemia associated with rest pain or tissue necro-sis was classed as **critical** when supine ankle systolic pressure was below 60 mmHg and **subcritical** when it was above. In patients with known tibial artery calcification elevation Doppler pressure (pole testing) was taken into account. Scoring for extent of occlusion was derived from duplex ultrasound images and arteriograms and is shown below (Table 1).

Table 1

Presentation	No. of grafts	No. of levels occluded (score)					
		1	1.5	2.0	2.5	3.0	Mean
Claudication	10	4	3	3	–	–	1.45
Subcritical	12	–	2	9	1	–	1.95
Acute on chronic	12	–	–	8	3	1	2.2
Critical	66	–	–	45	10	11	2.24

The number of levels occluded in patients with critical ischaemia was significantly greater than those with subcritical ischaemia or claudication (p=00.01). In addition, those with subcritical ischaemia had a higher number of occluded levels compared with claudicants (p=0.011-using the Kendall's Tau-b test).

The anatomic details of the 100 grafts analysed are as shown below (Table 2).

Table 2

Proximal inflow	No.	Distal anastomosis	Number
Axilla/Aorta/Common Iliac	13	Above-knee popliteal	10
External iliac	16	Below-knee popliteal	10
Common femoral	53	Tibioperoneal trunk	4
Superficial femoral	4	Anterior tibial	
Above-knee popliteal	14	Proximal third	15
		Middle third	6
Total	100	Distal third	4
		Posterior tibial	
		Proximal third	3
		Middle third	8
		Distal third	3
		Peroneal	
		Proximal third	3
		Middle third	15
		Distal third	5
		Dorsalis pedis	8
		Plantar	6
		Total	100

Table 3

Event	No	Eventual outcome
Early graft failure (9 occluded, 3 ruptured)	12	4 died, 6 amputated
Died with patent graft:	9	
Late graft occlusion	7	1 amputated
Alive with patent graft	72	
	Total	100

The clinical outcome in these 100 grafts at follow-up intervals of 1–24 months is as summarized below (Table 3).

This series is fairly representative of the experience of vascular units pursuing an active programme of intervention in patients with extensive PAOD. The relatively high rates of morbidity and mortality reflect the impact of complex reconstructive procedures in a high-risk clinical group.

Percutaneous interventions

The following data summarize the consecutive angioplasty experience of one of four interventional radiologists working at our centre over the period 2000–2002. As with the surgical bypass series, there was no formal selection protocol in operation and the treatment policy was based on clinical consensus between the referring surgeons and the radiologist. In a significant proportion of cases pre- and post-intervention recordings of ankle systolic pressure were not available so that it is not possible to distinguish critical from subcritical ischaemia by this parameter. The clinical presentations, levels of intervention and initial success rates are summarized below (Table 4).

A further analysis of the 42 subintimal angioplasties performed for conventional ischaemic indications is presented in Fig. 4 below, relating success/failure and clinical presentation to the numerical extent of arterial occlusion.

There is a significant gradation of numerical level of arterial block according to presenting symptom, with the mean for claudication of 1.35, for rest pain of 1.6, for ulceration of 1.74 and for gangrene of 2.4. The score was significantly higher

Table 4

Presentation	Subintimal	Crural	Iliac	Femoropop	Total
IC >200m	2	1	6	16	25
IC 50–200m	10	5	27	28	70
IC <50m	11	1	26	25	62
Rest pain	3	8	7	6	25
Ulcer	10	22	22	20	74
Gangrene	6	10	4	4	24
Other	3	5	20	9	37
Total	45	52	112	108	317
% Success	75.6	76.9	91.4	91.2	

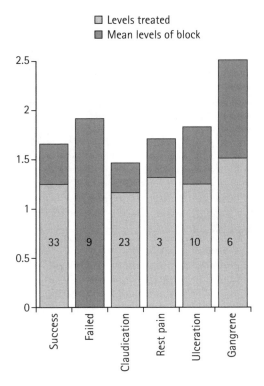

Figure 4. Levels of arterial block in subintimal angioplasty. The number of levels occluded in patients with critical ischaemia was significantly greater than those with claudication (p=0.003 Kendall's Tau-b test). The association between score and technical success did not reach significance.

in patients with rest pain or tissue loss compared with claudicants (p=0.003 Kendall's Tau-b test). These values refer to the total extent of occlusion in the ischaemic limb, including levels proximal and distal to the treated segment. Whereas in bypass reconstruction it is almost always essential to exclude proximal or distal occlusion in order to achieve graft patency, with angioplasty it is possible to treat the most significant stenosis and leave lesser areas of occlusion untreated without compromising the outcome. Thus in this series of SAP the mean numerical extent of arterial occlusion recanalized was 1.3. A typical example of a subintimal angioplasty extending from the distal popliteal to the distal peroneal artery is illustrated in Fig. 5.

Summary of local experience

Our local practice therefore suggests a policy of surgical bypass for limbs with more advanced grades of critical ischaemia and more extensive arterial occlusion. The angioplasty series contains a higher proportion of claudicants and although the incompleteness of ankle pressure data prevents any conclusions being drawn on the proportion of critical to subcritical ischaemia in the angioplasty series, the shorter levels of arterial block would suggest a prevalence of subcritical cases.

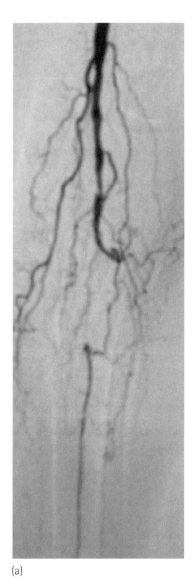

(a)

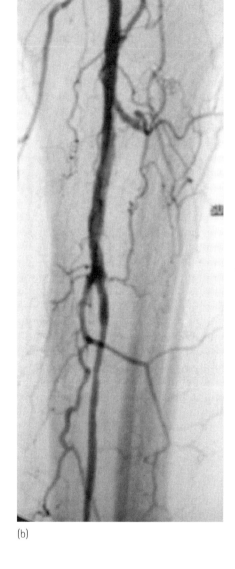

(b)

Figure 5a. Proximal peroneal occlusion.
Figure 5b. Subintimal recanalization.

Published experience

Recent reports suggest the increasing use of angioplasty as first-line treatment for critical limb ischaemia.[18] All series encompass a spectrum of presentations and it is seldom possible to distinguish between critical and subcritical ischaemia on the basis of the data supplied. The treatments offered will reflect not only the case mix but the opinions and skills of the clinicians involved. Table 5 summarizes seven published reports of infrainguinal vein bypass procedures for critical limb ischaemia with respect to clinical category, extent of bypass and outcome in terms of graft patency and limb salvage over time. In most of these reports, the diagnosis of critical ischaemia appears to be based on clinical criteria and ankle systolic pressure measurements are not supplied. Similarly, anatomical details of the extent of arterial occlusion are not furnished, so this has been inferred from the extent of grafting, making the assumption that the distal anastomosis marks the distal extent of the occlusive process and that from this point a patent artery extends into the foot.

Precise scoring of these series is therefore impossible but the majority of these surgical bypass procedures for critical limb ischaemia appear to extend over two or more anatomical levels.

Table 5. Surgical bypass for critical limb ischaemia

Author	No.	Presentation	AP	ABPI	Anatomy	Patency	Salvage	FU
Femoropop bypass								
Darke[26] 1989	34	34 CLI 16 rest pain 12 gangrene 6 ulcer	–	0.25	Length of crural disease not stated. Origin of calf vessel stenosis scored only	79	88	12
Femorodistal bypass								
Biancari[27] 2000	66	66 CLI 7 rest pain 45 ulcer 14 gangrene	–	–	Short grafts from popliteal to crural in 18 and pedal in 48	67	88	24
Shah[28] 1992	265	262 CLI 63 rest pain 199 tissue loss	–	–	All from groin to within 10cm from ankle	79	89	60
Londrey[29] 1991	253	233 CLI 103 rest pain 130 tissue loss	–	–	145 perimalloelar or pedal distal anastomosis	59	82	60
Hickey[30] 1991	329	329 CLI			Femoro-pop in 65 Femoro-crural/pedal in 239	80 82	80 82	60 60
Gloviczki[31] 1994	100	100 CLI TcPO$_2$<20mmHg 91 ulcer/gangrene in 78 9 rest pain		0.55	Pedal bypass.62 incomplete or no arch. Proximal anastomosis from ilio-fem in 52 and popliteal in 48	69	79	36
Panayiotopoulos[32] 1996	109 CLI	71 necrosis all had rest pain	–	–	100 from groin. Distal anastomosis at crural in 90 and pedal in 19	45	54	36

TcPO$_2$: transcutaneous oxygen tension. AP: ankle pressure. FU: follow-up (months). CLI: critical limb ischaemia.

Table 6a summarizes seven series of infrainguinal PTA procedures, analysing only those procedures purporting to be undertaken for critical limb ischaemia. Again, evidence to validate the diagnosis of critical ischaemia is incomplete. Assumptions as to the numbers of anatomic levels recanalized are based on the stated length of angioplasty. Table 6b presents the data from six series of SAP procedures for critical limb ischaemia and the data on level and length of angioplasty are again extrapolated to derive the number of levels recanalized. This would suggest that in the majority of cases in these series, angioplasty was used to treat disease extending over less than two anatomic levels according to our scoring system. As such it seems likely that most of these patients had subcritical ischaemia.

Direct comparisons of surgical bypass and angioplasty have been few due to the different indications for either modality depending on the pattern of the occlusive disease.[19,20] In 1989, Blair et al. reported that surgical bypass (2-year secondary patency of up to 68% and limb salvage rate of up to 90%) was superior to PTA (2-year patency of 18%).[19] However, infrapopliteal angioplasty was not employed in that series. In the presence of longer occlusions and diseased distal run-off, surgery was favoured over angioplasty. Infrapopliteal angioplasty has since yielded excellent results due to improvements through the 1990s in clinical experience combined with developments in catheter technology, reducing the risks of crural vessel thrombosis and embolism.

In another comparative study, angioplasty and surgery yielded similar limb salvage rates at 1-year follow-up in 135 patients.[20] In this series, 28 patients had surgical bypass traversing two levels of occlusion while in the angioplasty group, which included 37 crural lesions, only single levels were treated.

Although PTA is an effective tool in intermittent claudication and in selected patients with rest pain and tissue necrosis, it remains most effective in the correction

Table 6a. Percutaneous transluminal angioplasty

Author	No.	Presentation	AP	ABPI	Anatomy	Patency	Salvage	FU
PTA: Femoropop only								
Lofberg[33] 2001	121	94 CLI 30 rest pain 91ulcer/gangrene	91 had AP<40.	<0.30	Only <10cm length treated Length/extent of crural disease not given	34	86	60
Ray[34] 1995	29	29 CLI 15 rest pain 14 ulcer	TP 32–38	0.43–0.55	Single level treated only	45	100	6
PTA: Infrapopliteal								
Nasr[18] 2002	338	338 CLI	—	—	Crural and femoropop. But only single level treated. Series comprised bypass and PTA	—	—	60
London[35] 1995	54	54 CLI 19 rest pain 15 ulcer 19 gangrene	56% >50	0.43	41 one level 12 two levels 1 three levels	77	89	24
Brillu[36] 2001	37	37 CLI 13 rest pain 24 ulcer/gangrene	$TcPO_2$<30 in 13 and <40 in 24		No length given . Proximal PTA as well in 19.	—	87	24
Dorros[37] 2001	284	284 CLI 134 rest pain 150 ulcer/gangrene	—	—	169 had multi-level treated But no length given. Femoropop occlusions<35cm and crural <10cm only treated	—	91	60
Parsons[38] 1998	66	66 CLI (Fontaine II/III)	—	—	Occlusions longer than 7cm did worse	13	25	12

T: toe pressure. CLI: critical limb ischaemia.

of short and medium length occlusions. Randomized trials comparing surgical bypass and angioplasty have been marred due to the breadth of the inclusion criteria. Overall, both published trials showed that surgical bypass and angioplasty produced a similar outcome but mingled patients with intermittent claudication with those with purported critical limb ischaemia.[21,22]

Subintimal angioplasty was pioneered by Bolia from Leicester UK.[23] It allows angioplasty of extensive occlusions in the femoropopliteal and infrapopliteal arterial segments that would not be possible by transluminal angioplasty. Questions, however, remain over the true degree of the ischaemia quoted in these papers since severe multi-level disease has been excluded and measurements of ankle pressures are not quoted.[6,20] In addition, few reports evaluate late patency using duplex or angiography.[24] Varty et al. described the changes in the management of critical limb ischaemia in a single unit where surgical bypass reconstruction was carried out in only 24% of patients with critical limb ischaemia.[25] However, Doppler pressure criteria for defining critical limb ischaemia were not strictly adhered to. In this series of

Table 6b. Subintimal angioplasty

Author	No.	Presentation	AP	ABPI	Anatomy	Patency	Salvage	FU
Subintimal: Fem-pop								
McCarthy[39] 2000	69	43 CLI 26 IC	–	–	Average occlusion length 10cm 15 of CLI had 2 or more patent calf vessels but length not given	51	48	62
London[40] 1994	200	22 CLI 178 IC	–	>0.61	Femoropopliteal disease average occlusion length 11–12cm. 53 had 1 or no run-off. vessel. Crural disease excluded	58	61	36
Subintimal: Infrapopliteal								
Ingle[6] 2002	70	61 CLI: 34 ulcer 6 gangrene 21 rest pain 6 IC	–	–	Crural and popliteal disease included. Mean crural length 5–10cm (1–35). SFA occlusions extending to infrageniculates excluded	–	94	36
Nydahl[7] 1997	28	28 CLI 4 rest pain 17 ulcer 7 gangrene	–	–	19 prox procedures as well (subintimal) 16 had one vessel run-off. Median length 7cm	53	85	12
Vraux[24] 2000	40	40 CLI 31 ulcer/ gangrene 9 rest pain	–	–	27 occlusions were longer than 10cm, 10 were 5–10cm and 3 were less than 5cm. No run-off score given	56	81	12
Tisi[41] 2002	158	26 IC 122 CLI 28 rest pain 95 ulceration 6 gangrene	80	0.55	94/158 had femoropop level treated only	33	88	12

ICintermittent claudication. CLI: Critical limb ischaemia.

198 limbs presenting with rest pain (78), ulceration (89) and gangrene (55), only 71 required an infrapopliteal procedure (bypass in 28 and angioplasty in 43). Of the 94 limbs undergoing 108 angioplasty procedures only 30 had two levels treated. This would suggest that such patients had either subcritical ischaemia rather than true critical limb ischaemia or that multi-level disease was not fully treated. Data regarding the long-term patency of arteries treated by subintimal angioplasty would illuminate the argument in favour of a policy of employing angioplasty first in authenticated cases of critical limb ischaemia.

In a recent publication, Ingle *et al.* showed that subintimal infrageniculate angioplasty yielded a limb salvage rate of 94% at a follow-up of 3 years.[6] The use of the term 'limb salvage' implies that all patients were suffering from critical ischaemia but this cannot be established from the data presented. Patients with a proximal diseased femoropopliteal segment were excluded from this study. Furthermore, post-angioplasty patency data was not presented due to lack of duplex surveillance.

Reduced ankle systolic pressure is known to be a reliable prognostic indicator in critical limb ischaemia and used in conjunction with clinical information can be used to predict accurately the extent of arterial occlusion.[42] Its application is limited by the effect of reduced arterial wall compliance. The use of a simple index to describe the extent of infrainguinal occlusion appears to provide a valid index of comparison when evaluating therapeutic interventions from different centres.

Summary

- The term critical ischaemia should be restricted to limbs in which rest pain and/or tissue necrosis is associated with demonstrable arterial occlusive disease producing supine ankle systolic pressures below 60mmHg. It implies that without revascularization the limb will deteriorate and require amputation within a year. True critical limb ischaemia is usually associated with two or more anatomic levels of arterial occlusion, when surgical bypass is the most effective and durable treatment option.

- Skin necrosis and ulceration may affect limbs with ankle systolic pressures above 60mmHg and with short arterial occlusions, often because of trauma, sepsis or venous stasis. These limbs are unlikely to show progressive deterioration or require amputation but tissue healing requires revascularization, for which angioplasty is frequently effective. This condition could be termed 'subcritical ischaemia'. Once healing has been achieved, loss of angioplasty or graft patency may not precipitate relapse.

- Few series reporting surgical or radiological interventions for POAD supply sufficient information on ankle systolic pressure or length of arterial occlusion to determine whether they relate to cases of critical or subcritical ischaemia.

- Irrespective of the length of arterial occlusion, in a significant proportion of limbs suffering critical or subcritical ischaemia, endovascular techniques cannot be deployed for valid physiological or technical reasons.

- Angioplasty, though an indispensable weapon in the armament of POAD treatments, is seldom first in line for the treatment of authenticated critical limb ischaemia.

References

1. Wolfe JH, Wyatt MG. Critical and subcritical ischaemia. *Eur J Vasc Endovasc Surg* 1997; 13: 578–582.

2. Fontaine R, Kim M, Kieny R. Die chirurgische Behandlung der peripheren Durch-blutungsstorungen. Helvetia *Chirurgica Acta* 1054: 199–522.

3. Rutherford RB, Baker JD, Ernst C *et al*. Recommended standards for reports dealing with lower extremity ischemia: revised version. *J Vasc Surg* 1997; 26: 517–538.

4. Smith FC, Shearman CP, Simms MH, Gwynn BR. Falsely elevated ankle pressures in severe leg ischaemia: the pole test—an alternative approach. *Eur J Vasc Surg* 1994; 8: 408–412.

5. Gallino A, Mahler F, Probst P, Nachbur B. Percutaneous transluminal angioplasty of the arteries of the lower limbs: a 5-year follow-up. *Circulation* 1984; 70: 619–623.

6. Ingle H, Nasim A, Bolia A, Fishwick G *et al*. Subintimal angioplasty of isolated infragenicular vessels in lower limb ischemia: long-term results. *J Endovasc Ther* 2002; 9: 411–416.

7. Nydahl S, Hartshorne T, Bell PR *et al*. Subintimal angioplasty of infrapopliteal occlusions in critically ischaemic limbs. *Eur J Vasc Endovasc Surg* 1997; 14: 212–216.

8. Bolia A, Sayers RD, Thompson MM, Bell PR. Subintimal and intraluminal recanalisation of occluded crural arteries by percutaneous balloon angioplasty. *Eur J Vasc Surg* 1994; 8: 214–219.

9. Reekers JA, Bolia A. Percutaneous intentional extraluminal (subintimal) recanalization: how to do it yourself. *Eur J Radiol*. 1998; 28: 192–198.

10. Braithwaite BD, Davies B, Birch PA *et al*. Management of acute leg ischaemia in the elderly. *Br J Surg* 1998; 85: 217–220.

11. Korn P, Khilnani NM, Fellers JC *et al*. Thrombolysis for native arterial occlusions of the lower extremities: clinical outcome and cost. *J Vasc Surg* 2001; 33: 1148–1157.

12. Mahmood A, Salaman R, Sintler M *et al*. Surgery of popliteal artery aneurysms: a 12-year experience. *J Vasc Surg* (in press).

13. Ahn SS, Rutherford RB, Becker GJ *et al*. Reporting standards for lower extremity arterial endovascular procedures. Society for Vascular Surgery/International Society for Cardiovascular Surgery. *J Vasc Surg* 1993; 17: 1103–1107.

14. Robinson KD, Sato DT, Gregory RT *et al*. Long-term outcome after early infrainguinal graft failure. *J Vasc Surg* 1997; 26: 425–438.

15. Brewster DC, LaSalle AJ, Robinson JG *et al*. Femoropopliteal graft failures. Clinical consequences and success of secondary reconstructions. *Arch Surg* 1983; 118: 1043–1047.

16. Varty K, Bolia A, Naylor AR *et al*. Infrapopliteal percutaneous transluminal angioplasty: a safe and successful procedure. *Eur J Vasc Endovasc Surg* 1995; 9: 341–345.

17. Fowkes FG, Gillespie IN. Angioplasty (versus non surgical management) for intermittent claudication. *Cochrane Database Syst Rev* 2000; 2: CD000017.

18. Nasr MK, McCarthy RJ, Hardman J *et al*. The increasing role of percutaneous transluminal angioplasty in the primary management of critical limb ischaemia. *Eur J Vasc Endovasc Surg* 2002; 23: 398–403.

19. Blair JM, Gewertz BL, Moosa H *et al*. Percutaneous transluminal angioplasty versus surgery for limb-threatening ischemia. *J Vasc Surg* 1989; 9: 698–703.

20. Varty K, Nydahl S, Nasim A *et al*. Results of surgery and angioplasty for the treatment of chronic severe lower limb ischaemia. *Eur J Vasc Endovasc Surg* 1998; 16: 159–163.

21. Wolf GL, Wilson SE, Cross AP *et al*. Surgery or balloon angioplasty for peripheral vascular disease: a randomized clinical trial. Principal investigators and their Associates of Veterans Administration Cooperative Study Number 199. *J Vasc Interv Radiol* 1993; 4: 639–648.

22. Holm J, Arfvidsson B, Jivegard L *et al*. Chronic lower limb ischaemia. A prospective randomised controlled study comparing the 1-year results of vascular surgery and percutaneous transluminal angioplasty (PTA). *Eur J Vasc Surg* 1991; 5: 5175–22.

23. Bolia A, Miles KA, Brennan J, Bell PR. Percutaneous transluminal angioplasty of occlusions of the femoral and popliteal arteries by subintimal dissection. *Cardiovasc Intervent Radiol* 1990; 13: 357–363.

24. Vraux H, Hammer F, Verhelst R *et al*. Subintimal angioplasty of tibial vessel occlusions in the treatment of critical limb ischaemia: mid-term results. *Eur J Vasc Endovasc Surg* 2000; 20: 441–446.

25. Varty K, Nydahl S, Butterworth P, Errington M, Bolia A, Bell PR, London NJ. Changes in the management of critical limb ischaemia. *Br J Surg* 1996; 83: 953–956.

26. Darke S, Lamont P, Chant A *et al*. Femoro-popliteal versus femoro-distal bypass grafting for limb salvage in patients with an "isolated" popliteal segment. *Eur J Vasc Surg* 1989; 3: 203–207.

27. Biancari F, Kantonen I, Alback A *et al*. Popliteal-to-distal bypass grafts for critical leg ischaemia. *J Cardiovasc Surg (Torino)* 2000; 41: 281–286.

28. Shah DM, Darling RC 3rd, Chang BB *et al.* Is long vein bypass from groin to ankle a durable procedure? An analysis of a ten-year experience. *J Vasc Surg* 1992; **15**: 402–408.

29. Londrey GL, Ramsey DE, Hodgson KJ, Barkmeier LD, Sumner DS. Infrapopliteal bypass for severe ischemia: comparison of autogenous vein, composite, and prosthetic grafts. *J Vasc Surg* 1991; **13**: 631–636.

30. Hickey NC, Thomson IA, Shearman CP, Simms MH. Aggressive arterial reconstruction for critical lower limb ischaemia. *Br J Surg* 1991; **78**: 1476–1478.

31. Gloviczki P, Bower TC, Toomey BJ *et al.* Microscope-aided pedal bypass is an effective and low-risk operation to salvage the ischemic foot. *Am J Surg.* 1994; **168**: 76–84.

32. Panayiotopoulos YP, Tyrrell MR, Owen SE *et al.* Outcome and cost analysis after femorocrural and femoropedal grafting for critical limb ischaemia. *Br J Surg* 1997; **84**: 207–212.

33. Lofberg AM, Karacagil S, Ljungman C *et al.* Percutaneous transluminal angioplasty of the femoro-popliteal arteries in limbs with chronic critical lower limb ischemia. *J Vasc Surg* 2001; **34**: 114–121.

34. Ray SA, Minty I, Buckenham TM *et al.* Clinical outcome and restenosis following percutaneous transluminal angioplasty for ischaemic rest pain or ulceration. *Br J Surg* 1995; **82**: 1217–1221

35. London NJ, Varty K, Sayers RD *et al.* Percutaneous transluminal angioplasty for lower-limb critical ischaemia. *Br J Surg* 1995; **82**: 1232–1235.

36. Brillu C, Picquet J, Villapadierna F *et al.* Percutaneous transluminal angioplasty for management of critical ischemia in arteries below the knee. *Ann Vasc Surg* 2000; **15**: 175–181.

37. Dorros G, Jaff MR, Dorros AM *et al.* Tibioperoneal (outflow lesion) angioplasty can be used as primary treatment in 235 patients with critical limb ischemia: five-year follow-up. *Circulation* 2001; **104**: 2057–2062.

38. Parsons RE, Suggs WD, Lee JJ *et al.* Percutaneous transluminal angioplasty for the treatment of limb threatening ischemia: do the results justify an attempt before bypass grafting? *J Vasc Surg* 1998; **28**: 1066–1071.

39. McCarthy RJ, Neary W, Roobottom C *et al.* Short-term results of femoropopliteal subintimal angioplasty. *Br J Surg* 2000; **87**: 1361–1365.

40. London NJ, Srinivasan R, Naylor AR *et al.* Subintimal angioplasty of femoropopliteal artery occlusions: the long-term results. *Eur J Vasc Surg* 1994; **8**: 148–155.

41. Tisi PV, Mirnezami A, Baker S *et al.* Role of subintimal angioplasty in the treatment of chronic lower limb ischaemia. *Eur J Vasc Endovasc Surg* 2002; **24**: 417–422.

42. Shearman CP, Gwynn BR, Curran F *et al.* Non-invasive femoropopliteal assessment: is that angiogram really necessary? *Br Med J* 1986; **293**: 1086–1089.

Angioplasty is the first-line treatment for critical limb ischaemia

For the motion

Ian J Franklin, Alex Rodway

Introduction

Balloon angioplasty was introduced over 30 years ago. Given the obvious attractions of being able to improve blood flow through a narrowed or blocked vessel at surgically inaccessible sites via a small puncture site under local anaesthetic, it is surprising that the indications for angioplasty for lower limb ischaemia are still controversial. Opinions vary widely and in the month of writing, a study from the UK demonstrated much disagreement even between vascular specialists from one country.[1]

Part of this uncertainty stems from rapid changes in endovascular technology and a changing case-mix of patients. Technological advances include hydrophilic guidewires, low-profile high pressure balloons and drug eluting stents. Subintimal angioplasty pioneered by Amman Bolia in Leicester has expanded the indications for endovascular intervention. The population is aging and patients with critical limb ischaemia are increasingly frail with multifocal vascular disease. There is no doubt that angioplasty is being performed more and more often for patients with limb ischaemia. This rapidly changing environment makes it necessary to reappraise the role of endovascular surgery compared with surgical bypass procedures.

Definitions

It is easy to get bogged down defining the various forms of limb ischaemia, yet precise terminology is essential to evaluate different treatments. Critical limb ischaemia is generally accepted to be ischaemia that endangers all or part of a limb. Some definitions specify certain ankle pressures[2] but the value of these are questioned[3] as vascular calcification makes such measurements misleading.

The subdivision into acute and chronic critical leg ischaemia is more problematic. Chronic critical ischaemia is generally accepted to be rest pain for more than 2 weeks, ulceration, or gangrene of the foot. There is inevitably some overlap with acute ischaemia, which comprises previously stable limbs with sudden deterioration in arterial supply for less than 2 weeks.[4]

Evidence for vascular and endovascular treatment in critical limb ischaemia

There are no prospective randomized controlled trials comparing angioplasty with surgical bypass for patients with critical limb ischaemia. The Bypass versus Angioplasty in Severe Ischaemia of the Leg (BASIL) trial is not scheduled to report until 2004. There are, however, numerous publications demonstrating the shift away from surgical techniques towards endovascular procedures. In the Bath series of 526 patients (608 limbs),[5] angioplasty rates for critical limb ischaemia increased from 44% to 69% between 1994 and 1999. There was a corresponding drop in bypass procedures, and patient survival and limb salvage were not compromised. Similarly, in Leicester, a prospective study of 180 consecutive patients with critical limb ischaemia demonstrated that most patients could be treated successfully with angioplasty with 1-year survival and limb salvage rates of 75% and 71% respectively. In neither study was surgery found to be compromised by a previous endovascular procedure.

The role of angioplasty becomes more controversial further down the arterial tree. Short, proximal lesions are generally considered suitable for angioplasty without lengthy debate since the success rates are high and the complications low. Long occlusions towards and below the knee are much more controversial and the advent of subintimal angioplasty for these lesions has made the matter even more complex.

Transluminal angioplasty

In the aortoiliac segment, since aortic surgery is fairly high risk yet the results of angioplasty durable, endovascular techniques have found a secure place. The TransAtlantic InterSociety Consensus Document (TASC) divides aortoiliac lesions into four categories (see Table 1).[6] Endovascular treatment is recommended for type A lesions. There is uncertainty about the best option for type B and C lesions as

Table 1. TransAtlantic InterSociety Consensus (TASC) Document classification of aortoiliac artery lesions [6]

TASC classification of aortoiliac lesions	
TASC type A	Single stenosis <3cm in length of CIA or EIA
TASC type B	Single stenosis 3–10cm (excluding CFA)
	Total of 2 stenoses <5cm long in CIA
	Unilateral CIA occlusion
TASC type C	Bilateral 5–10cm stenoses of CIA/EIA
	Unilateral EIA occlusion
	Bilateral CIA occlusion
TASC type D	Diffuse multiple uni-iliac stenoses
	Unilateral occlusion of CIA and EIA
	Bilateral EIA occlusions
	Diffuse aortoiliac disease
	Iliac stenoses in a patient with aortic aneurysm or other problem requiring surgery

CIA: common iliac artery; EIA: external iliac artery; CFA: common femoral artery.

evidence is lacking, and firm recommendations cannot be made. The Cardiovascular and Interventional Radiological Society of Europe (CIRSE), however, indicates that technological advances allow the majority of such stenoses to be treated radiologically. Type D lesions still appear best treated by surgery if the patient is fit enough.

The success of transluminal angioplasty seen in the iliac arteries has not been as evident below the inguinal ligament. The Bristol team in 1994 found that transluminal dilatations of long occlusions of the femoropopliteal segment had poor durability and limb salvage after 2 years of 42%.[7] This was a particularly frail group of patients, all with critical ischaemia and only 60% survived for 2 years.

Two further studies from the USA published in the mid-1990s questioned the role of such procedures for treating severe limb ischaemia. The first focussed on distal lesions below the knee.[8] Twenty-five patients were studied, most (80%) of whom had severe critical limb ischaemia. No deaths or major morbidity resulted. Sixteen patients required a further procedure but only eight needed surgical bypass. The authors concluded that procedures should be restricted to patients with limited life expectancy or contraindications to operation. The second report was a much larger study of 307 procedures in 257 patients, all with limb threatening ischaemia.[9] Iliac angioplasties (85 of 307 procedures) produced limb salvage rates after 1 year of 96%. Superficial femoral artery procedures also produced good limb salvage (95% at 1 year). However, nearly half (30/67) of the patients with superficial femoral artery angioplasties required surgical bypass within 1 year.

Both these American studies questioned whether angioplasty had a place in acute limb ischaemia, especially below the inguinal ligament. The teams acknowledged that endoluminal techniques were useful for patients unfit for surgery, and in whom no autologous vein was available for bypass. Thus, even the teams advising caution in using angioplasty recommend its use on the type of patient that is becoming more and more common. Moreover, it has become increasingly clear that an attempt at angioplasty does not compromise the success of a subsequent operation and that there is little to lose, and much to gain, by using angioplasty as the first-line treatment.

This line of thought is borne out by several other studies. Angioplasty of the tibial arteries in a mixed group of patients with critical and non-critical ischaemia produced technical success in 96% of limbs with a sustained clinical improvement in over half over 21 months.[10] The authors recommended angioplasty, even of distal vessels, wherever feasible as the first-line treatment.

London et al. reported results of using transluminal angioplasty alone to treat critical limb ischaemia in a selected group of patients.[11] Patient survival and limb salvage rate after 7.5 months was 76% and 89% respectively. No death or limb loss was attributable to angioplasty and three embolic complications were treated successful by percutaneous aspiration.

Lofberg et al.[12] described 121 transluminal procedures in 92 patients, all with critical limb ischaemia; 51% of patients were alive after 5 years and the limb salvage rate for combined endovascular and surgical interventions was 86%. Again, angioplasty did not impair any subsequent surgical procedure.

Subintimal angioplasty

Transluminal angioplasty has thus found a place in the vascular repertoire, but has limited durability for long lesions, especially distally in the arterial tree. Subintimal angioplasty has broadened the indications for angioplasty beyond those patients with short and proximal occlusions. Lengthy blocks, even in the crural vessels, can now be tackled with a guidewire and balloon. One of the larger reported series in the UK came from Bournemouth where 148 patients and 158 limbs were treated with subintimal angioplasty.[13] Most (122) of the patients had critical limb ischaemia, the rest claudication. Median occlusion length was 10cm with most (77%) lesions in the femoropopliteal segment and the rest in the crural vessels. Technical success was achieved in 85%, 30-day mortality was 3% and 1-year limb salvage 88%. The authors concluded that morbidity was low and success of surgery was not prejudiced by technical failure or subsequent occlusion.

Another study from the southwest of England described 69 femoropopliteal subintimal procedures, 62% of which were for critical ischaemia.[14] The claudicants appeared not to derive great benefit from the procedure and the authors argued against its routine use for intermittent claudication. Nine of 42 patients treated for critical ischaemia were dead after 6 months and limb salvage rate was 21/43, perhaps reflecting the higher median age of this series (74 years) relative to other studies. Overall the procedural complication rate was low; however, one limb was amputated due to run-off being lost following the angioplasty. This failure is conspicuous by its isolation: such events are uncommon in the literature.

The Leicester group was the first to report success in using subintimal angioplasty to recanalize infrapopliteal arteries.[15] Half of their patients had intermittent claudication only and it is interesting to reflect how the importance of exercise has modified management of claudication in the seven years since this paper was published. In their series, half the limbs treated (20/40) were critically ischaemic and 77% of these were salvaged at 1 year; 30-day mortality was zero and no limbs were lost as a consequence of angioplasty. They conclude that attempts to recanalize occluded distal arteries in critically ischaemic limbs are worthwhile, especially in frail patients.[16]

Vraux and colleagues reported a series of 36 patients (40 limbs) with critical limb ischaemia treated by subintimal angioplasty of the crural vessels.[17] All patients had rest pain, ulceration or gangrene, and most (76%) were diabetic. Lesion length was longer than 10cm in 27 cases (68%). Technical success, defined by satisfactory angiographic appearance and duplex examination before discharge, was achieved in 31/40 cases (78%). All nine technical failures occurred in patients with long occlusions greater than 10cm. Clinical success (relief of rest pain, ulcer healing and limb salvage) was achieved in 27/40 (68%). Five complications were encountered and all but one was dealt with endovascularly. No complication prejudiced subsequent surgical bypass. Limb salvage at 1 year was 81%. Six of the seven deaths that occurred were of cardiac origin (1-year survival 78%). An important observation was that late reocclusion of a lesion usually did not lead to adverse clinical consequences. Five of eight late reocclusions required medical treatment only. The single patient who needed late femorodistal bypass grafting was not disadvantaged by the earlier angioplasty.

Boyer et al. from Clermont-Ferrand reported similar results.[18] Most (73%) of their patients were diabetic and all had critical limb ischaemia. Seventy-one consecutive procedures in 49 patients produced a limb salvage rate of 87%, with 75% of patients alive after 3 years. Again, late reocclusions did not cause major morbidity in the majority of patients and secondary surgery was not adversely affected by the prior angioplasty.

Discussion

Assessment of success of competing surgical or endovascular procedures often revolves around notions such as '1- and 5-year graft patency' and 'haemodynamic' and 'technical success'. The tendency to focus on the durability of the corrected arterial lesion is understandable but may mask more realistic considerations. Long-term patency rates may not concern an individual who has a low expectation of living for 1 full year, let alone 5. In such patients, the quality of the short remaining period of life is paramount and a minimally invasive procedure which relieves the immediate symptoms without prolonged convalescence may be more attractive, even at the expense of a lower expectation of long-term 'lesion patency'.

The studies highlighted above demonstrate that most cases of critical limb ischaemia can be managed using angioplasty techniques as the first-line treatment. Endovascular iliac interventions have largely replaced the old aortoiliac and aortofemoral bypass operations. Over time it has been shown that the longer the lesion or the more distal the artery, the more likely it is that subintimal angioplasty might be preferred over transluminal dilatation. Angioplasty appears not to prejudice subsequent surgical reconstruction when required, yet it spares many patients the ordeal of surgery. Long- term patency rates may appear low, but late reocclusions are often without serious clinical consequences and as previously emphasized, patients with severe limb ischaemia are increasingly frail with only a short life expectancy. The conclusion must be that angioplasty, transluminal or subintimal, offers a good chance of a favourable clinical outcome in severe limb ischaemia without adversely affecting subsequent surgery where it becomes necessary. Accordingly, it is logical to suggest that angioplasty should be used as a first-line treatment in critical limb ischaemia.

Summary

- There are no prospective randomized controlled trials comparing the use of angioplasty with the use of surgical bypass for patients with critical limb ischaemia.

- Patients with critical limb ischaemia are increasingly elderly, frail and unlikely to be fit for surgery. A growing proportion of such patients is being treated with angioplasty as a first-line treatment.

- Endovascular treatment of a critically ischaemic limb is unlikely to prejudice subsequent surgery should that become necessary.

- The durability of angioplasty is inferior to surgical bypass; however, late reocclusions tend not to have serious clinical consequences and many can be improved with a further endovascular procedure.

References

1. Bradbury AW, Bell J, Lee AJ et al. Bypass or angioplasty for severe limb ischaemia? A Delphi Consensus Study. *Eur J Vasc Endovasc Surg* 2002; **24**: 411–416.
2. Second European Consensus Document on Chronic Critical Leg Ischaemia. *EUR* 1992; 6(Suppl A): 1–4.
3. Thompson MM, Sayers RD, Varty K et al. Chronic critical leg ischaemia must be redefined. *EUR* 1993; **7**: 420–426.
4. Campbell WB, Ridler BM, Szymanska TH. Current management of acute leg ischaemia: results of an audit by the Vascular Surgical Society of Great Britain and Ireland. *Br J Surg* 1998; **85**: 1498–1503.
5. Nasr MK, McCarthy RJ, Hardman J et al. The increasing role of percutaneous transluminal angio-

plasty in the primary management of critical limb ischaemia. *Eur J Vasc Endovasc Surg* 2002; **23**: 398–403.

6. Management of Peripheral Arterial Disease (PAD), TransAtlantic Inter-Society Consensus (TASC). *Eur J Vasc Endovasc Surg* 2000; **19**: S182–S183.

7. Currie IC, Wakeley CJ, Cole SE *et al.* Femoropopliteal angioplasty for severe limb ischaemia. *Br J Surg* 1994; **81**: 191–193.

8. Treiman GS, Treiman RL, Ichikawa L, Van Allan R. Should percutaneous transluminal angioplasty be recommended for treatment of infrageniculate popliteal artery or tibioperoneal trunk stenosis? *J Vasc Surg* 1995; **22**: 457–463.

9. Parsons RE, Suggs WD, Lee JJ *et al.* Percutaneous transluminal angioplasty for the treatment of limb threatening ischemia: do the results justify an attempt before bypass grafting? *J Vasc Surg* 1998; **28**: 1066–1071.

10. Sivananthan UM, Browne TF, Thorley PJ, Rees MR. Percutaneous transluminal angioplasty of the tibial arteries. *Br J Surg* 1994; **81**: 1282–1285.

11. London NJ, Varty K, Sayers RD *et al.* Percutaneous transluminal angioplasty for lower-limb critical ischaemia. *Br J Surg* 1995; **82**: 1232–1235.

12. Lofberg AM, Karacagil S, Ljungman C *et al.* Percutaneous transluminal angioplasty of the femoropopliteal arteries in limbs with chronic critical lower limb ischemia. *J Vasc Surg* 2001; **34**: 114–121.

13. Tisi PV, Mirnezami A, Baker S *et al.* Role of subintimal angioplasty in the treatment of chronic lower limb ischaemia. *Eur J Vasc Endovasc Surg* 2002; **24**: 417–422.

14. McCarthy RJ, Neary W, Roobottom C *et al.* Short-term results of femoropopliteal subintimal angioplasty. [see comments.] *Br J Surg* 2000; **87**: 1361–5.

15. Varty K, Bolia A, Naylor AR *et al.* Infrapopliteal percutaneous transluminal angioplasty: a safe and successful procedure. *Eur J Vasc Endovasc Surg* 1995; **9**: 341–345.

16. Bolia A. Percutaneous intentional extraluminal (subintimal) recanalization of crural arteries. *Eur J Radiol* 1998; **28**: 199–204.

17. Vraux H, Hammer F, Verhelst R *et al.* Subintimal angioplasty of tibial vessel occlusions in the treatment of critical limb ischaemia: mid-term results. *Eur J Vasc Endovasc Surg* 2000; **20**: 441–446.

18. Boyer L, Therre T, Garcier JM *et al.* Infrapopliteal percutaneous transluminal angioplasty for limb salvage. *Acta Radiol* 2000; **41**: 73–77.

Angioplasty is the first-line treatment for critical limb ischaemia

Against the motion

Andrew Bradbury

Introduction

Before setting out the case against angioplasty as first-line treatment for critical limb ischaemia, three very important points regarding the motion need to be considered.

First, the motion asks us to consider patients with critical limb ischaemia, a term that has been precisely defined by the European Consensus[1] and recently endorsed by the Transatlantic Consensus[2] documents. Data relating to patients with lesser degrees of ischaemia that do not fulfil these criteria are not, therefore, germane to this debate.

Second, members of the floor should only vote for the motion if they are persuaded that level I data from randomized controlled trials support the use of angioplasty in true critical limb ischaemia. Uncontrolled, observational, single-centre data are not a basis for changing and informing modern practice. Vascular surgeons and intereventionalists have not accepted level III evidence in the context of abdominal aortic aneurysm or carotid interventions so why should critical limb ischaemia be different.

Third, as the motion includes the word 'first', the debate is only concerned with those patients who could be treated in another way. In other words, in reaching a conclusion, we must only consider the role of angioplasty in those patients who are suitable and fit for surgery.

Please, ladies and gentlemen, bear these important points in mind when reading or listening to the claims of the opposition as they 'side-track' you off the motion and try to persuade you to lower your critical threshold.

The literature and its deficiencies

In preparation for this debate, the author performed a Medline search of the literature since 1966 using the terms 'angioplasty', 'peripheral vascular disease' and 'critical limb ischaemia'. This resulted in the return of many hundreds of articles, most of which were concerned with intermittent claudication. Even those that do deal with non-claudicants are often impossible to interpret for various reasons (Table 1).[3-42] What follows, therefore, is a discussion of those papers where the authors report separately the results of infrainguinal angioplasty in non-claudicants. Papers from Leicester are considered separately section because their experience and outcomes are unique.

Table 1. Papers that consider angioplasty in patients with limb-threatening ischaemia but could not be used to inform this debate and why

Reviews, leading articles, opinion pieces and summaries of previously published data.[3-7]
Non-clinical endpoints.
Includes patients with claudication and or combines suprainguinal and infrainguinal interventions.[8-35]
Angioplasty combined with surgery or performed intraoperatively.[36-38]
Angioplasty combined with adjuvant techniques such as LASER, atherectomy, brachytherapy or stenting.[39,40]
Effect of angioplasty on healing of venous ulcers.[41]
Study combines angioplasty of native arteries and vein grafts.[42]

Zarins (1980)[43] treated six patients with rest pain and gangrene or ulceration by angioplasty. At 5 months, half the patients had undergone amputation.

Rush (1983)[44] attempted angioplasty in 97 limbs (86 patients) with end-stage occlusive disease. Major amputation was required in 22% following angioplasty. At 12 months, there was a 57% restenosis rate in the remainder.

Brown (1988)[45] performed infrapopliteal angioplasty in 11 patients. The immediate technical failure rate was 25% and at follow-up of only 1–22 months only two-thirds of remaining patients were still 'improved'.

Schwarten and Cutcliff (1988)[46] performed below-knee angioplasty in 98 patients (114 limbs) who were candidates for limb salvage surgery. Initial limb healing without amputation was achieved in 88% of limbs; 2 years after percutaneous transuminal angioplasty (PTA), 32 of 37 patients available for follow-up had viable pain-free extremities.

Bakal (1990)[47] retrospectively analysed the results of 57 procedures in 53 patients. Although 56 procedures were apparently performed for 'limb salvage' no further details are given and ankle pressures are not reported. In all, 76 infrapopliteal arteries were dilated and 33 patients had concomitant angioplasties of the femoropopliteal arteries or vein grafts. There were three major complications (6%) and 20 minor complications (37%). In the first 14 procedures the technical failure rate was 71% and, in remaining procedures, 14%. Immediate clinical improvement was observed in only 80% of 40 technically successful procedures giving an overall immediate clinical improvement rate of only 56%. No long-term data were presented.

Cooper and Welsh (1991)[48] reported the results of angioplasty in 24 patients with 'limb-threatening ischaemia'. Of these, ten were technically and/or clinically unsuccessful and required other treatment, two remained static and 12 improved.

Saab (1992)[49] undertook 17 tibial and four femoropopliteal 'limb salvage' angioplasties in 13 patients (14 limbs). At 2 months, only ten limbs had improved and at 6 months, three patients (23%) had undergone amputation.

Buckenham (1993)[50] performed 14 infrapopliteal angioplasties in 13 patients with critical limb ischaemia. Absolute pressures were not given. Improvement was seen in 11 patients (85%) with a mean (range) follow-up of 8 (1–18) months.

Currie (1994)[51] reported on 50 patients undergoing 51 femoropopliteal angioplasties for severe limb ischaemia. Eleven (22%) angioplasties were immediate technical failures, 25 failed in the first 6 months and only 14 were successful at 6 months follow-up. There were eight (16%) major complications after angioplasty, requiring amputation in five instances (10%).

Durham (1994)[52] studied 14 consecutive diabetic patients undergoing tibial angioplasty for treatment of limb-threatening ischaemia. All the patients had tissue loss but no ankle or toe pressures were given. The 30-day mortality (7%) and major morbidity (28%) were high and at a mean follow-up of only 17 months 23% of patients had required a major limb amputation.

Treiman (1995)[53] retrospectively examined the records of 25 patients undergoing below-knee popliteal artery angioplasty. Of these, 14 had rest pain and six had an ulcer with a mean ankle-brachial pressure index (ABPI) of 0.52. Absolute pressures were not given. At a mean follow-up of 44 months, success was 59%, 32% and 20% at 1, 2, and 3 years respectively.

Matsi (1995)[54] reported 103 consecutive patients (117 limbs) with rest pain and/or tissue undergoing iliac (n = 4), femoropopliteal (n = 121), or intrapopliteal (n = 84) angioplasty. Ankle pressures were not reported. The immediate technical success rate was 92% for stenosis and 80% for occlusion, there was a 11% major complication rate and the cumulative limb salvage rate at 1, 2 and 3 years was only 56%, 49% and 49% respectively.

Favre (1996)[55] performed 25 distal angioplasties in 24 patients of whom 20 were described as having critical limb ischaemia. The remaining four patients had asymptomatic graft stenoses. The mean (SD) ABPI was 0.61 (0.31) and absolute pressures were not given. There were four immediate failures and six patients had recurrent stenosis at mean follow-up of only 9 months. At 2 years, the cumulative primary and secondary patency rates were 46% and 64% respectively.

Lofberg (1996)[56] undertook crural (n = 39) and/or femoropopliteal (n = 55) angioplasty in 86 limbs (82 patients and 94 procedures) affected by rest pain and/or tissue loss. Absolute ankle or toe pressures were not given. The immediate technical failure was 12% and the cumulative primary clinical success rates at 6, 12, 24, and 36 months were 55%, 51%, 36%, and 36% respectively.

Hanna (1997)[57] performed angioplasty in 29 consecutive diabetic patients for limb salvage. Absolute pressures were not given. At 12-months follow-up, six had persistent and 40/50 infrapopliteal segments that had been successfully dilated had occluded.

Vraux (2000)[58] performed subintimal angioplasty in 36 patients with tibial artery occlusions. Forty limbs were treated of which 31 had tissue loss and nine had rest pain. Doppler pressures and ABPIs were not reported. The primary technical success rate was 78%, the primary clinical success rate 68% and the 12 months success rate 56%.

Boyer (2000)[59] performed a retrospective study of 71 consecutive infrapopliteal angioplasties in 49 patients with rest pain (n = 20) or ulceration (n = 29). In 18 patients, surgical minor amputation or debridement was also performed. Technical success was achieved in 45 patients. Four failures necessitated two amputations and one patient died. The morbidity rate was 16%, including minor complications in five patients and major vascular complications in three patients. After technical success during the follow-up (median duration 21 months), restenoses occurred in four patients, of whom three had a successful re-PTA (clinical success rate 72%). Survival, primary patency, secondary patency and limb salvage rates were, respectively, 75%, 81%, 88% and 87% after 3 years.

McCarthy (2000)[60] reviewed the results of 69 subintimal angioplasties performed for femoropopliteal occlusion in 66 patients suffering intermittent claudication (n=26) or critical limb ischaemia (n = 43). Median occlusion length was 10 (range 2–50) cm. Primary technical success was achieved in 51 occlusions (74%). There were 11 complications (16%) and surgical intervention was required in two patients (3%). At 6 months the cumulative symptomatic and haemodynamic primary patency rates were 60 and 51% respectively, analysed on an intention-to-treat basis. The symptomatic and haemodynamic patency rates for technically successful procedures were 80 and 77% respectively. The authors state 'In this series the short-term clinical success of subintimal angioplasty was poor because of a high incidence of re-occlusion and restenosis, despite a relatively high initial technical success rate'.

Dorros (2001)[61] reported that tibioperoneal vessel angioplasty for critical limb ischaemia was technically and clinically successful in over 90% of almost 300 limbs treated. At 5-year follow-up, bypass surgery was undertaken in 8% and amputations in 9% giving a limb salvage of 91%.

Melliere (2001)[62] reported that of 310 patients admitted over a 5-year period with tissue loss, only 26 diabetics (group 1) and 30 non-diabetics (group 2) were felt to have a pattern of disease that was amenable to angioplasty, of which 13 (23%) were iliac. In group 1, the primary cumulative patency rate at 1 and 3 years was 76%. In group 2, the primary cumulative patency rate at 1 and 3 years were 85% and 80%, respectively.

Clark (2001)[25] reported on the results of the US-based seven-centre Society for CardioVascular Interventional Radiology Transluminal Angioplasty and Revascularisation (STAR) registry. Of the 383 patients (397 limbs) who underwent femoropopliteal angioplasty, follow-up data were available in only 205 (53%), of whom 24 (11.7%) had rest pain and 52 (25.4%) had 'minor tissue loss'. The remaining patients had claudication. Clinical and ABPI outcome data are not presented separately for claudicants and non-claudicants. However, in a multivariate Cox proportional hazards model, the presence of diabetes (relative risk 3.5, p< 0.001) and poor tibial run-off (relative risk 5.8, p = 0.0001) were powerful and independent negative predictors of patency. Furthermore, when initial technical failures are included, the 12-month patency in patients with significant tibial run-off disease was approximately 30%.

Smith *et al.* (2002)[63] reported their experience with 43 consecutive patients (48 limbs) undergoing subintimal angioplasty for superficial femoral artery occlusions.

Table 2. Shortcomings of papers reporting on the results of angioplasty for limb-threatening ischaemia

---

Do the patients have CLI?
In none of the papers are absolute ankle or toe pressure reported so it is impossible to know whether the patients studied had true critical limb ischaemia or not; in many cases it seems likely that they did not.
Which patients are being studied?
Patients are highly selected.
Often only those not being considered for surgery are included.
In none of the papers are clear inclusion and exclusion criteria stated.
Numbers are usually small, often tiny, and patients recruited over long periods of time
Is follow-up adequate and credible?
Follow-up is almost universally short and incomplete.
In many papers initial technical and clinical failures are excluded from quoted long-term patency and clinical success rates.
Life table analysis is infrequently used.
Studies are usually retrospective
Even when follow-up is said to be complete it is often apparent that this was done indirectly via another doctor, relative, post or telephone.
Are the endpoints credible?
The choice and definition of endpoints, such as 'improved', is poor.
There is no quality of life analysis.
There is health-economic analysis.
There is no mention of out-of-hospital treatments and social care requirements.

There were 17 patients with critical limb ischaemia of median age 72 years and a median occlusion length of 10cm, in whom there was an 80% immediate technical success and a 12-month haemodynamic patency of only 25%. The authors concluded 'short and long-term patency in patients with critical limb ischaemia is poor. Subintimal angioplasty in the treatment of critical limb ischaemia should be reserved for those patients not suitable for surgical bypass'.

On the basis of these reports, one would have to conclude that:

1. the quality of reporting generally falls short of what is now expected and acceptable as an evidence-base for practice (Table 2);
2. the results are significantly worse than those that would be expected following femorodistal bypass.

The Leicester experience

The Leicester group is unique in maintaining that:

1. it is the majority of patients with critical limb ischaemia who can be treated with (subintimal) angioplasty
2. the results of sub-intimal angioplasty are superior to surgery.

As such, it is worth examining their data in some detail.

In 1994, Dr Bolia[64] described angioplasty of 29 occluded crural arteries in 21 patients with 24 ischaemic limbs; seven (29%) with claudication, five (21%) with rest pain and 12 (50%) with tissue loss. Ankle pressures and ABPI are reported for the group as a whole but not for the claudicants and non-claudicants separately. It is unclear, therefore, how many of these patients had true critical limb ischaemia. However, three of the 12 patients treated for tissue loss were immediate technical failures, and one re-occluded at 3 days and required a below-knee amputation. This represents a 33% immediate clinical failure rate in a group of patients the authors specifically point out would have been suitable for surgical bypass.

In the same year, the group reviewed the results of 200 attempted subintimal angioplasties for femoropopliteal artery occlusions of median (range) length 11 (2–37) cm.[65] Over 90% of the patients were claudicants. There was a 20% immediate technical failure rate and the haemodynamic patency of the remaining 80% was only 71% at 12 months (i.e. 51% if one includes the technical failures). These results are clearly inferior to those achievable by means of surgery. Furthermore, if the patency of subintimal angioplasty for single level femoropopliteal block in claudicants is this poor, it seems unlikely the technique could challenge surgical bypass in critical limb ischaemia patients with distal and multisegment disease.

The group published 2 years later a prospective study of 188 patients presenting to their unit with 'critical limb ischaemia' over a 12-month period.[66] The following treatments were offered: angioplasty (42%), surgery (24%), surgery and angioplasty (7%), primary major amputation (10%) and conservative therapy (17%). Importantly, the authors state that 'the Doppler pressure criteria of the European Consensus document were not adhered to' and, in fact, no ankle or toe pressures or ABPIs were reported.

The next year they retrospectively reviewed 28 consecutive limbs (27 patients) with what the authors describe as 'critical limb ischaemia' that had undergone subintimal angioplasty of 32 infrapopliteal artery occlusions.[67] No ankle or toe pressures or ABPIs were reported. Seventeen limbs (61%) were ulcerated, seven (25%) were gangrenous and four (14%) had rest pain only. The immediate technical failure rate was

16% and at 12-month follow-up the patency rate was only 53% (15 patients at risk). These figures appear to be worse that those anticipated for surgical bypass. Furthermore, despite the very disappointing haemodynamic patency, the authors report an 85% limb salvage at 12 months; it seems likely that most of these patients did not have true critical limb ischaemia.

More recently, in 2001, they retrospectively reviewed the case notes of 12 patients presenting with symptoms of lower limb ischaemia who presented with an occluded infrainguinal bypass graft.[68] Subintimal angioplasty of the occluded native vessels was attempted and was technically successful in seven patients. However, after a median follow up of only 4 weeks, only one case had persistent patency of the previously occluded segment. They concluded that the results were disappointing. Why are these patients so different from their other experience? Is it because the technique, in this circumstance, is being applied to a group of patients who for the most part had true critical limb ischaemia?

Most recently, the group reviewed their experience with subintimal angioplasty in treating isolated infragenicular disease in patients they now, interestingly, describe as having 'severe' as opposed to 'critical limb ischaemia'.[69] This was a retrospective study of 67 patients (70 limbs) treated between 1997 and 2000; 9% had claudication, 31% had rest pain, 51% had ulceration and 9% had gangrene (extent not specified). Ankle pressures and ABPI were not given either before or after intervention. The immediate technical and clinical success rates were only 86% and 80% respectively. Two patients developed acute limb-threatening ischaemia post-procedure, there were four (6%) groin haematomas and five (7%) intraprocedural arterial perforations.

What can we conclude from these data? No other individual interventionalist or unit in the world has been able to obtain such good results with subintimal angioplasty. No-one doubts the honesty of the reporting and I am sure we would all wish to be able to treat our patients in this way if we could. But, it remains difficult to explain why the Leicester group's experience is so uniquely favourable both in terms of the numbers of patients who appear suitable for the technique, the immediate technical success rate and complication rate[70] and the medium-term durability. While exceptional interventional skill is probably a factor, it seems likely that a significant proportion of the Leicester patients had subcritical limb ischaemia[71] as opposed to true critical limb ischaemia. Patients with subcritical limb ischaemia have:

1. rest pain with or without *limited* tissue loss;
2. ankle pressures that exceed 50mmHg;
3. a more limited arterial disease that lends itself more often to endovascular therapy;
4. a natural history that is more akin to claudication;
5. a low rate of limb loss (<50% at 12 months) whether or not they undergo surgical or endovascular intervention in addition to best medical therapy;[72]

As such patients do so much better than those with true critical limb ischaemia, to analyse critical limb ischaemia, subcritical limb ischaemia (and even claudicants) together is inappropriate. This is such a crucial point that in the Bypass versus Angioplasty in severe limb ischaemia (BASIL) trial (please see below), claudicants are specifically excluded and randomization of the admitted patients stratified by subcritical limb ischaemia versus critical limb ischaemia on the basis of clinical presentation (rest pain only versus rest pain and tissue loss) and ankle pressure (greater than versus less than or equal to 50mmHg)

The important point, however, is that a technique that only works in the hands of the few is of little use to the legs of the many. It also has to be respectfully pointed out that the Leicester group have never tested the results of subintimal angioplasty against those of surgery in a randomized, or even a non-randomized, controlled manner. And, in fact, at the time of writing the group have declined to enter their patients into the BASIL trial because they believe that angioplasty is so obviously superior to surgery in their hands that it would almost unethical to do so. However, the days when uncontrolled, single-centre data (level III evidence) could change the hearts and minds of vascular specialists are long gone.

Studies that try to compare surgery and angioplasty

As outlined above, there are mixed views as to whether angioplasty and surgery can, or even should, be compared within the rigorous confines of the randomized controlled trial, especially in the context of patients with critical limb ischaemia. [3,4] However, the fact remains that a proportion of patients with critical limb ischaemia could be treated by either method in the first instance. Although this proportion varies enormously between different units, even between different surgeons and radiologists working within the same unit, where there is 'clinical equipoise' the only way of making that decision is randomly until such time as the pros and cons of each strategy can be quantified more precisely.[73,74] Although, to date, there are no such randomized data available (please see below), it is worth reviewing the results of less rigorous comparative studies as these may provide the scientific and ethical basis for a randomized controlled trial.

Blair (1989)[75] retrospectively compared 54 patients undergoing transluminal angioplasty (54 procedures) and 56 patients undergoing 69 infrainguinal (29 femoropopliteal and 34 femorodistal) bypasses for critical limb ischaemia. Although this was not a controlled study, patients were comparable with respect to age, sex, and the presence of diabetes, hypertension, obesity, hypercholesterolaemia, and smoking. Mean follow-up was 40 months (4 to 88 months) for the PTA group and 28 months (6 to 78 months) for the surgery group. Thirty-nine of the 54 patients (72%) were initially improved after PTA. However, the 2-year patency determined by non-invasive Doppler studies was only 18%. By contrast, the 2-year patency for femoropopliteal and femorodistal bypasses was 68% and 47% respectively.

Wilson (1989)[76] conducted a randomized comparison of transluminal angioplasty (n = 129) and surgery (n = 126). The groups were comparable in terms of risk factors and distribution of disease. The immediate failure rate for PTA was 15.5%. Surgery was performed with one in-hospital death (0.8%) and 17 complications (13.5%). There were two late deaths ascribable to surgical complications and none to PTA. At 4.5 years, there were 50 deaths (20%) (28 from surgery; 22 with PTA) and 24 major amputations (13 with surgery; 11 with PTA). The ABPI, both before and 36-months after treatment, was not significantly different between the two groups. Unfortunately, patients with suprainguinal and infrainguinal disease, and patients with claudication (the majority) and severe limb ischaemia, were not analysed separately. As such, it is difficult to draw any firm conclusions from this trial.

Holm (1991)[77] reported on 102 patients with severe lower limb ischaemia or claudication who were randomized to PTA or surgery. Only patients who could be treated by both methods were included, constituting only 5% of the total number of patients treated during this period. The two groups were similar regarding age, severity of symptoms and diabetes. The immediate and 1-year results showed similar success and complication rates. Once again, the failure to analyse claudicants and patients with severe limb ischaemia separately hampers interpretation of the study.

Zdanowski (1998)[78] used Swedvasc to report on 3730 operations and 1199 angioplasties for 'critical limb ischaemia' due to infrainguinal disease between 1987 and 1995. Absolute Doppler pressures are not recorded in Swedvasc so it is not possible to determine how many of these patients had true critical limb ischaemia. Obviously this was not a randomized, or even controlled, study and it is not strictly appropriate therefore to compare the two groups. However, the mortality rate for the whole group was 5.3% at 1 month and 22.9% at 1 year, with no difference between the surgery and angioplasty groups. Significantly more patients were alive and improved after surgery than after angioplasty at 1 month (82.3% versus 77.7%) and at 1 year (49.6% versus 44.3%) (Fig. 1).

The BASIL trial

The author is the Principal Investigator for the UK-based, Health Technology Assessment (HTA)-funded Bypass versus Angioplasty in Severe Ischaemia of the Leg (BASIL) trial.[73,74] The aim of the study is to determine whether, in patients with severe limb ischaemia due to infrainguinal disease, angioplasty (transluminal or subintimal at the interventionalist's discretion) or bypass surgery as first-line therapy is associated with a superior amputation-free survival. As well as recording a full range of clinical end-points, the two treatment strategies will be compared in terms of health-related quality of life and in a full health economic analysis. The term severe limb ischaemia rather than critical limb ischaemia is used because the trial includes patients with both subcritical limb ischaemia and critical limb ischaemia. Claudicants and patients with uncorrected suprainguinal disease are specifically excluded.

In order to allow these two distinct clinical entities (critical limb ischaemia and subcritical limb ischaemia) to be differentiated, randomization is being stratified by ankle pressure and the presence/absence of tissue loss (Fig. 2). At the time of writing,

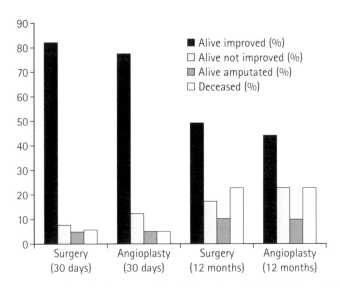

Figure 1. Outcome of infrainguinal surgery and angioplasty for critical limb ischaemia from Swedvasc registry.

over 300 patients have been randomized in almost 30 UK centres and the aim is to continue recruitment to 450 and then follow all of the patients for a minimum of 12 months. An audit of severe limb ischaemia patients being treated in the participating units outside the trial suggests that, overall, about 10–20% of patients are felt to be in 'clinical equipoise' i.e. they could be treated by either angioplasty or surgery (although this does vary considerably between different centres). The results of the trial should become available in 2005/6 and will provide, for the first time, a level I evidence-base on which to practice.

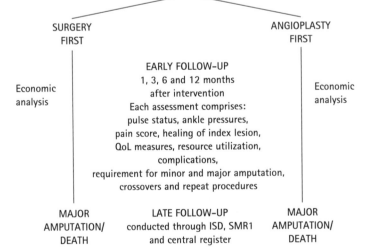

SEVERE LIMB ISCHAEMIA
Rest pain and/or tissue loss of presumed arterial aetiology for more than 2 weeks
Suprainguinal 'inflow' considered capable of supporting infrainguinal bypass or PTA
|
Research Nurse discusses trial with patient and distributes
PATIENT INFORMATION SHEET
|
Research Nurse completes **BASELINE ASSESSMENT FORM**
Patient completes **BASELINE QUALITY OF LIFE FORMS (SF–36 & VascuQol)**
|
Consultant surgeon or radiologist obtains informed consent
PATIENT CONSENT FORM is completed
|
ANGIOGRAPHY
Radiologist willing to perform infrainguinal angioplasty
AND Surgeon willing to perform infrainguinal bypass
RANDOMIZATION

Clinical presentation	Ankle pressure (mmHg)	
	<50	>50
Rest pain only	A	B
Tissue loss	C	D

Groups A, B, C and D also stratified by centre,

SURGERY FIRST		ANGIOPLASTY FIRST
Economic analysis	**EARLY FOLLOW-UP** 1, 3, 6 and 12 months after intervention Each assessment comprises: pulse status, ankle pressures, pain score, healing of index lesion, QoL measures, resource utilization, complications, requirement for minor and major amputation, crossovers and repeat procedures	Economic analysis
MAJOR AMPUTATION/ DEATH	LATE FOLLOW-UP conducted through ISD, SMR1 and central register	MAJOR AMPUTATION/ DEATH

QoL :Quality of life

Figure 2. Flow diagram of Bypass versus Angioplasty in Severe Ischaemia of the Leg (BASIL) trial.

Conclusion

With the notable exception of the Leicester data, the general world-wide consensus appears to be that only a minority of patients with true critical limb ischaemia are suitable for angioplasty and that even in these highly selected patient the immediate failure rate is high and the haemodynamic patency low (certainly lower than would be considered acceptable after surgery). Most authorities, therefore, seem to suggest that in patients with critical limb ischaemia, angioplasty should be reserved for those who are too unfit for surgery. However, the literature would suggest that the results in such patients are abysmal and rarely delay the need for major limb amputation or death. Such patients may be best served by a primary amputation but this difficult decision has to be made on a case-by-case basis

Although not, of course, germane to the present debate, there may be a role for angioplasty in patients with:

1. subcritical limb ischaemia, who usually have less extensive disease, and may be concerted back into claudicants by a combination of aggressive best medical therapy and limited angioplasty;
2. venous ulcers and limited arterial disease in order to relieve pain and/or permit compression therapy;
3. neuroischaemic tissue loss in diabetics where the primary problem is neuropathy but where endovascular treatment of limited arterial disease may improve blood flow and speed healing;

However, at the present time, there is absolutely no credible evidence to suggest that in patients with true critical limb ischaemia and who are suitable for femorodistal bypass, angioplasty is the preferred option.

Summary

- Surgery provides long-term anatomic patency.

- Angioplasty has limited anatomic patency.

- Only a minority of patients suitable with transluminal technique.

- An inability of most radiologists to reproduce subintimal results.

References

1. Second European Consensus Document. *Eur J Vasc Surg* 1992; **6** (Suppl A): 1–32.
2. TransAtlantic Inter-Society Consensus (TASC). Management of peripheral arterial disease (PAD). Section D: chronic critical limb ischaemia. *Eur J Vasc Endovasc Surg* 2000; **19** Suppl A: S144–243.
3. Becquemin JP, Allaire E, Cavillon A *et al.* Conventional versus endovascular surgical procedures: a no choice option. *Eur J Vasc Endovasc Surg* 1995; **10**: 1–3.
4. Bradbury AW, Ruckley CV. Angioplasty for lower limb ischaemia: time for randomised controlled trials. *Lancet* 1996; **347**: 277–278.
5. Dondelinger RF. Chronic critical limb ischemia: what is the benefit of radiological intervention? Indications and results. *J Belge Radiol* 1998; **81**: 96–100.
6. Huntington FM, Prentis F, Hildreth AJ, Holdsworth J. Lower limb occlusive arterial disease in the North of England: workload and development of management guidelines. The Northern Regional Vascular Surgeons. *Eur J Vasc Endovasc Surg* 2000; **20**: 260–7.

7. Jackson MJ, Wolfe JH. Are infra-inguinal angioplasty and surgery comparable? *Acta Chirurg Belg* 2001; **101**: 6–10.

8. van der Lugt A, Gussenhoven EJ, Pasterkamp G *et al*. Intravascular ultrasound predictors of restenosis after balloon angioplasty of the femoropopliteal artery. *Eur J Vasc Endovasc Surg* 1998; **16**: 110–119.

9. Roller RE, Janisch S, Carroll V *et al*. Changes in the fibrinolytic system in patients with peripheral arterial occlusive disease undergoing percutaneous transluminal angioplasty. *Thromb Res* 1999; **94**: 241–247.

10. Collins RH, Voorhees AB, Reemtsma K *et al*. Efficacy of percutaneous angioplasty in lower extremity arterial occlusive disease. *J Cardiovasc Surg* 1984; **25**: 390–394.

11. Lally ME, Johnston KW, Andrews D. Percutaneous transluminal dilatation of peripheral arteries: an analysis of factors predicting early success. *J Vasc Surg* 1984; **1**: 704–709.

12. Morin J, Johnston KW, Wasserman L, Andrews D. Factors that determine the long-term results of percutaneous transluminal dilatation for peripheral arterial occlusive disease. *J Vasc Surg* 1986; **4**: 68–72.

13. Horvath W, Oertl M, Haidinger D. Percutaneous transluminal angioplasty of crural arteries. *Radiology* 1990; **177**: 565–569.

14. Jeans WD, Armstrong S, Cole SE *et al*. Fate of patients undergoing transluminal angioplasty for lower-limb ischemia. *Radiology* 1990; **177**: 559–564.

15. Jeans WD, Cole SE, Horrocks M, Baird RN. Angioplasty gives good results in critical lower limb ischaemia. A 5-year follow-up in patients with known ankle pressure and diabetic status having femoropopliteal dilations.*Br J Radiol* 1994; **67**: 123–128.

16. Flueckiger F, Lammer J, Klein GE, Hausegger K, Pilger E, Waltner F, Aschauer M. Percutaneous transluminal angioplasty of crural arteries. *Acta Radiol* 1992; **33**: 152–5.

17. Arfvidsson B, Davidsen JP, Persson B, Spangen L. Percutaneous transluminal angioplasty (PTA) for lower extremity arterial insufficiency. *Acta Chirurgic Scand* 1983; **149**: 43–47.

18. Dorros G, Lewin RF, Jamnadas P, Mathiak LM. Below-the-knee angioplasty: tibioperoneal vessels, the acute outcome. *Cathet Cardiovasc Diag* 1990; **19**: 170–178.

19. Dacie JE, Daniell SJ. The value of percutaneous transluminal angioplasty of the profunda femoris artery in threatened limb loss and intermittent claudication. *Clin Radiol* 1991; **44**: 311–6.

20. Sivananthan UM, Browne TF, Thorley PJ, Rees MR. Percutaneous transluminal angioplasty of the tibial arteries. *Br J Surg* 1994; **81**: 1282–1285.

21. Martin DR, Katz SG, Kohl RD, Qian D. Percutaneous transluminal angioplasty of infrainguinal vessels. *Annl Vasc Surg* 1999; **13**: 184–187.

22. Golledge J, Ferguson K, Ellis M *et al*. Outcome of femoropopliteal angioplasty. *Annl Surg* 1999; **229**: 146–153.

23. Soder HK, Manninen HI, Jaakkola P *et al*. Prospective trial of infrapopliteal artery balloon angioplasty for critical limb ischemia: angiographic and clinical results. *J Vasc Intervent Radiol* 2000; **11**: 1021–1031.

24. Karch LA, Mattos MA, Henretta JP *et al*. Clinical failure after percutaneous transluminal angioplasty of the superficial femoral and popliteal arteries. *J Vasc Surg* 2000; **31**: 880–887.

25. Clark TW, Groffsky JL, Soulen MC. Predictors of long-term patency after femoropopliteal angioplasty: results from the STAR registry. *J Vasc Intervent Radiol* 2001; **12**: 923–933.

26. Saha S, Gibson M, Magee TR *et al*. Early results of retrograde transpopliteal angioplasty of iliofemoral lesions. *Cardiovasc Intervention Radiol* 2001; **24**: 378–382.

27. Bucek RA, Hudak P, Schnurer G *et al*. Clinical long-term results of percutaneous transluminal angioplasty in patients with peripheral arterial occlusive disease. *Vasa* 2002; **31**: 36–42.

28. Nasr MK, McCarthy RJ, Hardman J *et al*. The increasing role of percutaneous transluminal angioplasty in the primary management of critical limb ischaemia. *Eur J Vasc Endovasc Surg* 2002; **23**: 398–403.

29. Waltman AC, Greenfield AJ, Novelline RA *et al*. Transluminal angioplasty of the iliac and femoropopliteal arteries. Current status. *Arch Surg* 1982; **117**: 1218–1221.

30. Campbell WB, Jeans WD, Cole SE, Baird RN. Percutaneous transluminal angioplasty for lower limb ischaemia. *Br J Surg* 1983; **70**: 736–739.

31. Gallino A, Mahler F, Probst P, Nachbur B. Percutaneous transluminal angioplasty of the arteries of the lower limbs: a 5 year follow-up. *Circulation* 1984; **70**: 619–623.

32. Jones BA, Maggisano R, Robb C, Saibil EA, Witchell SJ, Harrison AW. Transluminal angioplasty: results in high-risk patients with advanced peripheral vascular disease. *Can J Surg* 1985; **28**: 150–152.

33. Spence LD, Hartnell GG, Reinking G, Gibbons G, Pomposelli F, Clouse ME. Diabetic versus non-diabetic limb-threatening ischemia: outcome of percutaneous iliac intervention. *American Journal of Roentgenology* 1999; **172**: 1335–1341.

34. Siskin G, Darling RC 3rd, Stainken B, Chang BB, Paty PSK, Kreienberg PB, Papanicolaou G, Shah DM. Combined use of iliac artery angioplasty and infrainguinal revascularization for treatment of multilevel atherosclerotic disease. *Annl Vasc Surg* 1999; 13: 45–51.

35. Powell RJ, Fillinger M, Bettmann M, Jeffery R, Langdon D, Walsh DB, Zwolak R, Hines M, Cronenwett JL. The durability of endovascular treatment of multisegment iliac occlusive disease. *J Vasc Surg* 2000; 31: 1178–1184.

36. O'Donohoe MK, Sultan S, Colgan MP, Moore DJ, Shanik GD. Outcome of the first 100 femoropopliteal angioplasties performed in the operating theatre. *Eur J Vasc Endovasc Surg* 1999; 17: 66–71.

37. Balas P, Pangratis N, Ioannou N *et al.* Open sub-intimal angioplasty of the superficial femoral and distal arteries. *J Endovasc Ther* 2000; 7: 68–71.

38. Schneider PA, Caps MT, Ogawa DY, Hayman ES. Intraoperative superficial femoral artery balloon angioplasty and popliteal to distal bypass graft: an option for combined open and endovascular treatment of diabetic gangrene. *J Vasc Surg* 2001; 33: 955–962.

39. Sanborn TA, Mitty HA, Train JS, Dan SJ. Infrapopliteal and below-knee popliteal lesions: treatment with sole laser thermal angioplasty. Work in progress. *Radiology* 1989; 172: 89–93.

40. Cheng SW, Ting AC, Wong J. Endovascular stenting of superficial femoral artery stenosis and occlusions: results and risk factor analysis. *Cardiovasc Surg* 2001; 9: 133–140.

41. Treiman GS, Copland S, McNamara RM, Yellin AE, Schneider PA, Treiman RL. Factors influencing ulcer healing in patients with combined arterial and venous insufficiency. *J Vasc Surg* 2001; 33: 1158–1164.

42. Lofberg AM, Karacagil S, Ljungman C *et al.* Distal percutaneous transluminal angioplasty through infrainguinal bypass grafts. *Eur J Vasc Endovasc Surg* 2002; 23: 212–219.

43. Zarins CK, Lu CT, McDonnell AE, Whitehouse WM Jr. Limb salvage by percutaneous transluminal recanalization of the occluded superficial femoral artery. *Surgery* 1980; 87: 701–708.

44. Rush DS, Gewertz BL, Lu CT *et al.* Limb salvage in poor-risk patients using transluminal angioplasty. *Archives of Surgery* 1983; 118: 1209–1212.

45. Brown KT, Schoenberg NY, Moore ED, Saddekni S. Percutaneous transluminal angioplasty of infrapopliteal vessels: preliminary results and technical considerations. *Radiology* 1988; 169: 75–78.

46. Schwarten DE, Cutcliff WB. Arterial occlusive disease below the knee: treatment with percutaneous transluminal angioplasty performed with low-profile catheters and steerable guide wires. *Radiology* 1988; 169: 71–74.

47. Bakal CW, Sprayregen S, Scheinbaum K *et al.* Percutaneous transluminal angioplasty of the infrapopliteal arteries: results in 53 patients. *Am J Roent* 1990; 154: 171–174.

48. Cooper JC, Welsh CL. The role of percutaneous transluminal angioplasty in the treatment of critical ischaemia. *Eur J Vasc Surg* 1991; 5: 261–264.

49. Saab MH, Smith DC, Aka PK *et al.* Percutaneous transluminal angioplasty of tibial arteries for limb salvage. *Cardiovasc Intervent Radiol* 1992; 15: 211–216.

50. Buckenham TM, Loh A, Dormandy JA, Taylor RS. Infrapopliteal angioplasty for limb salvage. *European J Vasc Surg* 1993; 7: 21–25.

51. Currie IC, Wakeley CJ, Cole SE *et al.* Femoropopliteal angioplasty for severe limb ischaemia. *Br J Surg* 1994; 81: 191–193.

52. Durham JR, Horowitz JD, Wright JG, Smead WL. Percutaneous transluminal angioplasty of tibial arteries for limb salvage in the high-risk diabetic patient. *Annl Vasc Surg* 1994; 8: 48–53.

53. Treiman GS, Treiman RL, Ichikawa L, Van Allan R. Should percutaneous transluminal angioplasty be recommended for treatment of infrageniculate popliteal artery or tibioperoneal trunk stenosis? *J Vasc Surg* 1995; 22: 457–463.

54. Matsi P. Percutaneous transluminal angioplasty in critical limb ischaemia. *Annl Chirurg Gynaecol* 1995; 84: 359–362.

55. Favre JP, Do Carmo G, Adham M, Gournier JP, Barral X. Results of transluminal angioplasty of infra-popliteal arteries. *J Cardiovasc Surg* 1996; 37(Suppl 1): 33–37.

56. Lofberg AM, Lorelius LE, Karacagil S *et al.* The use of below-knee percutaneous transluminal angioplasty in arterial occlusive disease causing chronic critical limb ischemia. *Cardiovasc Intervent Radiol* 1996; 19: 317–322.

57. Hanna GP, Fujise K, Kjellgren O *et al.* Infrapopliteal transcatheter interventions for limb salvage in diabetic patients: importance of aggressive interventional approach and role of transcutaneous oximetry. *J Am Coll Cardiol* 1997; 30: 664–669.

58. Vraux H, Hammer F, Verhelst R *et al.* Subintimal angioplasty of tibial vessel occlusions in the treatment of critical limb ischaemia: mid-term results. *Eur J Vasc Endovasc Surg* 2000; 20: 441–446.

59. Boyer L, Therre T, Garcier JM *et al.* Infrapopliteal percutaneous transluminal angioplasty for limb salvage. *Acta Radiol* 2000; 41: 73–77.

60. McCarthy RJ, Neary W, Roobottom C *et al*. Short-term results of femoropopliteal subintimal angioplasty. *Br J Surg* 2000; **87**: 1361–1365.

61. Dorros G, Jaff MR, Dorros AM *et al*. Tibioperoneal (outflow lesion) angioplasty can be used as primary treatment in 235 patients with critical limb ischemia: five-year follow-up. *Circulation* 2001; **104**: 2057–2062.

62. Melliere D, Berrahal D, D'Audiffret A *et al*. Percutaneous transluminal angioplasty in patients with ischemic tissue necrosis is worthwhile. *Cardiovasc Surg* 2001; **9**: 122–1226.

63. Smith BM, Stetchman M, Gibson M *et al*. Sub-intimal angioplasty for superficial femoral artery occlusion: poor outcome in critical ischaemia. *Vascular Surgical Society of Great Britain and Ireland Yearbook*. 2002: 74 (abstract).

64. Bolia A, Sayers RD, Thompson MM, Bell PR. Subintimal and intraluminal recanalisation of occluded crural arteries by percutaneous balloon angioplasty. European *J Vasc Surg* 1994; **8**: 214–219.

65. London NJ, Srinivasan R, Naylor AR *et al*. Subintimal angioplasty of femoropopliteal artery occlusions: the long-term results. *Eur J Vasc Surg* 1994; **8**: 148–155.

66. Varty K, Nydahl S, Butterworth P *et al*. Changes in the management of critical limb ischaemia. *Br J Surg* 1996; **83**: 953–956.

67. Nydahl S, Hartshorne T, Bell PR *et al*. Subintimal angioplasty of infrapopliteal occlusions in critically ischaemic limbs. *Eur J Vasc Endovasc Surg* 1997; **14**: 212–216.

68. Walker SR, Papavassiliou VG, Bolia A, London N. Subintimal angioplasty of native vessels in the management of occluded vascular grafts. *Eur J Vasc Endovasc Surg* 2001; **22**: 41–43.

69. Ingle H, Nasim A, Bolia A *et al*. Sub-intimal angioplasty of isolated infragenicular vessels in lower limb ischaemia: long-tern results. *J Endovasc Ther* 2002; **9**: 411–416.

70. Axisa B, Fishwick G, Bolia A *et al*. Complications following peripheral angioplasty. *Annl Roy Coll Surg Engl* 2002; **84**: 39–42.

71. Wolfe JHN, Wyatt MG. Critical and sub-critical limb ischaemia. *Eur J Vasc Endovasc Surg* 1997; **13**: 578–582.

72. Burns P, Lima E, Bradbury AW. Second best medical therapy. *Eur J Vasc Endovasc Surg* 2002; **24**: 400–404.

73. Bradbury AW, Bell J, Lee AJ *et al*. Bypass or angioplasty for severelimb ischaemia? A Delphi consensus study. *Eur J Vasc Endovasc Surg* 2002; **24**: 411–4116.

74. Bell J, Papp L, Bradbury AW. Bypass or angioplasty for severe ischaemia of the leg: the BASIL trial In: *Vascular and Endovascular Opportunities* Greenhalgh RM, Powell JT, Mitchell AW (eds). London: Saunders, 2000: 485–494.

75. Blair JM, Gewertz BL, Moosa H *et al*. Percutaneous transluminal angioplasty versus surgery for limb-threatening ischaemia. *J Vasc Surg* 1989; **9**: 698–703.

76. Wilson SE, Wolf GL, Cross AP. Percutaneous transluminal angioplasty versus operation for peripheral arteriosclerosis. Report of a prospective randomized trial in a selected group of patients. *J Vasc Surg* 1989; **9**: 1–9.

77. Holm J, Arfvidsson B, Jivegard L *et al*. Chronic lower limb ischaemia. A prospective randomised controlled study comparing the 1-year results of vascular surgery and percutaneous transluminal angioplasty (PTA). *Eur J Vasc Surg* 1991; **5**: 517–522.

78. Zdanowski Z, Troeng T, Norgren L. Outcome and influence of age after infrainguinal revascularisation in critical limb ischaemia. The Swedish Vascular Registry. *Eur J Vasc Endovasc Surg* 1998; **16**: 137–141.

Angioplasty is the first-line treatment for critical limb ischaemia

Charing Cross Editorial Comments towards Consensus

This is a very 'hot topic'.

Amman Bolia has certainly started something and from personal experience of subintimal angioplasty has seen radiologists and surgeons learn the technique and reproduce it with considerable ease. Others are having difficulty with it. There is certainly a knack to it but only time will tell whether it will be universally adopted. It has already been taken on by some in the United States and at the time of writing it would seem that this is a technique which is expanding rapidly and finding a place for the long lesions in the superficial femoral artery in particular, and especially in patients with critical ischaemia. This does not determine whether it should supersede bypass surgery but frequently a patient is frail, elderly and at high risk of an imminent cardiovascular event.

The proposers make the case but the Birmingham group, opposing the motion, argue very effectively in favour of the surgical option. The group lead by Malcolm Simms has long been energetic in limb salvage surgery and Andrew Bradbury speaks in favour of long-term anatomic papers that have been achieved better by surgery and stresses that only a minority of patients are suitable for transluminal angioplasty and feels that the promising results reported with subintimal angioplasty may not be reproducible in the hands of most radiologists.

Roger M Greenhalgh
Editor

There is no evidence for the effectiveness of tibioperoneal angioplasty

For the motion

K Paula M Murphy, Marcus D Bradley, Roger N Baird

Introduction

At first sight, tibioperoneal angioplasty is an attractive arterial reconstruction for atherosclerotic occlusions of the calf arteries on the grounds that it is less invasive and is quicker to perform than open surgical infrapopliteal bypass. However, the tibioperoneal segment is the least commonly performed site of angioplasty for four good reasons. First, its efficacy and durability are unproved. Many have a concurrent above-knee angioplasty, which is a confounding factor. Good short-term results are offset by high restenosis rates. In consequence, it is generally done as a 'last ditch' effort to save a critically ischaemic limb, often in a poorly mobile patient who is elderly and infirm with significant co-morbidity. Surgical bypass is the preferred option in younger, fitter patients. Second, not all lesions are suitable and the appropriate procedure can be technically challenging. These very small vessels have the tendency to develop spasm when guidewires and catheters are passed. Third, the risk of post-angioplasty complications at calf vessel level is greater than when the wider popliteal and femoral arteries are dilated. Finally, randomized trials have not been done and solid scientific evidence of quality is not available in the literature to allow the clinician to draw reliable conclusions.

There are certain circumstances in which the risk/benefit ratio may be acceptable, including the presence of a technically feasible lesion and the lack of a realistic surgical alternative in a patient who would otherwise be facing an amputation. There are anecdotal cases of triumphs in this area but disasters are also encountered.

The clinical dilemma

Surgical distal bypass is the preferred option if the inflow and outflow are acceptable, a suitable vein is available, and the patient is fit for a 3–4 hour operation. The clinical dilemma is whether an unproven tibioperoneal angioplasty should be attempted in a higher risk patient with digital gangrene and ischaemic rest pain.

Developments in angioplasty

The advent in the 1980s of low profile balloon catheters and steerable hydrophilic guidewires has allowed for less traumatic access to the distal vessels in the calf. Cardiology angioplasty technology did not transfer easily to the low flow, very small calibre of the calf vessels, and the tendency of intraluminal guidewires and catheters to cause spasm, compounded difficulties with this procedure. The number and quality of the distal run-off vessels and especially the presence of pedal outflow are all important.

The evidence

Most reports of tibioperoneal angioplasty are series of patients with critical limb ischaemia[1-4,6,8-9,11-18,20,23] several of which include patients with diabetes.[4,8,14,15] Critical limb ischaemia in these patients presented clinically as rest pain, ulcers and gangrene. Many of these patients were facing the prospect of a major amputation because no surgical revascularization was feasible. In these circumstances, a successful distal angioplasty is a triumph when the alternative is amputation. In patients with critical ischaemia who can be treated by both modalities, surgical bypass and percutaneous transluminal angioplasty (PTA) are reported to have similar outcomes.[14]

In a series of 215 successful tibioperoneal angioplasties, 91% of limbs were salvaged, 8% requiring surgical bypass after PTA.[1] The 5-year survival was 56%, reflecting the significant co-morbidity of many of these patients. Those with milder disease had better survival. In another series,[2] there was an 87% limb salvage rate with below-knee PTA in 37 patients with limb-threatening ischaemia, which is probably comparable with the results of surgical bypass. A retrospective comparison[4] of PTA and surgical bypass in diabetic patients with critical limb ischaemia showed similar limb salvage rates. Bypass in 125 patients led to 95% limb salvage at 30 days, 80% at 1 year and 63% at 7 years. PTA in 89 limbs resulted in 95% limb salvage at 30 days, 82% at 1 year and 63% at 6 years. As this was not a randomized controlled trial, patients in each arm of the study are not strictly comparable. Another study[20] compared surgery with tibial PTA with similar results. However, PTA was only suitable for those 20-30% of patients who had isolated tibial disease with short occlusions or few stenoses.

Although initial technical success can be high, the long-term outlook is not so good, due to the high stenosis recurrence rate[5,7,10,21] The highest rate reported is 40% at 9 months.[21] A study of 82 patients with critical ischaemia had an initial 88% PTA success rate dropping to 55% at 6 months and 36% at 2 years;[9] 40 limbs having subintimal angioplasty to tibial vessels had an early technical success of 78% falling to 56% at 2 years.[3] There is evidence that technical failure does not preclude bail-out bypass if surgery was possible before angioplasty undertaken,[3,17] but this still remains a concern.

One of the confounding variables is the concurrent angioplasty to more proximal lesions, particularly in the popliteal and superficial femoral arteries. Many series report high rates of inflow PTA ranging from 33% to 88%.[1,13,18-19,21-22] This makes it difficult to be sure that the distal vessel PTA was the most crucial in the patients' management.

There are very few reports of tibioperoneal angioplasty on patients with claudication.[6,11,19,21] These are simple descriptions of results following angioplasty in distal leg vessels. In one paper there was high recurrence rate needing treatment,[21] another only looked at 'disabling claudication'[19] and a third looked at severe cases with favourable anatomy for angioplasty.[6] The last report did not report separately the results in claudicants.[11] Even though the rate of serious complications was modest, it was sufficiently worrying to preclude calf vessel PTA for mild to moderate claudication. The complication rate in a group of patients of whom half were claudicants included contrast induced renal failure in 4%, distal embolization in 4%, entry site arterial repair or embolectomy in 2%, and dissection or occlusion in 2%.[21]

The largest series of recent years comes from St Lukes Medical Centre Milwaukee Wisconsin.[21] There are over 100 patients with 168 below-knee vessels and lesions. However, 47% of them are claudicants, traditionally not considered for angioplasty at this level; 27% had a non-healing ulcer or gangrene and 26% had rest pain. Interestingly 56% of them had an above-knee vessel dilatation pre-distal angioplasty. Their success rate of angioplasty was 90%, but on further analysis of their results 64% had disease progression with symptoms. The complication rate, though not high, was serious particularly in a group of patients of whom half were simply claudicants, i.e. contrast-induced renal failure 4%, distal embolization 4%, entry site arterial repair or embolectomy 2%, dissection or occlusion 2%. A combined complication rate of 3% included death, emergency bypass surgery or just an embolization. The conclusion of this paper was that below-knee angioplasty should not be restricted to limb salvage situations so therefore many of these patients would have been suitable for distal bypass and it did not address the group of ischaemic and limb threatened patients who are more obviously candidates for tibioperoneal angioplasty, particularly if there is no surgical alternative for them.

Technique

The intention to treat is usually decided jointly by the interventional radiologist and vascular surgeon who consider the following:

1. Is a surgical distal bypass technically feasible?
2. If unsuitable, is the reason (a) the lack of an adequate distal vessel to anastomose to or (b) general co-morbidity with additional risk factors?
3. Could (a) a distal angioplasty be considered pre-bypass and (b) could a failed procedure compromise the possibility of a surgical approach?
4. Is there good inflow to the area and is there a need for a preliminary angioplasty at the above-knee level?

Procedure

An antegrade puncture of the ipsilateral common femoral artery is the usual approach as there is more control of the catheter tip than if a contralateral approach is used. A contralateral approach may be more advisable if there has been thrombolysis from the contralateral groin, in which case a second needle puncture is best avoided because of the risks of bleeding and haematoma formation. Proximal calf run-off vessels can be dilated with a 0.035 guidewire and a standard 5 French PTA balloon catheter. Smaller more distal calf vessels need a 0.018-inch guidewire of lower profile, with small 2mm-diameter balloons. Pre-angioplasty anti-coagulation with a bolus dose of 5000 international units of heparin is vital. Anti-spasmodic agents also are very usual as spasm in below-knee vessels is not uncommon and, apart from the extreme discomfort to the patient, can greatly diminish the chance of technical success. A guidewire is left across the lesion at all times pre- and post-angioplasty until a check angiogram shows patency.

Occlusions are more of a challenge. The subintimal technique described by Bolia may be employed, although this is very dependent on the experience of the operator. Re-entry into the distal vessel can be difficult, particularly if there is heavy calcification. Heparinization should continue post-angioplasty, particularly in very tiny calibre vessels and in circumstances where there are many complex lesions and also where an occlusion has been opened. Long- term treatment with anti-platelet agents such as aspirin and clopidogrel is routine, and anticoagulation with warfarin should be considered.

Complications

1. *Thrombosis*
If this occurs thrombolysis can be very successful either by bolus injection or by an infusion.

2. *Dissection at the site of angioplasty*
Re-dilatation of the dissection flap may prove sufficient to remedy this situation but in a single vessel it may have a catastrophic outcome with loss of all blood flow to the limb, thereby worsening the already limb threatened situation. This is the main reason for the reluctance of many vascular radiologists to perform these distal angioplasties.

3. *Perforation or rupture*
Arterial perforation and rupture are rare but can occur. There is often no serious consequence. The procedure should be discontinued.

Balloon angioplasty combined with surgery

There are two scenarios for consideration.

1. *Angioplasty in conjunction with more proximal bypass*
When the angioplasty is done in conjunction with a more proximal bypass. This of course makes provision of evidence of the success of the balloon angioplasty itself difficult to provide.

2. *Bypass graft with distal stenosis*
The use of balloon angioplasty may be unhelpful in improving the patency of a bypass graft with a distal stenosis.[17,19] It is more successful when a new stenosis develops at the site of the distal anastomosis than where there is intimal hyperplasia or progression of atherosclerotic disease. If a new stenosis occurs soon after surgery then further surgical correction is indicated and PTA is unlikely to correct the problem.

Summary

Anecdotal evidence of success of tibioperoneal angioplasty is available but hard supportive evidence of its value is difficult to find because:

- Successful distal bypass grafting is frequently offered.

- Few below-knee, compared with above-knee angioplasties are performed.

- The mixed indications for tibioperoneal angioplasty, including patients with high co-morbidity, stenotic and occlusive lesions, and variable foot arch and 1, 2 and 3 vessels run-off lead to differences in outcome.

- Tibioperoneal angioplasty is usually done in a pre-amputation situation in the frail and elderly, where the clinical features include critical ischaemia, gangrene and severe rest pain. During follow-up, death from the cardiovascular disease often intervenes.

- Randomized trials are difficult to perform in this group of patients.

- This procedure has high technical demands and the opportunities to gain experience are limited.

References

1. Dorros G, Jaff MR, Dorros AM *et al*. Tibioperoneal (outflow lesion)angioplasty can be used as primary treatment in 235 patients with critical limb ischemia: five-year follow-up. *Circulation* 2001; 104: 2057–2062.

2. Brillu C, Picquet J, Villapadierna F, Papon X, L'Hoste P, Jousset Y, Enon B. Percutaneous transluminal angioplasty for management of critical ischemia in arteries below the knee. *Annl Vasc Surg* 2001; 15: 175–181.

3. Vraux H, Hammer F, Verhelst R *et al*. Subintimal angioplasty of tibial vessel occlusions in the treatment of critical limb ischaemia: mid-term results. *Eur J Vasc Endovasc Surg* 2000; 20: 441–446.

4. Wolfle KD, Bruijnen H, Reeps C *et al*. Loeprecht tibioperoneal arterial lesions and critical foot ischaemia: successful management by the use of short vein grafts and percutaneous transluminal angioplasty. *Vasa* 2000; 29: 207–214.

5. Desgranges P, Kobeiter K, d'Audiffret A *et al*. Acute occlusion of popliteal and/or tibial arteries: the value of percutaneous treatment. *Eur J Vasc Endovasc Surg* 2000; 20: 138–145.

6. Dorros G, Jaff MR, Murphy KJ, Mathiak L. The acute outcome of tibioperoneal vessel angioplasty in 417 cases with claudication and critical limb ischemia. *Cathet Cardiovasc Diagn* 1998; 45: 251–256.

7. Wagner HJ, Rager G. [Infrapopliteal angioplasty: a forgotten region?].[Review: German]. ROFO-Fortschritte auf dem Gebiet der Rontgenstrahlen und der Bildgebenden V. 1998; 168: 415–420.

8. Hanna GP, Fujise K, Kjellgren O *et al*. Infrapopliteal transcatheter interventions for limb salvage in diabetic patients: importance of aggressive interventional approach and role of transcutaneous oximetry. *J Am Coll Cardiol* 1997; 30: 664–339.

9. Lofberg AM, Lorelius LE, Karacagil S, Westman B, Almgren B, Berqgvist D. The use of below-knee percutaneous transluminal angioplasty in arterial occlusive disease causing chronic critical limb ischemia. *Cardiovasc Intervent Radiol* 1996; 19: 317–322,

10. Treiman GS, Treiman RL, Ichikawa L, Van Allan R. Should percutaneous transluminal angioplasty be recommended for treatment of infrageniculate popliteal artery or tibioperoneal trunk stenosis? *J Vasc Surg* 1995; 22: 457–465.

11. Varty K. Bolia A. Naylor AR. Bell PR. London NJ. Infrapopliteal percutaneous transluminal angioplasty: a safe and successful procedure. *Eur J Vasc Endovasc Surg* 1995; 9: 341–345.

12. Motarjeme A. PTA and thrombolysis in leg salvage. *J Endovasc Surg* 1994; 1: 81–7.

13. Sivananthan UM, Browne TF, Thorley PJ, Rees MR. Percutaneous transluminal angioplasty of the tibial arteries. *Br J Surg* 1994; 81: 1282–1285.

14. Durham JR, Horowitz JD, Wright JG, Smead WL. Percutaneous transluminal angioplasty of tibial arteries for limb salvage in the high-risk diabetic patient. *Annl Vasc Surg* 1994; 8: 48–53.

15. Wack C, Wolfle KD, Loeprecht H *et al.* [Percutaneous balloon dilatation of isolated lesions of the calf arteries in critical ischemia of the leg]. [German] *Vasa* 1994; 23: 30–34.

16. Lang EV, Stevick CA. Transcatheter therapy of severe acute lower extremity ischemia. *J Vasc Intervent Radiol* 1993; 4: 481–488.

17. Brown KT, Moore ED, Getrajdman GI, Saddekni S. Infrapopliteal angioplasty: long-term follow-up. *J Vasc Intervent Radiol* 1993; 4: 139–144.

18. Saab MH, Smith DC, Aka PK *et al.* Percutaneous transluminal angioplasty of tibial arteries for limb salvage. *Cardiovasc Intervent Radiol* 1992; 15: 211–216.

19. Bull PG, Mendel H, Hold M, Schlegl A, Denck H. Distal popliteal and tibioperoneal transluminal angioplasty: long-term follow-up. *J Vasc Intervent Radiol* 1992; 3: 45–53.

20. Schwarten DE. Clinical and anatomical considerations for nonoperative therapy in tibial disease and the results of angioplasty. *Circulation* 1991; 83(2 Suppl): I86–90.

21. Dorros G, Lewin RF, Jamnadas P, Mathiak LM. Below-the-knee angioplasty: tibioperoneal vessels, the acute outcome. *Catheter Cardiovasc Diagn* 1990; 19: 170–178.

22. Bakal CW, Sprayregen S, Scheinbaum K, Cynamon J, Veith FJ. Percutaneous transluminal angioplasty of the infrapopliteal arteries: results in 53 patients. *Am J Roent* 1990; 154: 171–174.

23. Schwarten DE, Cutcliff WB. Arterial occlusive disease below the knee: treatment with percutaneous transluminal angioplasty performed with low-profile catheters and steerable guide wires. *Radiology* 1988; 169: 71–74.

There is no evidence for the effectiveness of tibioperoneal angioplasty

Against the motion
Peter RF Bell

Introduction

Arterial disease of the tibioperoneal vessels frequently presents with critical ischaemia. A recent audit in our unit of 133 limbs presenting with critical ischaemia showed that nearly 30% were due to isolated crural lesions, a figure published by other authors some years ago.[1] In such cases where limb loss or amputation is likely, the results of intraluminal angioplasty are poor as many of the lesions are not suitable for that treatment.[2,3] Because of this, historically, femorodistal bypasses using vein has become the standard treatment for such lesions.

These procedures carry a mortality in the region of 10% with a 2-year primary patency rate of about 50% at 2 years and a 12% amputation rate.[4] Many of these patients are diabetics and the mortality at 3 years is often as high as 50%, which is normal for this age group. Such cases therefore are at risk after surgery with a high mortality and the long-term outcome is not necessarily very good.

Although intraluminal angioplasty is of limited benefit in these cases subintimal angioplasty has much more to offer. This technique was described by Bolia and his colleagues many years ago and has been shown to be effective in the femoropopliteal segment where a primary patency rate of about 50% at 6 years can be achieved.[5] The use of this technique in the tibioperoneal and crural vessels has been more recent but the initial and late results indicate that outcomes are excellent with a low mortality and high limb salvage rates.[6]

The technique depends on the creation of a channel (Fig. 1) in the subintimal space using a wire which has to be looped to produce that channel (Fig. 2). Re-entry normally occurs into the relatively normal lumen below the obstruction. Any length of lumen can be treated (Figs 3,4).

In a recent 1-year prospective audit in our unit of 133 limbs presenting with critical ischaemia 42% were due to superficial femoral occlusion, 26% to crural occlusion, 18% due to popliteal occlusion and 14% due to ileofemoral occlusion. Subintimal angioplasty was used in 80% of the procedures with a mean length of occlusion of 21.6 cm. Technical success was achieved in 79% of these cases. The initial results of subintimal angioplasty of the tibioperoneal trunk and crural vessels provided 1-year limb survival of 79% and a patency rate of 70%.[6] More recently we have followed 67 consecutive patients with 70 treated limbs for 3 years. The mean crural artery occlusion was 6 cm in these cases. The technical success rate in these patients was 86%. Of the remaining 14% (ten patients) three had a successful bypass, four had an amputation, one a lumbar sympathectomy and two were treated conservatively. The cumulative limb salvage rate and freedom from pain in those patients where angioplasty was possible was 94% at 3 years (Figs 5, 6). Mortality was as expected, 19% at 1 year, 43% at 2 years and 41% at 3 years; 46% of these patients were diabetic[7] (Fig. 7).

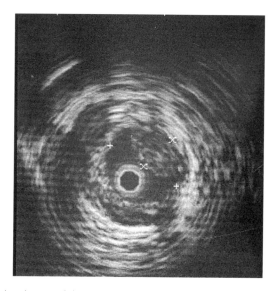

Figure 1. Intravascular ultrasound demonstrating a subintimal channel caused by the guidewire.

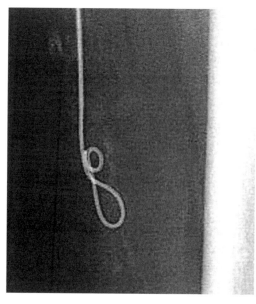

Figure 2. The wire is looped prior to forming the channel.

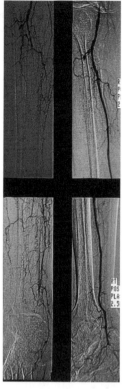

Figure 3. Successful recanalization of crural vessels.

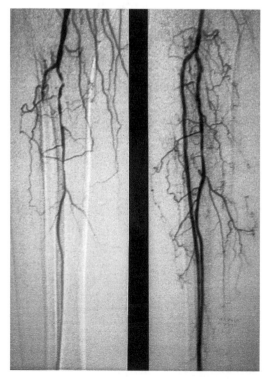

Figure 4. Successful recanalization of crural vessels.

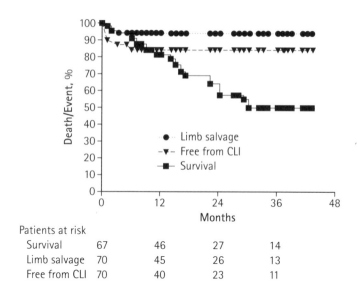

Figure 5. Kaplan-Meier life-table analysis demonstrating survival, cumulative limb salvage, and cumulative freedom from severe ischaemia at 12, 24 and 36 months in the 67-patient cohort. Reproduced with permission from *Journal of Endovascular Therapy* 2002; **9**(4): 411–416.

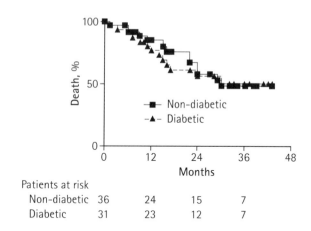

Figure 6. Kaplan-Meier life-table analysis demonstrating the cumulative limb salvage in diabetic versus non-diabetic patients (p=0.26). Reproduced with permission from *Journal of Endovascular Therapy* 2002; **9**(4):411–416.

Patients with critical limb ischaemia caused by occlusion of the tibioperoneal and crural vessels are an ill group with many additional cardiovascular problems. Few of them have lesions which can be dealt with by intraluminal angioplasty which means that a bypass graft is all that is available. If surgery is undertaken, which is the usual treatment in many centres, there is a significant mortality of around 10% and a graft patency of 55% at 2 years.[4] In our series of 70 patients the 30-day mortality was 1.4%

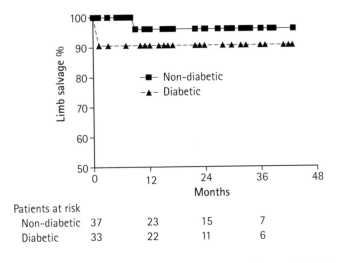

Figure 7. Kaplan-Meier life-table analysis demonstrating the cumulative survival of diabetic versus non-diabetic patients. Reproduced with permission from *Journal of Endovascular Therapy* 2002; **9**(4):411–416.

as all patients were dealt with under local anaesthesia. This figure is much better than can be achieved with surgery. Although specialized centres have reported excellent graft patency and salvage rates of 88% at 2 years[8] these procedures cause far more morbidity than subintimal angioplasty and have a higher death rate. In conclusion subintimal angioplasty has now been shown to be effective in the long-term in patients with tibioperoneal disease, many of them diabetics.

The procedure has a low mortality, is very cost-effective and leads to ulcer healing and the abolition of rest pain with limb salvage rates at 3 years in over 90% of survivors. Angioplasty using the subintimal route should be the primary treatment of such patients so much so that in our unit the first line of treatment is always subintimal angioplasty in such cases.

Failures can occur and in our last 300 tibioperoneal procedures we have had seven patients who deteriorated acutely after the procedure and required emergency surgery to try and save the limb. In three cases the leg was saved but in the remainder it was not. These were, however, cases where the limb was going to be lost in any event. If the procedure fails, surgery can still be undertaken as in the majority of cases where failure occurs no deterioration in the patient's condition is seen. The effect of this on surgical practice in our unit has been that femorodistal bypass which used to be performed in all such patients is now performed in relatively few (17%).

The remainder of our patients are successfully dealt with by subintimal angioplasty. If the technique fails, acute deterioration is rare and bypass surgery can be carried out. There is no question that subintimal tibioperoneal angioplasty is an excellent and durable treatment, so much so that a randomized prospective trial is almost impossible to perform now as equipoise is not present.

Summary

- Subintimal angioplasty is acceptable.

- It has a low mortality and is performed under a local anaesthetic.

- Bypass is required in only 17% of patients.

- The results are so good that equipoise is lost and a trial is unethical.

References

1. Haimovici H. Patterns of arteriosclerotic lesions of the lower extremity. *Arch Surg* 1967; **95**: 918–933.
2. Schwart E, Cutcliff WP. Arterial occlusive disease below the knee. Treatment with percutaneous transluminal angioplasty performed with low profile catheters and steerable guidewires. *Radiology* 1988; **169**: 71–74.
3. Lofberg AM, Lorelius LE, Karacagil S *et al*. The use of below-knee percutaneous transluminal angioplasty in arterial occlusive disease causing chronic critical limb ischaemia. *Cardiovasc Intervent Radiol* 1996; **19**: 317–22.
4. Biancri F, Kantonen L, Alback A *et al*. Popliteal to distal bypass grafts. Critical Leg Ischaemia. *J Cardiovasc Surg (Tereno)* 2000; **41**: 281–286.
5. Bolia A, Miles KA, Brennan J *et al*. Percutaneous transluminal angioplasty of occlusions of the femoropopliteal arteries by subintimal dissection. *Cardiovascular Intervention Radiol* 1990; **13**: 357–363.
6. Nydahl S, Hartshorne T, Bell PRF *et al*. Subintimal angioplasty of infrapopliteal occlusions in critically ischaemic limbs. *Surgery* 1997; **14**: 212–216.
7. Ingle H, Nasin A, Bolia A *et al*. Subintimal angioplasty of isolated infragenicular vessels in lower limb ischaemia. Long term results. *J Vasc Surg* 2002; **35**: 411–417.
8. Kalra M, Gloviczki P, Bower TC *et al*. Limb salvage – a successful pedal bypass grafting is associated with improved long term survival. *J Vasc Surg* 2001; **33**: 6–16.

There is no evidence for the effectiveness of tibioperoneal angioplasty

Charing Cross Editorial Comments towards Consensus

The proposers offer distal bypass frequently and so there is little opportunity in their practice for angioplasty. They argue that randomized trials are difficult to perform and the opposition naturally paints a completely different picture. Essentially the opposition argues that subintimal angioplasty has 'stolen the show'. This has occurred in their practice to the extent that only 17% of patients are available for consideration of surgical reconstruction. This group believes that subintimal angioplasty is so good that equipoise is lost and a randomized controlled trial is no longer possible for that reason. How can both views be correct?

Roger M Greenhalgh
Editor

Arterial stents are not required for femoropopliteal angioplasty

For the motion
Dierk Vorwerk

Introduction

Percutaneous intervention in the femoral arteries is widely performed for lesions as defined below.

Introduction of stent technology brought about a major improvement in the treatment of iliac arteries. There was also major interest in use of those stents in the femoral arteries.

It has been agreed for a long time that a vascular surgical approach to peripheral vascular disease requires major clinical symptoms such as severe claudication or rest pain.

Endovascular versus surgical treatment

Endovascular therapy is known to be of low invasiveness with good technical success and a fair overall patency. In iliac percutaneous transluminal angioplasty (PTA) (taken from five publications reporting on 1264 procedures), there was an average complication rate of 3.6% with a 95% success rate shows a 61% patency after 5 years.[1] In iliac stenting for stenoses (taken from nine publications reporting on 1365 patients), the results are a little better with a 99% technical success and 72% 5-year patency. Weighted average complication rate was 6.3%.[1]

In femoropopliteal endovascular interventions (taken from eight publications reporting on 1469 procedures), however, weighted average technical success was 90%. The complication rate was 4.3% and the 3-year patency rate was 51%.

In contrast, surgery offers a limb-based 5-year-patency of 91% for aortobifemoral bypasses; weighted average mortality was 3.3%. For distal reconstruction, an average 5-year patency of 80% for vein bypasses and 65–75% for expanded polytetraflouroethylene (ePTFE) bypasses has been reported. Combined mortality and amputation risk was calculated to be about 2.2 % for aortobifemoral reconstructions and 1.4% for femoropopliteal reconstructions.[1]

Despite better clinical outcome for surgery, TransAtlantic Inter-Societies Concensus (TASC) recommendation 37, recommends surgery only as a treatment for intermittent claudication in case other forms of medical therapy have been recommended but have been either failed or rejected for good reasons.[1] Furthermore, there should be a high benefit-to-risk ratio given.[1]

This is difficult to achieve in patients with mild to moderate claudication. Thus, endovascular therapy appears to be the method of choice – if applicable - in this sub-group of patients with intermittent claudications.

It is therefore fair to consider, whether use of modern techniques in percutaneous peripheral stents and stent-grafts may help to improve the overall results even in femoral arteries.

Type of lesion

The morphology of a lesion treated will have an influence on the technical outcome, follow-up results and also risk of treatment. The TASC document introduced a classi-fication system that tries to categorize lesions with regard to their accessability to either percutaneous treatment or surgery with type A lesions ideal for percutaneous approach, type B lesions where percutaneous approach is still the preferred technique, type C lesions where surgical approach should be preferred and type D lesions where surgery is the option of choice. The TASC classification overrules older classifications since it takes into account all available and published techniques including stent-technology which offer a much wider variation of treatment and also an effective tool to deal with current acute complications of balloon angioplasty such as occluding dissection or vascular rupture.

In the femoropopliteal arteries, type A lesions are single stenoses up to 3 cm in length not involving the very proximal superficial femoral and the distal popliteal artery. Type B lesions are stenoses 3–5 cm in length, heavily calcified stenoses, mul-tiple lesions (each up to 3 cm) and lesions with no sufficient tibial run-off (the latter are unlikely to meet the criteria of mild or moderate claudication). Type C lesions are classified as stenoses or occlusions longer than 5 cm and multiple mid-size lesions (3–5 cm). Total common femoral, superficial femoral and popliteal occlusions are clas-sified as type D lesions. There was some dissenting discussion on the definition of type B lesions since interventional radiologists representing the Cardiac and Interventional Radiological Society of Europe (CIRSE) wished to express their assumption that it may be justified to classify even longer lesions up to 10 cm as type B instead of type C claiming that the results reported are mainly due to underdeveloped techniques and instruments which have greatly improved in the meantime and no evidence exists comparing efficacy of PTA with bypass surgery for lesions between 4 and 10 cm.

Other than in the iliac area, fewer lesions will meet the criteria of type A and B especially if limited to 5 cm in length. Thus, fewer patients with mild and moderate claudications due to femoropopliteal lesions will become ideal candidates for percu-taneous treatment. Moreover – without limiting the importance of the TASC document which certainly means a step forward in the joint approach to peripheral vascular disease – the morphological classification does not take into account some technical considerations that depend on the age and composition of a lesion. Particularly in femoral occlusions, the degree of organization of the occluding throm-bus or the composition of the lesion with the original stenosis at proximal and distal end or in the middle are factors which are not very predictable but may influence the technical outcome of the intervention or also its complication rate i.e. distal embolization which might cause an aggravation of symptoms.

The TASC classification is predominantly morphological not taking into account that even in simple lesions complications may occur after balloon angioplasty that lead to dissection, acute occlusion or extravasation which might start other periph-eral interventions such as stent placement.

Cost-effectiveness

Muradin and Hunink[2] tried to determine the criteria that would make use of an endovascular device cost-effective compared with bypass surgery and PTA in the treatment of femoropopliteal arterial disease. They found that use of a device that costs $3000 would be cost-effective compared with bypass surgery for critical ischaemia if the 5-year patency rate was 29%–46%. Use of the same device would be cost-effective compared with angioplasty for disabling claudication and stenosis if the 5-year patency rate was 69%–86%. The target combinations of costs and patency rates found in this study are probably attainable, and further development of such endovascular devices seems warranted.

This trial shows that there is obviously a place for even more costly developments if they can show a benefit over simple balloon angioplasty.

Evidence

Stents had been used in a relatively early stage to treat femoropopliteal arteries. Rousseau et al. [3] reported the results of 40 femoropopliteal implantations of self-expanding stents in 36 patients; the follow-up period was greater than 6 months in all patients. Lesion length exceeded 7 cm in 25% of cases and was 3–7 cm in 75%; 30% of lesions were total occlusions.

In patients not receiving orally administered anticoagulants, six thromboses occurred early; no early thromboses were noted in the nine patients treated with acenocoumarol. Restenosis occurred in 10% of cases (maximum follow-up, 2 years) and was noted even in lesions longer than 7 cm.

Since then, combined use of antiplatelet drugs drastically reduced the risk of early thrombosis so the key question became the question of patency.

Other reports with modern stents followed. Lugmayr et al.[4] evaluated the effectiveness of self-expanding nitinol stents in patients with short, complex lesions in the superficial femoral and popliteal arteries and to assess midterm results. Self-expandable nitinol stents were implanted in 54 extremities in 44 patients to treat complex stenoses (n = 32) and occlusions (n = 22) in the superficial femoral and popliteal arteries. Follow-up was performed for 5–51 months to evaluate early thrombosis and midterm patency rates. Mid-term patency rates were compared between the following: stenoses and occlusions, proximal and distal locations, good and poor run-off, and diabetic and non-diabetic patients. All patients underwent clinical investigation and colour Doppler sonography after 1 month and 6 months and at 6-month intervals thereafter. If restenosis or stent thrombosis was suspected, intra-arterial digital subtraction angiography of the superficial and popliteal arteries was performed.

Percutaneous stent implantation was successful in all patients. The mean duration of follow-up was 27 months (range, 5–51 months). No thrombotic occlusion occurred within the first 4 weeks of stent implantation. The primary 3-year patency rate was 76%, and the secondary patency rate was 87%; 3-year primary patency rates were 65% for diabetic patients and 82% for non-diabetic patients.

From these data the authors concluded that in patients with short, complex stenoses and occlusions, implantation of nitinol stents may have a positive impact on midterm results.

Jahnke et al.[5] reported on the use of a spiral nitinol stent (Intracoil) in patients with femoropopliteal obstructive disease. The IntraCoil nitinol stent was used in 37 patients presenting with high-grade stenoses (n = 23) or short (<3 cm) occlusions (n = 17) of the superficial femoral artery (SFA; n = 33) or popliteal artery (n = 4). Indications for stent placement were significant residual stenosis (>30%) or dissection after angioplasty. Follow-up evaluations with measurement of the Doppler ankle-brachial index (ABI), assessment of Rutherford clinical stage, and colour-coded duplex sonography were performed at discharge and 1, 3, 6, 12, and 18 months thereafter. Primary endpoints of the study were immediate technical and clinical success and 1-year patency. Initial technical success was achieved in all patients. In ten patients (27%), more than one 40-mm long device had to be implanted for total lesion coverage; in three patients (8.1%), stents were placed in two separate segments of the SFA simultaneously. The total number of stents deployed was 50. Follow-up data for 12 months after treatment are available for 29 of 37 patients (78.4%); mean follow-up was 15.6 months (range, 1–26 months). Primary patency rates at 6 and 12 months were 97.1% (SE=2.9) and 86.2% (SE=6.5). The primary assisted patency rate was 100% at 12 months. The authors concluded that endovascular placement of the IntraCoil self-expanding nitinol coil stent for salvage of failed angioplasty in patients with femoropopliteal obstructive disease is an effective and safe procedure with promising mid-term results.

Evidence data are, however, rare. Cejna et al.[6] performed a randomized trial to evaluate if stent-placement is superior to PTA in the treatment of chronic symptoms in short femoropopliteal arterial lesions. In 141 patients who ranged in age from 39 to 87 years (mean age, 67 years) 154 limbs were randomized to PTA (n=77) versus PTA followed by implantation of Palmaz stents (n=77). Inclusion criteria were patients with intermittent claudication (n=108, Society of Vascular Surgery/International Society of Cardiovascular Surgery [SVS-ISCVS] categories 1–3) or chronic critical limb ischaemia (n=46 with either ischaemic rest pain [category 4] or minor tissue loss [category 5]), short stenosis or occlusion (lesion length < or = 5 cm), and at least one patent run-off vessel at angiography. Follow-up included clinical assessment, measurement of ABI, colour duplex ultrasound, and/or angiography at 6 or 12 months. Angiographic follow-up between 12 and 36 months was available in 46 limbs (29.9%).

In the PTA group, initial technical success was achieved in 65 of 77 limbs (84%) versus 76 of 77 (99%) limbs in the stent group which was significantly better. Overall, major complications occurred in 3.9% (n = 6); n = 4 in the PTA group compared with n = 2 in the stent group. There was no difference between groups of treatment: haemodynamic/clinical success at 1 and 2 years in the PTA group was 72% and 65% versus 77% and 65% in the stent group. The cumulative 1- and 2-year angiographic primary patency rates were 63% and 53%, respectively, for both groups. The secondary 1- and 2-year angiographic patency rates were 86% and 74% in the PTA group versus 79% and 73% in the stent group. The conclusion from this data after 1 year was that angiographic and clinical/haemodynamic success was not improved after stenting compared with PTA alone.

Muradin et al.[7] tried to perform a meta-analyis to find benefits of stenting over PTA. They searched the English-language literature for studies published between 1993 and 2000. Inclusion criteria for articles were presentation of long-term primary patency rates, standard errors (explicitly reported or derivable), and baseline characteristics of the study population. Two reviewers independently extracted data, and discrepancies were resolved by consensus. Primary patency rates were combined by using a technique that allows adjustment for differences across study populations. Analyses were adjusted for lesion type and clinical indication. Nineteen studies met the inclusion criteria, representing 923 balloon dilations and 473 stent implantations.

Combined 3-year patency rates after balloon dilation were 61% (SE=2.2%) for stenoses and claudication, 48% (SE=3.3%) for occlusions and claudication, 43% (SE=4.1%) for stenoses and critical ischaemia, and 30% (SE=3.7%) for occlusions and critical ischaemia. The 3-year patency rates after stent-implantation were 63%–66% (SE=4.1%) and were independent of clinical indication and lesion type. Funnel plots demonstrated an asymmetric distribution of the data points associated with stent studies. From this analysis they concluded that balloon dilation and stent-implantation for claudication and stenosis yield similar long-term patency rates. For more severe femoropopliteal disease, the results of stent-implantation seem more favourable.

From these data it is pretty clear that – other than in the iliac arteries – liberal use of stents and stent grafts may help to overcome acute technical problems of a failed balloon angioplasty and to solve the technical outcome but does not achieve an improved long-term efficacy or may start up a life-time dependency on recurrent interventional or surgical procedures. Moreover, after restenosis, instent stenosis is more difficult to treat with more costs involved.

These considerations mainly restrict use of endovascular stents for technical bail-out cases to prevent worsening of the symptoms.

New developments

Since the clinical outcome with femoropopliteal stents is rather poor and no better than with PTA alone, many new technologies were clinically tested to improve the outcome of percutaneous work in the femoropoliteal arteries. They include covered stent-grafts and drug eluting stents and of course each modern type of stent coming along.

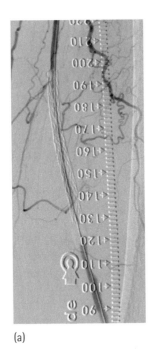 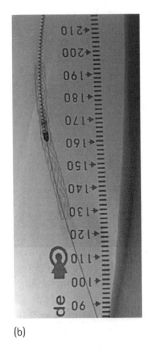 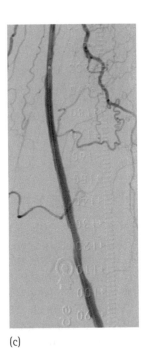

(a)   (b)   (c)

Figure 1.   Stent reocclusion and recanalization.
Figure 1a.   Complete reocclusion of a femoral nitinol stent 5 months after placement.
Figure 1b.   Mechanical recanalization using a new mechanical thrombectomy device (Rotarex, Straub Medical).
Figure 1c.   After thrombectomy and PTA stent patency is regained.

Stent-grafts

The results with stent-grafts depend on what type of covering was used. Ahmadi *et al.*[8] reported on the immediate and long-term outcome after femoropopliteal implantation of a Dacron-covered stent-graft in patients with peripheral arterial disease. They included 30 consecutive patients who underwent Dacron-covered stent-graft implantation because of recurrent stenosis after PTA in the femoropopliteal segment. Patients were followed up with ABI measurement, colour-coded duplex ultrasonography, and angiography: initial technical success was achieved in all 30 patients, with significant improvement of ABI from a pre-intervention mean of 0.5 +/- 0.14 (SD) to a post-intervention mean of 0.8 +/- 0.17 (p <0.001). Post-implantation non-infectious fever and leukocyte and C-reactive protein level elevation occurred in 12 patients (40%), and 17 patients (57%) reported persistent pain at the site of implantation for a mean of 5 days (range, 2–28 days). Early recurrent occlusion within the first 24 hours was found in five patients (17%). Within the mean follow-up period of 60 months +/-10, restenosis occurred in 25 patients (83%). At 6, 12, 36, and 72 months, respectively, primary patency rates were 27%, 23%, 17%, 17%, and secondary patency rates were 63%, 60%, 34%, 34%. They concluded that Dacron-covered stent-grafts are not suitable for femoropopliteal lesions.

Lammer *et al.*[9] evaluated the results from a multicentre trial using a self-expanding endoprosthesis with an expanded PTFE tube inside a nitinol support structure that was implanted in 127 patients with symptomatic PAOD in the iliac (61 limbs) and femoral arteries (80 limbs). Complications occurred in 24 of 141 procedures and included three major complications. Early thrombosis (within 30 days) occurred in one iliac and three femoral arteries. Late restenosis or reocclusion was observed in five iliac and 14 femoral arteries within the 1st year. Primary patency rates in iliac arteries were 98% +/- 3% (standard error) and 91% +/- 4%, respectively, at 6 and 12 months after treatment. Primary patency rates in femoral arteries were 90% +/- 3% and 79% +/- 5%, respectively, at 6 and 12 months.

These multicentre data were encouraging compared with PTA alone but many other centres working with this device could not experience such positive long-term results (personal communication).

Coated stents

While radiating stents never played a role in the femoral arteries, Duda *et al.*[10] reported on the first results using a drug eluting stent in femoral. They evaluated the effectiveness of shape memory alloy recoverable technology (SMART) nitinol self-expanding stents coated with a polymer impregnated with Sirolimus (rapamycin) versus uncoated SMART stents in superficial femoral artery obstructions: Thirty-six patients with chronic limb ischaemia and femoral artery occlusions (57%) or stenoses (average lesion length, 85+/-57 mm) were included.

Eighteen patients received Sirolimus-eluting SMART stents and 18 patients received uncoated SMART stents. The primary endpoint of the study was the in-stent mean percent diameter stenosis, as measured by quantitative angiography at 6 months. This was 22.6% in the sirolimus-eluting stent group versus 30.9% in the uncoated stent group (p=0.294). The in-stent mean lumen diameter was significantly larger in the sirolimus-eluting stent group (4.95 mm versus 4.31 mm in the uncoated stent group; p=0.047). No serious adverse events (death or prolonged hospitalization) were reported. They concluded that the use of sirolimus-eluting stents for superficial femoral artery occlusion is feasible, with a trend toward reducing late loss compared with uncoated stents but a statistical significant change is still missing.

Conclusion

Despite many hopes stents failed to improve the outcome of subinguinal interventions. The only randomized trial including only short lesions did not show a significant difference between PTA and stenting but experienced a much better technical outcome if stents were used.

Experiences with new developments are scarce and do not rely on randomized data or fail to show significance. Thus, the old rule is still in power: Do not use stents in the femoropopliteal arteries on a regular base, try your best to avoid them and use them only if no alternative remains.

Summary

- There are no data proving a benefit of stents over PTA in the femoropopliteal arteries.

- Stents do not fare better than PTA in short lesions and there are no data testing their benefit in complex lesions

- There is nothing but hope that new technologies might overcome this problem

- Stents remain a bail-out case tool in infrainguinal arteries

References

1. The TASC Working Group. Management of peripheral arterial disease (PAD). TransAtlantic Inter-Society Consensus (TASC). *J Vasc Surg* 2000; **31**: S1–S296.
2. Muradin GS, Myriam Hunink MG. Cost and patency rate targets for the development of endovascular devices to treat femoropopliteal arterial disease. *Radiology* 2001; **218**: 464–469.
3. Rousseau HP, Raillat CR, Joffre FG *et al*. Treatment of femoropopliteal stenoses by means of self-expandable endoprostheses: midterm results. *Radiology* 1989; **172**: 961–964.
4. Lugmayr HF, Holzer H, Kastner M *et al*. Treatment of complex arteriosclerotic lesions with nitinol stents in the superficial femoral and popliteal arteries: a midterm follow-up. *Radiology* 2002; **222**: 37–43.
5. Jahnke T, Voshage G, Muller-Hulsbeck S *et al*. Endovascular placement of self expanding nitinol coil stents for the treatment of femoropopliteal obstructive disease. *J Vasc Interv Radiol* 2002; **13**: 257–266.
6. Cejna M, Thurnher S, Illiasch H *et al*. PTA versus Palmaz stent placement in femoropopliteal artery obstructions: a multicenter prospective randomized study. *J Vasc Interv Radiol* 2001; **12**: 23–31.
7. Muradin GS, Bosch JL, Stijnen T, Hunink MG. Balloon dilation and stent implantation for treatment of femoropopliteal arterial disease: meta-analysis. *Radiology* 2001; **221**: 137–145.
8. Ahmadi R, Schillinger M, Maca T, Minar E. Femoropopliteal arteries: immediate and long-term results with a Dacron-covered stent-graft. *Radiology* 2002; **223**: 345–350.
9. Lammer J, Dake MD, Bleyn J *et al*. Peripheral arterial obstruction: prospective study of treatment with a transluminally placed self-expanding stent-graft. International Trial Study Group. *Radiology* 2000; **217**: 95–104.
10. Duda SH, Pusich B, Richter G *et al*. Sirolimus-eluting stents for the treatment of obstructive superficial femoral artery disease: six-month results. *Circulation* 2002; **106**: 1505–1509.

Arterial stents are not required for femoropopliteal angioplasty

Against the motion

Jim A Reekers

Introduction

In a recent published paper about a randomized study of sirolimus-eluting stents for treatment of obstructive superficial femoral artery (SFA) disease the authors conclude:' Interestingly, the restenosis rates for the uncoated stent were much lower than what had been expected from results reported in the published literature'.[1] This raises the question about the validity of the published literature on this topic. The TransAtlantic Inter-Society Consensus Group (TASC) summarized the results of femoropopliteal stenting as follows: in a comparison of 11 trials involving femoropopliteal artery stenting in 585 patients, the primary patency rate was 67% (range, 22%–81%) at 23 months and 58% at 36 months.[2] However, there were no randomized trials and most follow-up data were incomplete. There is a publication about a group of 55 patients, most of whom were treated with femoral Wallstents, which showed a primary 6-month patency rate of only 47%.[3] In the sirolimus-eluting stents trial the 6-months patency rate of the uncoated stent was 95%.[1] Is this due to the randomization, patient selection, the careful follow-up or have we been biased by the general opinion that: 'Stents are no good in the SFA'?

The technique of SFA stenting

The technique for SFA stenting is more or less uniform. After crossing a lesion, long stenotic segment or occlusion, with a guidewire, a stent is introduced. In most reports there is no pre-dilatation before stent deployment recommended. Both the balloon-expandable and the self-expanding stents are vulnerable to bending or forces from outside. Therefore they should not be placed in those areas where bending is likely to occur.

The groin and the popliteal artery below the patella are therefore excluded. Using overlapping stents is reported to show early breaking of struts, so when avoidable this should not be done. Using one stent of the appropriate length, which are currently available up to 15 cm through a 5 French sheath, is the correct technique. To stent 'as short as possible', might not be a real advantage; maybe restoration of laminar flow with a long stent is more optimal. With balloon-expandable stents overdilatation is not recommended; however we feel that a 2-mm increase in nominal stent diameter for a self-expanding stent is an advantage. So we do not pre-dilate, always use a 7-mm diameter self-expanding nitinol stent, with 5-mm balloon dilatation post-placement. When good flow is established follow-up with asprin and 3 months of clopidogel will prevent early reocclusion in most cases. Over- and pre-dilatation might be one of the key factors in early restenosis.

Indication for stent placement in the SFA

Currently only a failed percutaneous transluminal angioplasty (PTA) in the SFA is accepted as an indication to place a stent, where a failed PTA can be saved by stenting to the patency of a successful PTA. However, this is also based on literature with no clear definition of failed PTA. And if there is no difference between PTA and stenting, the poor results of PTA of long SFA occlusions may for that reason warrant a stent just to achieve a 'normal' PTA result. The unpublished data from our trial comparing intraluminal PTA of long SFA occlusions (>10 cm long) with bypass surgery show a very poor 1-year PTA result, with a 1-year primary patency after PTA of 43% and 82% after bypass surgery. For that reason the results from PTA in long SFA could only benefit from stenting.

Evidence

Over the years, from 1995 to 2002, there have been several publications showing favourable results from stenting in the SFA, both with the Palmaz-stent and nitinol stents.[4-10] However, none of these publications have the scientific power needed to settle the argument. There are three papers, all published more than a decade ago, which show promising results, mid-term and long-term, with the use of Palmaz stents in the SFA.[4-6] However, small numbers and poor study design mean that these papers cannot meet the current demands for evidence-based medicine, although they should not be disregarded.

There are several recent papers which also show a positive impact on the mid-term results.[7-10] Again the study designs were not optimal, using either historical controls or no controls. The lesions treated were both stenosis and occlusions in patients with either simple claudication and others with severe ischaemia with poor run-off. The number of patients in these latter publications were higher and the follow-up was better. Again the general message from these papers was that stenting could have an advantage over PTA alone.

A meta-analysis

In a recent published meta-analysis by Muradin et al.[11] the purpose was to look at the long-term results of balloon dilation and stent implantation in the treatment of femoropopliteal arterial disease. The 3-year patency rates after stent implantation were 63%-66% (SE=4.1%) and were independent of clinical indication and lesion type. In comparison the combined 3-year patency rates after balloon dilation were 61% (SE=2.2%) for stenoses and claudication, 48% (SE=3.3%) for occlusions and claudication, 43% (SE=4.1%) for stenoses and critical ischaemia, and 30% (SE=3.7%) for occlusions and critical ischaemia. They conclude that for more severe femoropopliteal disease, the results of stent implantation seem more favourable than for PTA. However, publication bias could not be ruled out.

Costs

But, even if we agree that stents in the SFA might improve the patency, we still have to consider whether the extra costs of stenting will be cost-effective. Stenting all superficial femoral arteries will in most cases double the costs of the materials used, which has to be earned back by fewer re-interventions and occlusions. So, the primary patency is the only endpoint to look at. However, costs of the materials are only about 20% of the total in-hospital costs. By simple calculation it is clear that, in this model, a gain of more than 25% in primary patency after stenting is cost-effective. Comparing the known poor patencies after PTA of long SFA lesions and the good outcome of the uncoated stent in the sirolimus trial, this 25% is easily achieved.[1-2]

Conclusion

There is a constant message from the literature that stenting of the SFA might be beneficial. However, there is currently no scientific evidence to give definitive advice. Calculating with our own data from PTA of long SFA occlusions and the break-even point of costs, a randomized study with 80 patients to prove 25% increase in primary patency will have enough power to settle the debate. In the light of these data showing good results from uncoated stents, it is very doubtful if drug eluting stents in the SFA will ever be cost-effective.

Summary

- There are no randomized trials concerning stenting in the SFA and most follow-up data are incomplete.

- Using overlapping stents is reported to show early breaking of struts, so when avoidable this should not be done.

- Currently only a failed PTA in the SFA is accepted as an indication to place a stent.

- A recent meta-analysis shows that for more severe femoropopliteal disease, the results of stent implantation seem more favourable than for PTA.

- A gain of more than 25% in primary patency after stenting compared with PTA is cost-effective.

- A randomized study of PTA versus stenting in the SFA still has to be performed.

References

1. Duda SH, Pusich B, Richter G *et al.* Sirolimus-eluting stents for the treatment of obstructive superficial femoral artery disease. *Circulation* 2002; **106**: 1505–1509.
2. TransAtlantic Inter-Society Consensus (TASC). Management of peripheral arterial disease (PAD), section B: intermittent claudication. *Eur J Vasc Endovasc Surg* 2000; **19**(Suppl A): S47–S114.
3. Gray BH, Sullivan TM, Childs MB *et al.* High incidence of restenosis/reocclusion of stents in the percutaneous treatment of long segment superficial femoral artery disease after suboptimal angioplasty. *J Vasc Surg* 1997; **25**: 74–83.

4. Bergeron P, Pinot JJ, Poyen V *et al*. Long-term results with the Palmaz stent in the superficial femoral artery. *J Endovasc Surg* 1995; 2: 161–167.
5. Chatelard P, Guibourt C. Long-term results with a Palmaz stent in the femoropopliteal arteries. *J Cardiovasc Surg* 1996; 37 Suppl 1: 67–72.
6. Muller-Hulsbeck S, Schwarzenberg H, Steffens JC *et al*. Treatment of arterial femoropopliteal obstructions with Palmaz midsize stents. *Rofo* 1998; 168: 604–609.
7. Gordon IL, Conroy RM, Arefi M *et al*. Three-year outcome of endovascular treatment of superficial femoral artery occlusion. *Arch Surg* 2001; 136: 221–228.
8. Cheng SW, Ting AC, Wong J. Endovascular stenting of superficial femoral artery stenosis and occlusions: results and risk factor analysis. *Cardiovasc Surg* 2001; 9: 133–140.
9. Jahnke T, Voshage G, Muller-Hulsbech S *et al*. Endovascular placement of self-expanding nitinol stents for the treatment of femoropopliteal obstructive disease. *J Vasc Interv Radiol* 2002; 13: 257–266.
10. Lugmayr HF, Holzer H, Kastner M *et al*. Treatment of complex arteriosclerotic lesions with nitinol stents in the superficial femoral and popliteal arteries:a midterm follow-up. *Radiology* 2002; 222: 37–43.
11. Muradin GSR, Bosch JL, Stijnen T, Hunink MGM. Balloon dilatation and stent implantation for treatment of femoropopliteal arterial disease: meta-analysis. *Radiology* 2001; 221: 137–145.

Arterial stents are not required for femoropopliteal angioplasty

Charing Cross Editorial Comments towards Consensus

Two distinguished radiologists lock horns and wrangle vehemently about stenting or not stenting the superficial femoral artery. They each make a strong case, one for need of stent and the other for angioplasty alone, and both slate the TransAtlantic Inter-Societies Consensus! So here you have it.

The two radiologists have the floor and both kill off vascular surgery and put it behind them and argue the toss about whether there should be angioplasty with or without stent.

Dr Vorwerk places great importance upon the morphology of the lesion and clearly relates strictly to the precise morphology. He and his senior colleagues in CIRSE clearly want to have a category of femoral artery lesion agreed so that audit in the future can give more accurate results by combining the data.

Dr Reekers largely rests his argument upon the absence of present data to argue the toss one way or the other. In essence he is saying that as we are uncertain about whether arterial stents are required for femoropopliteal bypass, they may be, so you cannot say that they are not required.

Time will tell and, as Dr Reekers says, we will await the first randomized controlled trial results to tell us.

A surgeon would like both of these treatment modalities compared with an alternative. It is likely that if very mild lesions are chosen, the alternative will be best medical and supervised exercise, smoking cessation advice, control of diabetes etc., against all of that plus angioplasty with or without stents. This is exactly what the proposed MIMIC trial seeks to test and there will also be useful data on the different modalities of exercise in the so-called EXACT trial.

Roger M Greenhalgh
Editor

Drug eluting stents will revolutionize stent outcome

For the motion

Barry T Katzen

Introduction

During the past decade the use of intravascular stents has increased significantly and become an important part of the armamentarium of the vascular interventionist and vascular surgeon. Both balloon-expandable and self-expanding stents are widely used in diverse anatomic beds for treatment of disease in the aortoiliac, femoral, popliteal, renal, brachiocephalic and carotid regions, in addition to other less commonly employed applications. Restenosis rates of percutaneous transluminal angioplasty (PTA) and/or stenting in these areas varies to some extent by location, with relatively low rates in the aortoiliac region, and higher rates in the renal and superficial femoral locations.[1] Most peripheral restenosis rates tend to be less that those in the coronary applications where rates of 25% are typical.

Restenosis has been long recognized as the 'Achilles heel' of vascular intervention but understanding of the underlying process has been increasing.[2] Numerous efforts to address this problem have been made. These include alternative revascularization techniques such as atherectomy or laser to debulk, as well as the use of stents, brachytherapy and other techniques. Most investigations regarding restenosis reduction have occurred in the coronary application, where stents have a proven efficacy in improving outcomes.[3,4] Peripheral application of stents has proven value in the iliac circulation.[5-6] At this time, there has been increasing use and enthusiasm for use of stents in the superficial femoral artery.[7,8] However, there is evidence from clinical trials to support efficacy of bare stents in reducing restenosis in the periphery[9] although they may provide benefit in improving initial outcomes. A diverse group of techniques for reducing restenosis is being developed for infrainguinal intervention, including drug eluting stents.

However, the bulk of our knowledge and understanding of drug eluting stents comes from animal research, feasibility and controlled trials for coronary applications, and the preceding pre-clinical work in animals. Data from these trials have produced encouraging results in reducing the incidence of restenosis and events secondary to that process, namely delayed MACE (Major Adverse Cardiovascular Events) and target lesion revascularization.

Based on current data, the author believes drug eluting stents will revolutionize vascular intervention by improving the results of revascularization for occlusive disease through delivery of therapeutic agents in conjunction with stent delivery.

Peripheral vascular stents

Stents have proved to be efficacious in the iliac arteries, where both self-expanding and balloon-expandable stents have been widely used. In the United States, two devices (Palmaz Balloon Expandable Stent, Cordis Johnson and Johnson, and Wallstent, Boston Scientific) have label indications for use in suboptimal angioplasty. For infrainguinal applications, the most recent consensus statement[1] indicated that data was insufficient for a recommendation on efficacy regarding stents in the superficial femoral artery. Most studies regarding stents in the superficial femoral artery failed to clearly demonstrate benefits in long-term patency over angioplasty alone, but the TASC document did acknowledge benefit of stents for improvement of immediate outcomes of vascular intervention. Much of the early data on efficacy of stents for superficial femoral artery applications involved a variety of self-expanded woven stents, but there was relatively little about the more recent self-expanding nitinol stents. Although small series have suggested that these stents may result in improved outcomes,[9,10] no large well-controlled studies have addressed the issue.

Most series of superficial femoral artery stenting have produced results similar to those reported with angioplasty alone. In fact, both techniques of infrainguinal revascularization suffer from problems of restenosis with 12 month patency rates of approximately 50–60%.[8]

In-stent and angioplasty restenosis is primarily the result of neointimal hyperplasia resulting from injury related to either technique. A cascade resulting from vascular injury begins with platelet activation and mural thrombus formation, which in turn activates inflammatory cells which then release cytokines and growth factors that activate smooth muscle cells, and subsequent proliferation. Extracellular matrix is also produced which in addition to the smooth muscle cell proliferation around the injury sites, results in luminal narrowing over time.[2]

Stents can result in improvement in restenosis rates in the coronary vessels and improve the outcome of PTA in the renal arteries by overcoming elastic recoil, but none-the-less the injury model still exists. Restenosis remains a significant limitation in peripheral angioplasty and stenting in the superficial femoral artery, and therefore a possible solution would have great benefit in this anatomic distribution, particularly for superficial femoral artery application.

Principles of drug eluting stents

Stents have proven efficacy in treating one of the limitations of angioplasty, namely elastic recoil. Although balloon-expandable stents have been most effective, deformability in exposed areas makes them less desirable for application in the exposed areas such as the lower extremities, or the carotid artery. Self-expanding nitinol stents provide good radial force, flexibility and are not permanently deformable by external forces, making them more suitable for exposed applications.

Stents also offer the potential for delivery of drugs to the biologically active part of the vessel wall, actively interfering with the cellular process associated with in-stent restenosis. They can function not only as structural scaffolding but as a platform for delivery of drugs to the vessel wall or to the circulation depending on agent and treatment goals. Although stents provide the platform for drug delivery, other critical factors include the specific agent and its mechanism of action, the polymer necessary for binding and controlled delivery, and the stent geometry which will have both an independent effect on restenosis as well as provide the surface area for contact and delivery to tissue.

Problems associated with drug delivery include, but are not limited to, binding of the agent to the device, controlled release, dosing and distribution of release, identifying optimal agent, balancing efficacy against toxicity.

Well-defined restenosis models have been developed in both porcine and rabbit models. Attempts to moderate restenosis have been directed at the injury event, inflammatory component, or proliferative response, and there is rationale for various approaches. Stent geometry may be important in differentiating patency in coronary stenoses, but has not been proven to be significant in peripheral trials. Most drugs intended for therapeutic benefit must be placed in polymers necessary for binding to the metallic surface of the stents. Frequently the coatings themselves may be associated with an inflammatory process and induce intimal hyperplasia. Additionally some coatings themselves may have some benefit in reducing the restenosis process.

Agents evaluated on drug eluting stents

A variety of agents have been considered for use as restenosis lowering agents (Table 1).

Table 1. Substances that have been examined as stent coating

Coating	Mechanism of action
Biocompatible coatings	
Carbon	Chemically inert and potentially non-inflamatory
Gold	Chemically inert and potentially non-inflammatory
Silicon carbide	Inert semi-conductor potentially less thrombogenic and inflammatory
Phosphorylcholine	Organic polymer potentially less thombogenic and inflammatory
Drug coatings	
Anticoagulants	
Heparin	Anti-thrombotic and possible direct inhibition of smooth muscle cell proliferation
Incomplete apposition	
Hirudin	Anti-thrombotic and potentially anti-proliferative
Iloprost	Prostacyclin analogue that is anti-thrombotic and potentially anti-proliferative
Corticosteroids	
Dexamethasone	Corticosteroid and potent anti-inflammatory properties
Methylprednisolone	Coticosteroid with potent anti-inflammatory properties
Anti-mitotic agents	
Paclitaxel	Interferes with microtubule function and thereby inhibits a variety of intracellular processes including mitosi and cell migration
Sirolimus	Inhibits production of proteins essential for cell division; has potent immunosuppressive and anti-mitotic properties
Angiopeptin	Somatostatin analogue that inhibits many cytokines and growth factors, and potentially has anti-proliferative effects
Tyrosine kinase inhibitors	Interfere with intracellular cell signalling that regulate cell proliferation and differentiation

From Ref. 20.

They include anticoagulants, antimicrobial agents, antiproliferative agents, anti-inflammatory agents, and others including some polymer coatings. The mechanisms of actions and comparative aspects of different approaches towards drug coatings are beyond the scope of this discussion, but the reader is referred to the bibliography for further information.

Results of drug eluting stent trials

Several clinical trials have been completed, in the coronary circulation and more recently in the peripheral circulation. Some have confirmed lack of efficacy, e.g. gold[11,12] and heparin,[13] but others more recently using agents such as sirolimus[14] and paclitaxel[15,16] have shown striking efficacy based on MACE rates at 6 months, as well as reduction in restenosis (Fig. 1) Some have produced marked differences compared with control with 80–90% reduction in adverse event rates and restenosis (Tables 2, 3).

In the superficial femoral artery, benefit at 6 months in superficial femoral artery applications with sirolimus coating of self-expanding stents for a diverse group of superficial femoral artery lesions were shown.[17] This randomized, prospective controlled study was well designed, but small and intended to be a feasibility study. A diverse group of variables including lesion length, total number of stents and others have made conclusions difficult other than to say that overall improvement over historic controls for angioplasty and stenting seem to be conferred by the coated stent group. Other trials in the periphery are planned or in early stages of feasibility using a variety of stent platforms, and a variety of active agents.

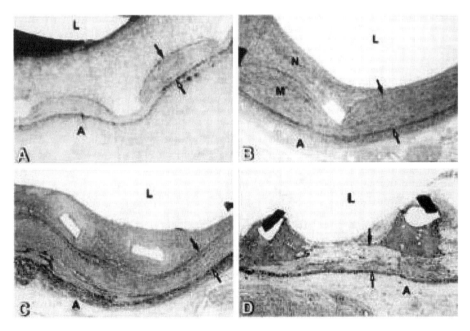

Figure 1. Photomicrographs of stented porcine arteries (magnification x 32). A: No paclitaxel (control); B: low-dose paclitaxel (0.2 µg/stent); C: intermediate-dose paclitaxel (15 µg/stent); and D: high-dose paclitaxel (187 µg/stent). Black material partially filling lumen in A is barium gelatin dye contrast medium. Solid and open arrows indicate boundaries formed by internal and external elastic laminae, respectively. L: lumen; N: neointima; M: tunica media; and A: tunica advetitia. Reprinted with permission from Ref. 19.

Table 2. Human observational studies investigating stent eluting anti-mitotic agent

Study	Coating	No	Restenosis risk	Follow-up (months)	MACE (%)	Mean late loss (mm)	Mean late stenosis (%)	Binary re-stenosis (%)
Sousa et al.[41]*	Sirolimus (fast release)	15	Low	4	0	(-)0.10 +/- 0.3	4.6 +/- 5.7	0
	Sirolimus (slow release)	15	Low	4	0	0.09 +/- 0.3	5.0 +/- 6.7	0
Sousa et al.[42]+	Sirolimus (fast release)	15	Low	12	0	0.09	8.9 +/- 6.1	0
	Sirolimus (slow release)	15	Low	12	0	0.07	6.7 +/- 7.0	0
Rensing et al.[43]	Sirolimus (slow release)	15	Low	6	0	0	13.7	0
Honda et al.[44]	QP2	14	Low	8	10	0.1	13.3 +/- 15.1	0
de la Fuente et al.[46]	QP2	32	Intermediate	11	0	0.42 +/- 0.36	6.3 +/- 9.3	0
Listro et al.[47]	QP2	15	High	12	87	1.36 +/- 0.94	NR	62

NR indicates not reported

*These are the 4- and 12-month follow-up results of the same cohort of 30 patients

From Ref. 20. [References 41–44,46 and 47 cited in this table can be found in Ref 20.]

Table 3. Clinical trial investigating coated stents

Study	Coating	No	Restenosis risk	Follow-up (months)	MACE (%)			Binary restenosis (%)		
					Coated	Un-coated	p Value	Coated	Un-coated	p Value
Kastrati et al.[48]	Gold	731	Intermediate	12*	37.1	26.1	0.0001	49.7	38.1	0.003
Gvom Dahl et al.[49]	Gold	204	Low	6	3	2	NS	36	24	0.13
Park et al.[50]	Gold	216	Intermediate	9*	23.6	15.1	0.113	46.7	26.4	<0.05
Worle et al.[51]	Heparin	277	Intermediate	9*	25.2	25.7	NS	33.1	30.3	NS
Morice et al.[52]	Sirolimus	238	Low	12*	5.8	28.8	0.001	0	26.6	0.001
Park et al.[54]	Paclitaxel (high dose)	s	Low	6	NA	NA	NA	4	27	<0.001
	Paclitaxel (low dose)	s	Low	6	NA	NA	NA	12	27	NA
Gershlick et al.[55]	Paclitaxel	192	Low	6	11	11	NS	3	21	0.055 t
Grube et al.[56]	Paclitaxel	61	Low	6	NA	NA	NA	0	11	0.106
Grube et al.[57]	QP2	266	Low	6	NA	NA	NA	10.1 tt	36.9	<0.001

NS: not significant; NA: data not availabe.

*Angiographic follow-up at 6 months.

t The values given here for the highest-dose paclitaxel group (2.7 µg/mm).

tt 9.4% due to subacute and delayed stent thrombosis.

s The total number for this three-arm trial 177.

From Ref. 20. [References 48–52, 54–57 cited in this table can be found in Ref. 20.]

Attempts at using systemic agents of a variety of types including anti-inflammatory agents, anti-platelet agents and others have not been successful to date. Recently Farb[18] reported successful suppression of restenosis in a rabbit model using everolimus with systemic delivery. This method of drug delivery has the potential disadvantage of affecting endothelial function throughout the circulation, whereas targeted drug delivery has the benefit of controlled and targeted drug release, in theory increasing efficacy and decreasing undesirable secondary systemic effects.

Discussion and basis for optimism for drug eluting stents in the peripheral circulation

Peripheral intervention is a broad area of therapy as opposed to treatment of coronary artery lesions, which represent a more homogenous area for target lesions. Within peripheral intervention, angioplasty and stenting has differing long-term results, some of which are superior to those described in the coronary circulation (i.e. iliac artery), and some quite worse (i.e. superficial femoral artery). In peripheral intervention, treatment of the superficial femoral artery has been the least effective in terms of long-term patency and in particular the development of restenosis as a cause of treatment failure. Additionally, despite numerous advances in technology that have improved outcome in other vessels and lesion types, such as stents, atherectomy, and adjunctive medical therapy such as use of Plavix, little improvement in superficial femoral artery intervention has been documented.

The results of SIRROCO trial as well as an increasing body of evidence in animals and the coronary circulation provide abundant reasons to be optimistic that drug eluting stents will have great impact on peripheral intervention, particularly in the superficial femoral artery, a vessel that has resisted effective therapy using other technologies to date. While much needs to be learned, and controlled trials need to be designed and completed, the author feels that sufficient data exists to be optimistic that drug eluting stents will change the face of peripheral intervention, improving results in many patients with peripheral arterial occlusive disease.

Summary

- Restenosis limits the efficacy of peripheral angioplasty and stenting.
- The highest rates of restenosis are in the superficial femoral artery.
- Drug eluting stents have proven efficacy in animal models and early human clinical coronary trials.
- Initial evaluation of drug-coated stents in superficial femoral artery applications are favourable.
- Drug eluting stents will prove to be as valuable in peripheral applications as in coronary applications.
- Drug eluting stents will increase the durability of peripheral stenting.

References

1. TransAtlantic Inter-Society Consensus (TASC). Management of Peripheral Artery Disease. *J Vasc Surg* 2000; **31**: No 1, Part 2.

2. Virmani R, Farb A. Pathology of in-stent restenosis. *Curr Opin Lipidol* 1999; **10**: 499–506.

3. Edelman ER, Rogers C. Stent-versus-stent equivalency trials: are some stents more equal than others? *Circulation.* 1999; **100**: 896–898.

4. Bauters C, Hubert E, Prat A *et al.* Predictors of restenosis after coronary stent implantation. *J Am Coll Cardiol.* 1998; **31**: 1291–1298.

5. Palmaz JC, Garcia O, Schatz RA *et al.* Placement of balloon expandable stents in iliac arteries: First 171 patients. *Radiology* 1990; **174**: 969–975.

6. Palmaz JC, Richter GM, Noeldge G *et al.* Intraluminal stents in atherosclerotic iliac artery stenosis: Preliminary report of a multicenter trial. *Radiology* 1988; **168**: 727–731.

7. Benenati JF, Becker GJ, Katzen BT *et al.* Chronic iliac artery occlusions: treatment with percutaneous endoluminal stents [abstract]. *Radiology* 1991; **181**(P): 162.

8. Martin EC, Katzen BT, Benenati JF *et al.* Multicenter trial of the wallstent in the iliac and femoral arteries. *J Vasc Interv Radiol* 1995; **6**: 843–849.

9. Gray BH, Sullivan TM, Childs MB *et al.* High incidence of restenosis/reocclusion of stents in the percutaneous treatment of long segment superficial femoral artery disease after suboptimal angioplasty. *J Vasc Surg* 1997; **25**: 74–83.

10. Do-dai-Do, Triller J, Walpoth BH et al. A comparison study of self-expandable stents vs balloon angioplasty alone in femoropopliteal artery occlusions. *Cardiovascular Intervent Radiol* 1992; **15**: 306–312.

11. Kastrati A, Schomig A, Dirschinger J *et al.* A randomized trial comparing stenting with balloon angioplasty in small vessels in patients with symptomatic coronary artery disease. ISAR-SMART Study Investigators: Intracoronary Stenting or Angioplasty for Restenosis Reduction in Small Arteries. *Circulation* 2000; **102**: 2593–2598.

12. Park SJ, Lee CW, Hong MK *et al.* Comparison of gold-coated NIR stents with uncoated NIR stents in patients with coronary artery disease. *Am J Cardiol.* 2002; **89**: 872–875.

13. Wohrle J, Al-Khayer E, Grotzinger U *et al.* Comparison of the heparin coated vs the uncoated Jostent: no influence on restenosis or clinical outcome. *Eur Heart J* 2001; **22**: 1808–1816.

14. Morice M-C, Serruys PW, Sousa JE *et al.* A randomized comparison of a Sirolimus-eluting stent with a standard stent for coronary revascularization. *N Engl J Med* 2002; **346**: 1773–1780.

15. Park SJ, Shim WH, Ho DS *et al.* The clinical effectiveness of paclitaxel-coated coronary stents for the reduction of restenosis in the ASPECT trial. *Circulation.* 2001; **104**(Suppl II): II-464. Abstract.

16. Drachman DE, Edelman ER, Seifert P *et al.* Neointimal thickening after stent delivery of Paclitaxel: change in composition and arrest of growth over six months. *J Am Coll Cardiol.* 2000; **36**: 2325–2332.

17. Duda SH, Pusich B, Richter G *et al.* Sirolimus-eluting stents for the treatment of obstructive superficial femoral artery disease: six-month results. *Circulation* 2002; **106**: 1505–1509.

18. Farb A, John M, Acampado E *et al.* Oral everolimus in-stent neointimal growth. *Circulation.* 2002; **106**: 2379–2384.

19. Heldman AW, Cheng L, Jenkins GM *et al.* Paclitaxel stent coating inhibits neointimal hyperplasia at 4 weeks in a porcine model of coronary restenosis. *Circulation* 2001; **103**: 2289–2295.

20. Babapulle MN, Eisenberg MJ. Coated stents for the prevention of restenosis: Part I: *Circulation* 2002; **106**: 2734–2740.

Drug eluting stents will revolutionize stent outcome

Against the motion
Dominic Fay, Phil Davey, Michael Wyatt, John Rose

Introduction

The recanalization of diseased infrainguinal arteries poses unique problems. Endovascular techniques are able to yield technically impressive results in the short term but the durability of patency is limited. An analysis of pooled results for percutaneous transluminal angioplasty (PTA) of femoropopliteal stenoses and occlusions in 1469 limbs (1241 patients) showed primary patency rates of 61% at 1 year and 51% at 3 years.[1] The analysis of the results of conventional metal stents in similar groups yielded only slightly improved results with 67% 1-year and 58% 3-year primary patency rates. This was despite initial technical success rates of 90% for PTA and 98% for stent placement.

Currently in the United Kingdom, the use of stents in the femoropopliteal arteries is largely reserved for those patients in whom PTA has yielded a haemodynamically sub-optimal result. It may be argued that stent deployment for salvage of failed angioplasty is subject to an inherently higher likelihood of re-occlusion. But data from randomized trials of femoropopliteal PTA versus primary stent placement have also shown stents to be of no benefit.[2,3,4] PTA is often part of the routine management of patients with critical limb ischaemia but remains controversial for the treatment of intermittent claudication in the UK. Many clinicians promote lifestyle modification and exercise rather than PTA.[5]

In order to predict that drug eluting stents will revolutionize stent outcomes in the management of femoropopliteal disease, two basic assumptions have to be made:

1. that lesions requiring recanalization in the femoropopliteal segment are analagous to those coronary artery lesions which are typically suitable for stenting;
2. that drug eluting stents will offer more advantage in large vessels than all other novel types of stent.

There is currently little evidence for either of these two assumptions.

Physical effects of angioplasty and stenting

The generally accepted mechanism of balloon angioplasty[6,7] indicates that the adventitia and media are stretched and the diseased intima and plaque fractured, displaced and partially separated. Although the potential increase of luminal diameter is offset by immediate elastic recoil, the local division of the diseased intima allows dynamic remodelling by removing the restraining effect of the relatively hard atheromatous intimal lining. The additional effects of platelet adhesion, causing migration of smooth muscle cells and deposition of a neointimal layer, are to further reduce luminal gain. The introduction of a stent is known to prevent elastic recoil and will also improve the early results of angioplasty by smoothing away intimal flaps. However, there is greater intimal proliferation after stent insertion which is responsible for much of the late lumen loss and will accentuate any tendency to restenosis.

Drug eluting stents

Stent placement in coronary artery lesions was shown in large randomized trials performed in the 1990s[8,9] to improve outcome and thus stent insertion has become standard practice in non-surgical coronary revascularization. However, moderate rates of restenosis in the coronary vessels have driven interest in the development of novel drug impregnated stents. These typically employ a polymer coating from which an anti-inflammatory or anti-proliferative agent can leach into the adjacent tissues in order to modify the local foreign body response.

Trials have been conducted in coronary arteries using stents that elute rapamycin (sirolimus)[10,11] and paclitaxel (Taxol).[12] An uncontrolled study examining the use of sirolimus eluting stents showed low restenosis rates up to 12 months after stent implantation.[10] While similar work with paclitaxel-derivative eluting stents showed reduced restenosis rates at 6 months this benefit was not sustained at 12 months.[12] Preliminary data presented from randomized trials of both paclitaxel and rapamycin eluting stents have shown results in favour of drug elution although these are yet to be published. The coronary experience of drug eluting stents is therefore limited to short-term follow-up and further evaluation is required before firm conclusions can be reached.

Efficacy of stents in the peripheral vasculature

The best results in the coronary arteries and the peripheral circulation will accrue from the treatment of a single stenosis with no tandem lesions. However, the typical symptomatic patient enrolled for endovascular treatment in the UK will have an extensive femoropopliteal lesion. The effects of angioplasty and stenting on occluded large vessels are likely to be different from those taking place during and after treatment of a stenotic coronary artery. In contrast to the coronary arteries, the use of bare metal stents in the femoropopliteal segments has not been demonstrated to improve long-term angiographic or clinical results although improved immediate patency was shown.[1-4] This crucial difference in post-stent behaviour between these anatomical regions means that assumptions cannot be made that the coronary experience will apply to the femoropopliteal vessels, even if the longer term experience of drug eluting stents in the coronary arteries shows an unequivocal benefit. The use of drug eluting stents in the femoropopliteal arteries therefore requires evaluation with separate randomized controlled trials.

Current evidence for the efficacy of drug eluting stents in peripheral vessels

A trial of dexamethasone eluting stents has been performed in canine femoral arteries[13] but to date only one study has been published comparing the effects of drug eluting and bare metal stents on human femoropopliteal disease.[14] This double-blind prospective multicentre study sponsored by Cordis randomized 36 patients to receive either rapamycin (sirolimus) eluting or bare metal Cordis SMART stents to femoral artery stenoses or occlusions. The sirolimus-treated lesions differed from the controls in that they exhibited greater levels of calcification but otherwise there was close correlation between the groups. Up to three 80mm stents were deployed in each patient (mean 2.2 in each group) and 33 patients were followed up with quantitative angiography at 6 months. At this early point statistically significant differences were not shown in the primary end point of in-stent mean percentage diameter stenosis. There was a moderate improvement in the absolute in-stent mean lumen diameter (4.95mm in the sirolimus group versus 4.31 mm in the uncoated group, p=0.047). This small study has not yet demonstrated the use of the sirolimus eluting stent to be beneficial although the authors claim a trend in its favour. Clearly larger numbers of patients will need to be recruited into longer term studies before meaningful data are available and significant conclusions can be made.

Covered stents

The use of metal stents covered with or lined by graft material is an established method in the treatment of aneurysms, pseudoaneurysms, dissections and breaches in the vessel wall throughout the arterial tree. Intuitively, the presence of a membrane between the restored vascular lumen and the diseased vessel wall should act as a barrier against tissue encroachment and help to reduce in-stent restenosis. There are animal studies to support this concept.[15,16] The additional thickness of the graft material has perhaps limited the application of 'first-generation' stent-grafts to the large vessels of the aortoiliac segments. However, there are covered stents designed for smaller vessels which include more flexible stents with fine layers of polytetrafluoroethylene (PTFE) (Fig. 1).

A recent report of a prospective clinical trial of a covered stent system in peripheral arterial disease[17] is promising but long-term follow-up and randomized trials are required.

Other avenues

There are several other incompletely evaluated techniques with the common aim of providing durable minimally invasive infrainguinal revascularization. Subintimal angioplasty provides good initial technical and clinical results[18] although long-term data are lacking. Endoluminal irradiation using gamma sources was debated in these pages last year and a randomized study comparing the effect of brachytherapy and stenting versus stenting alone should report in the near future. Recently there has been interest in the use of gene therapy, namely the infusion of mutant genes at the site of angioplasty and stenting in order to modify the endothelial response and prevent restenosis.[19]

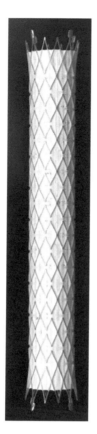
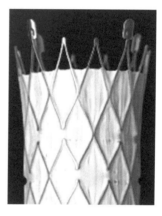

(a)   (b)

Figure 1. (a) ePTFE encapsulated Nitinol stent with highly radiopaque Tantalum spoons (b) at either end. Both ends of the stent are flared. Currently in experimental use (diameters: 6–10mm, lengths: 40–100mm).

Conclusion

Until more reliable data emerges the use of drug eluting stents in the infrainguinal vessels must be regarded as unproven. It will be important to ensure that this application is backed by randomized trials in individual target vessels and weighed against the likely cost. Other techniques are also being examined and in the case of covered stents, subintimal angioplasty and brachytherapy there is already substantial experience awaiting corroboration by ongoing trials.

Summary

- The pitfalls of extrapolating data from the coronary literature to the peripheral vessels are illustrated by the differing results of bare stents in the coronary arteries compared with the femoropopliteal vessels.

- The coronary trials of drug eluting stents are short term and there may be a loss of benefit at 12 months follow-up despite promising early results.

- There are insufficient data to support the use of drug eluting stents in the peripheral vessels.

- Alternative stent platforms, including endovascular stent grafts, may also have an impact on restenosis rates in the near future.

References

1. TASC. TransAtlantic Inter-Society Consensus (TASC) document on management of peripheral arterial disease. *J Vasc Surg* 2000; 31: S1–S296.
2. Vroegindewiej D, Vos LD *et al*. Balloon angioplasty combined with stent placement versus balloon angioplasty alone in femoropopliteal obstructions: A comparative randomised study. *Cardiovasc Intervent Radiol* 1997; 20: 420–425.
3. Cejna M, Thurnher S *et al*. PTA versus Palmaz stent placement in femoropopliteal obstructions; a multicenter prospective randomised study. *J Vasc Intervent Radiol* 2001; 12: 23–31.
4. Grimm J, Muller-Hulsbeck S *et al*. Randomised study to compare PTA alone versus PTA with Palmaz stent placement for femoropopliteal lesions. *J Vasc Intervent Radiol* 2001; 12: 935–941.
5. Whyman MR, Fowkes FG *et al*. Is intermittent claudication improved by percutaneous transluminal angioplasty? A randomised controlled trial. *J Vasc Surg* 1997; 26: 551–557.
6. Castenada-Zuniga WR, Formanek A, Tadavarthy M *et al*. The mechanism of balloon angioplasty. *Radiology* 1980; 135: 565–571.
7. Lammer J. Femoropopliteal artery obstructions: from the balloon to the stent-graft. *Cardiovasc Intervent Radiol* 2001; 24: 73–83.
8. Fischman DL, Leon MB *et al*. A randomized comparison of coronary-stent placement and balloon angioplasty in the treatment of coronary artery disease. Stent Restenosis Study Investigators. *N Engl J Med* 1994; 331: 496–501.
9. Serruys PW, de Jaegere P *et al*. A comparison of balloon-expandable-stent implantation with balloon angioplasty in patients with coronary artery disease. Benestent Study Group. *N Engl J Med* 1994; 331: 489–495.
10. Sousa JE, Costa MA *et al*. Lack of neointimal proliferation after implantation of sirolimus-coated stents in human coronary arteries. A quantitative coronary angiography and three dimensional intravascualr ultrasound study. *Circulation* 2001; 103: 192–195.
11. Sousa JE, Costa MA *et al*. Sustained suppression of neointimal proliferation by sirolimus-eluting stents. One year angiographic and intravascular ultrasound follow-up. *Circulation* 2001; 104: 2007–2011.
12. Liistro F, Stankovic G *et al*. First clinical experience with a paclitaxel derivative eluting polymer stent system implantation for in-stent restenosis. *Circulation* 2002; 105: 1883–1886.
13. Strecker EP, Gabelmann A *et al*. Effect on intimal hyperplasia of dexamethasone released from coated metal stents compared with non-coated stents in canine femoral arteries. *Cardiovasc Intervent Radiol* 1998; 21: 487–496.
14. Duda SH, Pusich BP *et al*. Sirolimus eluting stents for the treatment of obstructive superficial femoral artery disease: six month results. *Circulation* 2002; 106: 1505–1509.
15. Vermani R, Kolodgie FD, Dake MD *et al*. Histopathologic evaluation of an expanded PTFE - nitinol stent endoprosthesis in canine ilio-femoral arteries. *J Vasc Intervent Radiol* 1999; 10: 445–456.
16. Schurmann K, Haage P, Meyer J *et al*. Comparison of two stent grafts with different porosity: *in-vivo* studies in a sheep model. *J Vasc Intervent Radiol* 2000; 11: 493–502.
17. Duda SH, Bosiers M, Pusich B *et al*. Endovascular treatment of peripheral artery disease with expanded PTFE-covered nitinol stents: interim analysis from a prospective controlled study. *Cardiovasc Intervent Radiol* 2002; 25: 413–418.
18. Varty K, Nasim A, Bolia A *et al*. Results of surgery and angioplasty for the treatment of severe lower limb ischaemia. *Eur J Vasc Endovasc Surg* 1998; 16: 159–163.
19. Laukkanen, MO, Kivela, A, Yla-Herttuala S *et al*. Adenovirus-mediated extracellular superoxide dismutase gene therapy reduces neointima formation in balloon-denuded rabbit aorta. *Circulation* 2002; 106: 1999–2003.

Drug eluting stents will revolutionize stent outcome

Charing Cross Editorial Comments towards Consensus

Drug eluting stents are the rage for 2003. Drug eluting stents will change the current paradigm for vascular intervention according to Barry Katzen. Re-stenosis has dogged these stents. He assesses that the results of the Sirocco Trial as well as an increasing body of evidence in animals and the coronary circulation provide abundant reason to be optimistic that drug eluting stents will have great impact on peripheral intervention.

Dr Thomas Fogarty is stated to doubt the value of drug eluting stent above the popliteal artery in the peripheral circulation. He is due to comment at the Symposium and it will be interesting to hear his views.

Jon Rose draws attention to the pitfalls of extrapolating data from the coronary literature to the peripheral vessels. He stresses that coronary trials of drug eluting stents are short term. There could be loss of benefit at 12 months. He also believes that the data are insufficient to support the use of drug eluting stents in the peripheral vessels.

This subject is in its infancy. There is a wide spectrum of opinion. No-one knows for sure. Just wait for evangelism on the day.

Thrombolysis is irrelevant in the treatment of acute arterial graft occlusion

For the motion
Alun H Davies, Alexander Rodway,
Richard Gibbs

Introduction

The standard open surgical treatment for the occluded bypass graft is open thrombectomy with graft revision, or a new bypass procedure. Treatment of thrombosis by enzymatic breakdown was developed over 30 years ago, and advances in technique, particularly catheter directed intra-arterial thrombolysis have provided a further therapeutic pathway in the treatment of graft occlusions.

Systemic venous infusion of high dose thrombolytic agents in acute arterial occlusion was pioneered in the 1960s.[1] Patency of recently occluded arteries was achieved in two-thirds of cases, although this was at the cost of major haemorragic complications. Catheter-directed intra-arterial thrombolysis evolved in the 1980s, and became a recognized therapeutic modality in the treatment of arterial occlusions.

Thrombolysis has been advocated in the treatment of acute graft thrombosis because of the theoretical advantages it offers compared with immediate open surgery. Thrombolysis is less invasive, and general anasthaesia is avoided in the emergency situation. Perfusion is restored, and the underlying aetiological lesion responsible for the thrombosis is unmasked by angiography. Further elective endovascular or open surgical treatment can then be planned. The magnitude of open surgical procedure may well be less than an immediate emergency procedure. However, there are also disadvantages associated with thrombolysis. Recognized complications can be drug-related (haemorrhage, distal embolization, allergic reactions) or catheter-related (pericatheter thrombosis, pseudoaneurysm at puncture site). The technique is perceived to be expensive in terms of time and cost.

Technique

Guidewire penetration of the occlusion is an important indicator of the likelihood of success; if the guidewire passes, intrathrombus lysis is more likely to be successful. If the guidewire cannot pass the occlusion, it is because the degree of underlying atherosclerosis or neointimal hyperplasia, or the presence of calcified, organized thrombus means the chances of successful lysis are low.[2] When the occlusion is infrainguinal in position the artery or graft to be lysed is usually approached from the contralateral femoral artery over the aortic bifurcation.

Once the catheter tip has penetrated the thrombus, there are various techniques in the infusion of the thrombolytic agent. *Stepwise infusion*[3] involves infiltrating the proximal part of the thrombus with small fixed volumes of thrombolytic agent and then advancing the catheter every 5–15 minutes until the thrombus has lysed and the catheter tip has reached open distal lumen. The patient has to remain in the angiography suite until this is achieved. *Continuous infusion* is the current standard method for catheter-directed thrombolysis. A steady flow infusion pump delivers a constant infusion of the thrombolytic agent. Higher initial doses followed by a tapering down of the volume of the thrombolytic agent is a varient called *graded infusion*. Continuous infusions can be preceded by intrathrombus lacing, in which the catheter is slowly withdrawn up the length of the thrombus whilst the thrombolytic agent is infused, hence 'lacing' the entire thrombus to hasten breakdown. *Pulse spray* infusion involves forceful injection of the agent into the thrombus in order to break down the thrombus, hence increasing the available surface area for action by the thrombolytic agent.[4] Mechanical devices such as balloons or pulse spray delivery systems can be combined with thrombolysis, techniques referred to as *pharmacomechanical thrombolysis*.

Thrombolytic agents

The basic mode of action of the thrombolytic agents is to activate fibrin-bound plasminogen in the thrombus to generate a high local concentration of the active enzyme plasmin which breaks down fibrin. The most commonly used plasminogen activators were streptokinase, urokinase, recombinant tissue plasminogen activator, prourokinase and acylated streptokinase. More recently the highly fibrin specific recombinant staphylokinase[5] has been used in an attempt to reduce systemic fibrinogen depletion, and other agents such as the platelet inhibitor abciximab[6] have been added to the thrombolytic agents in an attempt to improve thrombus breakdown.

Evidence

There have been a number of studies reporting on thrombolysis as an alternative intervention in occluded lower limb bypass grafts,[7,8] but only four prospective randomized trials comparing intra-arterial thrombolysis with surgery in the management of acute limb-threatening ischaemia. The working party on thrombolysis in lower limb arterial occlusion published a consensus document, which suggested that these prospective randomized trials provided the evidence for suggestions on the treatment of these patients.[2] Three of these trials included bypass grafts, both autogenous and prosthetic. Two of the trials were large multicentre studies, and one was a smaller single unit study. The final trial was a small single unit study of 20 patients only, and graft occlusions were not specified.[9]

The Rochester study compared operative revascularization (n=57, 30 grafts) with catheter-directed urokinase thrombolysis (n=57, 33 grafts) for patients presenting with limb-threatening ischaemia of less than 7 days duration.[10] The primary endpoints were survival and limb salvage. Patency was achieved in 70% of the thrombolytic group. No subgroup analysis was made of graft compared with native vessel, so the results reflect a heterogenous group.

Early results (30 days) demonstrated no difference in either amputation (9% versus 14%) or mortality (12% versus 18%), but there was a significant increase in major bleeding episodes in the thrombolysis group (11% versus 2%), with one intracerebral bleed leading to death. At 1 year the amputation rate for both groups was the same at 18%, but there was a significant improvement in survival in the thrombolysis group (84% versus 58%, p=0.01) compared with the operative group. The authors attributed this observed difference to an increase in cardiorespiratory complications in the operative group (49% versus 16%).

The STILE trial[11] (Table 1) included 124 graft occlusions within the overall remit of comparing optimal surgical procedure with thrombolysis in non-embolic arterial and graft occlusion causing lower limb ischaemia.

A total of 78 patients were randomized to catheter-directed thrombolysis with either urokinase or recombinant tissue plasminogen activator, and 46 to surgery in the form of graft thrombectomy and graft revision or placement of a new bypass graft.[12] Thrombolytic success was defined by the achievement of angiographically demonstrable graft patency. The aetiological lesion causing the graft thrombosis was subsequently dealt with by endovascular or open intervention, and this was considered part of successful thrombolysis. The endpoint of the trial was a composite clinical outcome of at least one specified adverse 'event' occurring during the first 30 days. Events included ongoing or recurrent ischaemia, major amputation, death and life threatening haemorrage.

Results demonstrated a significantly better outcome in patients randomized to surgery compared with thrombolysis, both at 30 days (p=0.02) and 1 year (p=0.04). This was ascribed to a reduction in ongoing or recurrent ischaemia in the surgery group. In the thrombolysis group patency was established in 47% of occluded grafts on an intention-to-treat basis. In all, 81% of the successfully lysed grafts required subsequent endovascular or open surgery to correct the aetiological lesion. In the thrombolysis group, the magnitude of the surgical procedure required was reduced in 39% of vein grafts, and 44% of prosthetic grafts, compared with a lesser procedure than that indicated at randomization in 8% of the group randomized to surgery.

Subgroup analysis suggested that the time period from the onset of ischaemia was important.

Patients presenting with acute ischaemia (0-14 days) who were randomized to lysis had a significantly lower major amputation rate at 1 year (p=0.026) than the group randomized to surgery. In those patients with a duration of ischaemia exceeding 14 days, the lytic group had a higher ongoing or recurrent ischaemia rate than the surgery group (p<0.001). Graft type was important, with prosthetic grafts having a significantly greater major morbidity than vein grafts (p=0.038).

The TOPAS trial (Table 2) enrolled 548 patients into a head-to-head comparison of surgery versus 'best dose' thrombolysis with recombinant urokinase.[13] Both native

Table 1. Results in bypass graft occlusions (n=124) at 1 year, from the STILE study

	Surgery		Lysis		p value
	No	%	No	%	
Composite clinical outcome (adverse outcome)	28	61	61	78	0.04
Death	0	0	5	6	0.29
Amputation	14	30	14	18	0.11
Ongoing/recurrent ischaemia	23	50	57	73	0.01
Major morbidity	7	15	17	22	0.37

Table 2. Results in bypass graft occlusions (n=302) at 6 months and 1 year, from the TOPAS study

Intervention	Lysis (n=150)	Surgery (n=152])	p value
Clot dissolution-no/total no patients	100/134 (75%)	N/A	
Increase in ABPI	0.48	0.5	0.76
% Mortality			
6 months	12.1	9.4	0.45
1 year	16.2	15.0	0.77
% Amputation-free survival			
6 months	75.2	73.9	0.79
1 year	68.2	68.8	0.91

arterial and graft occlusions due to thrombosis or embolism were included. The limb-threatening ischaemia had to be 14 days or less in duration. A total of 272 patients were randomized to surgery, of whom 152 had graft occlusions; 272 were randomized to lysis, of whom150 had graft occlusions. The primary endpoint chosen was amputation-free survival at 6 months, with a range of secondary endpoints including ankle brachial pressure index, adverse treatment effects, amputation-free survival at 1 year, and in the lysis group, the degree of clot lysis and survival free of open surgical procedure at 6 months.

There were no significant differences in the mortality and amputation-free survival at both 6 months and 1 year between the treatment groups. This was also true of the native arterial occlusion group. Although the investigators did not report the sub-group analyses for number of operative interventions, overall during the first 6 months patients randomized to the surgery group underwent 551 open procedures, whilst the thrombolysis group underwent 315 open procedures.

The STILE and TOPAS studies represent the only large multicentre trials in which prospective and randomized methodology has been applied to answering the question of whether there is a convincing difference in outcomes between primary surgery versus initial thrombolysis in the management of lower limb ischaemia secondary to thrombotic or embolic occlusions. The STILE trial is particularly useful in that outcomes specifically for both vein and prosthetic grafts are subjected to subgroup analysis. Both trials randomized a total of 426 occluded bypass grafts. Can an unequivocal answer be drawn from the results?

The consensus document on thrombolysis in the management of lower limb peripheral arterial occlusion recommends that the primary endpoint that defines either success or failure of therapy should be amputation-free survival of the patient. This endpoint has been used by the TOPAS study, whilst the STILE study used a composite clinical outcome that included mortality and major amputation. Whether the primary endpoint of amputation-free survival adequately answers the question is debatable. Patient survival is as much a function of disease status at entry to the trial as the treatment given. In the TOPAS trial 14% of the patients had congestive cardiac failure, and 12% had cancer; 6- and 12-month survival was probably based upon the coincidental pathology the patients had, rather than their intervention The amputation rate as the other component to the primary endpoint is also problematic. The underlying assumption is that all of the occluded grafts would have inevitably have led to limb loss if either surgery or thrombolysis had not been performed. However it has been shown that anticoagulation alone can save two-thirds of acutely ischaemic limbs.[14] Nonetheless, using these primary endpoints, which modality was superior? (See Fig. 1).

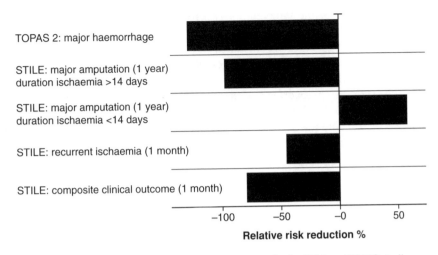

TOPAS 2: major haemorrhage

STILE: major amputation (1 year)
duration ischaemia >14 days

STILE: major amputation (1 year)
duration ischaemia <14 days

STILE: recurrent ischaemia (1 month)

STILE: composite clinical outcome (1 month)

Relative risk reduction %

−100   −50   −0   50

Figure 1. Relative risk reduction for thrombolytic treatment in the STILE and TOPAS studies. Adapted from the meta-analysis of Palfreyman *et al.* [15]

There were no significant differences in either mortality or amputation rates at 1 year in either study. The exception to this was the subgroup of patients with duration of ischaemia of less than 14 days in the STILE trial, who had a greater risk of amputation in the surgery group (relative risk 0.42). It must be remembered that the 14-day duration of ischaemia was not part of the original study design. Within this arbitary time-frame limbs with especially acute onset (i.e. days) of ischaemia were more likely to reflect embolic events, with a concomitant higher success rate in terms of thrombolysis.

The primary endpoints do not clearly discriminate between the two treatment options. Do secondary endpoints help? The consensus document recommends a range of different secondary endpoints including graft patency substantiated by objective imaging, restoration of useful limb function, relief of ischaemic symptoms, the reduction in magnitude of surgical procedures and complication rates.

An assessment of graft patency after discharge, together with an estimation of limb function, would certainly help in the comparison of the two treatments. The TOPAS study reported on initial patency rates after thrombolysis, with 75% success in clot dissolution, whilst the STILE study reported 47% initial patency. No follow-up estimation of patency rates was made, yet follow-up data from the NATALI database suggests 33% patency at 12 months and 27% patency at 18 months following successful lysis with or without additional treatments.[16] Initial patency rates are thus meaningless unless followed-up and compared with grafts treated by primary surgery.

Limb function was indirectly followed up in the TOPAS study by ABPI estimation, which increased by virtually the same in both groups. The STILE trial was more stringent in follow-up by assessing ongoing or recurrent ischaemia as part of the composite clinical outcome. This showed that at 30 days (p=0.017) and at 1 year (p=0.01) the lysis group had a significantly higher rate of ischaemia than the surgical group. The whole trial was stopped early because of the significantly increased risk of adverse events in the lysis group, and the major component of this was recurring ischaemia. The only conclusion that can be made from these data is that initial surgery is better than initial thrombolysis in preventing limb ischaemia both at early (30 days) and later (1 year) follow-up.

Complication due to the intervention is a further secondary endpoint that helps discriminate between surgery and thrombolysis.

In the TOPAS study there were four episodes of intracerebral bleeding, one of which led to death, in the lysis group compared with none in the surgical group (Table 3). In the STILE study three patients receiving lytic therapy had intracerebral bleeds. The TOPAS study reported on other complications occurring in the lysis group including distal embolization of partially thrombolysed material (n=36), pericatheter thrombosis (n=13), and the development of false aneurysms at the catheter site (n=7). Based on the tendency of serious bleeding problems alone, primary surgery is significantly safer than thrombolysis.

Table 3. Major haemorrhage in the TOPAS and STILE studies*

Study	Primary surgery (%)	Thrombolysis (%)	p-value
TOPAS	5.5	12.5	0.005
STILE	0.7	5.6	0.014

*These figures are for both native arteries and grafts

A further secondary endpoint is the concept of reduction in magnitude of surgery. All patients had a planned surgical procedure prior to randomization, and this was compared with the actual procedure carried out post- thrombolysis. The TOPAS study showed that at 6 months 31.5% of patients in the thrombolysis group had not needed open surgery, whilst the STILE trial reported a reduction in magnitude of surgical procedure in 39% of vein grafts and 44% of prosthetic grafts.

Further issues to be considered include costs and length of patient stay. These trials did not specifically report on the difference in cost between the two groups, but the Rochester study showed that thrombolysis was 25% more expensive than open surgery. In a urokinase comparative study of primary surgery and thrombolysis there was little overall difference, with attempted limb salvage costing £3429 for surgery and £3230 for thrombolysis.[17] However, if further surgical adjunctive procedures in the primary thrombolysis group are factored into the analysis, the costs rise to twice that of surgery.[18]

Deciding on whether initial thrombolysis should be the first-line treatment of choice in acute bypass graft occlusion is not an easy task based upon the evidence offered by the two major multicentre trials of thrombolysis versus surgery undertaken to date. A heterogenous group of patients were enrolled, including acute and chronically ischaemic limbs, occluded native arterial, autogenous and prosthetic grafts in supra and infrainguinal positions. Only the STILE trial analysed graft data separately. The investigators' conclusions drawn from their own data are intriguing.

The interpretation of the TOPAS trial was that an initial policy of thrombolysis reduced the need for surgery without an increase in mortality or amputation rate. An alternative conclusion might be that in the chosen primary endpoint of amputation-free survival there were no significant differences between the groups, but the patients randomized to thrombolysis had a significant increase in major haemorrhage including intracranial bleeds and a fatality.

The STILE trial is more relevant in so far as graft occlusions were dealt with as a separate group, and the data is more transparent in the context of answering this debate. The authors concluded that proper catheter positioning limits the 'potential' of thrombolysis. The overall trial was halted early due to the significant increase in adverse events in the group assigned to thrombolysis. The primary range of endpoints chosen, the composite clinical outcome, was significantly better at both 1 month and 1 year in the surgical group, and this was largely due to the reduction in ischaemia. Although a post-study analysis suggested a significantly higher amputation rate in the surgery group at 1 year for patients presenting with acute ischaemia, this was not part of the original study design, and may have been subject to confounds such as acute embolic events masquerading as *in situ* thromboses.

The only meaningful conclusion that can be drawn is that not only is thrombolysis irrelevant in the initial management of graft thrombosis, but it is significantly associated with prolonged and recurrently ischaemic 'treated' limbs and an increased risk of major haemorrhage.

Summary

- There is no difference in published survival rates at 1 year between initial surgery and thrombolysis for graft occlusion.

- There is no difference in published amputation rates at 1 year between initial surgery and thrombolysis for graft occlusion.

- Thrombolysis is associated with a significantly greater rate of both early and late limb ischaemia compared with initial surgery.

- Thrombolysis is associated with a significantly greater rate of major haemorrhage compared with initial surgery.

References

1. Amery A, Deloof W, Vermylen J, Verstraete M. Outcome of recent thromboembolic occlusions of limb arteries treated with streptokinase. *Br Med J* 1970; 4: 639–644.
2. Anonymous. Thrombolysis in the management of lower limb peripheral arterial occlusion–a consensus document. Working Party on Thrombolysis in the Management of Limb Ischemia. *Am J Cardiol* 1998; 81: 207–218.
3. Hess H, Ingrisch H, Mietaschk A, Rath H. Local low-dose thrombolytic therapy of peripheral arterial occlusions. *N Engl J Med* 1982; 307: 1627–1630.
4. Valji K, Roberts AC, Davis GB, Bookstein JJ. Pulsed-spray thrombolysis of arterial and bypass graft occlusions. *AJR* 1991; 156:617
5. Heymans S, Vanderschueren S, Verhaeghe R *et al.* Outcome and one year follow-up of intra-arterial staphylokinase in 191 patients with peripheral arterial occlusion. *Thromb Haem* 2000; 83: 666–671.
6. Duda SH, Tepe G, Luz O *et al.* Peripheral artery occlusion: treatment with abciximab plus urokinase versus with urokinase alone–a randomized pilot trial (the PROMPT Study). Platelet Receptor Antibodies in Order to Manage Peripheral Artery Thrombosis. *Radiology* 2001; 221: 689–696.
7. Belkin M, Donaldson MC, Whittemore AD *et al.* Observations on the use of thrombolytic agents for thrombotic occlusion of infrainguinal vein grafts. *J Vasc Surg* 1990; 11: 289–294.
8. Sullivan KL, Gardiner GAJ, Kandarpa K *et al.* Efficacy of thrombolysis in infrainguinal bypass grafts. *Circulation* 1991; 83: 199–105.
9. Nilsson L, Albrechtsson U, Jonung T *et al.* Surgical treatment versus thrombolysis in acute arterial occlusion: a randomised controlled study. *Eur J Vasc Surg* 1992; 6: 189–193.
10. Ouriel K, Shortell CK, DeWeese JA *et al.* A comparison of thrombolytic therapy with operative revascularization in the initial treatment of acute peripheral arterial ischemia. *J Vasc Surg* 1994; 19: 1021–1030.
11. Anonymous. Results of a prospective randomized trial evaluating surgery versus thrombolysis for ischemia of the lower extremity. The STILE trial. *Annl Surg* 1994; 220: 251–266.

12. Comerota AJ, Weaver FA, Hosking JD *et al.* Results of a prospective, randomized trial of surgery versus thrombolysis for occluded lower extremity bypass grafts. *Am J Surg* 1996; **172**: 105–112.

13. Ouriel K, Veith FJ, Sasahara AA. A comparison of recombinant urokinase with vascular surgery as initial treatment for acute arterial occlusion of the legs. Thrombolysis or Peripheral Arterial Surgery (TOPAS) Investigators. *N Engl J Med* 1998; **338**: 1105–1111.

14. Blaisdell FW, Steele M, Allen RE. Management of acute lower extremity arterial ischemia due to embolism and thrombosis. *Surgery* 1978; **84**: 822–834.

15. Palfreyman SJ, Booth A, Michaels JA. A systematic review of intra-arterial thrombolytic therapy for lower-limb ischaemia. *Eur J Vasc Endovasc Surg* 2000; **19**: 143–157.

16. Galland RB, Magee TR, Whitman B *et al.* Patency following successful thrombolysis of occluded vascular grafts. *Eur J Vasc Endovasc Surg* 2001; **22**: 157–160.

17. Braithwaite BD, Jones L, Heather BP *et al.* Management cost of acute limb ischaemia. *Br J Surg* 1996; **83**: 1390–1393.

18. Hoch JR, Tullis MJ, Archer CW. Thrombolysis versus surgery as the initial management for native artery occlusion; efficacy, safety, and cost. *Surgery* 1994; **116**: 649–657.

Thrombolysis is irrelevant in the treatment of acute arterial graft occlusion

Against the motion
Kenneth Ouriel

Introduction

Patients who experience acute thrombosis of a peripheral arterial bypass graft present with symptoms that equal or surpass those that were present at the time the graft was placed. Symptoms are usually no more severe than they were prior to the initial revascularization procedure if the occlusion is not accompanied by propagation of thrombus into the native arterial system. In other words, symptoms merely return to the baseline symptoms that were present prior to the initial revascularization when the thrombotic process remains confined to the graft itself. In some cases, however, the symptoms develop from graft occlusion are substantially worse than the baseline symptoms. In these cases, the thrombus propagates into the outflow or inflow vessels; an event that is more common when the graft is prosthetic.[1]

Acute occlusion of a bypass graft is associated with significant risks to the patient's life.[2] Whether from *in situ* thrombosis of a native artery or bypass graft or from embolization, acute limb ischaemia is associated with significant risks of amputation and death (Table 1). The classic study by Blaisdell documented amputation and mortality rates in excess of 25% each following open surgical repair for acute leg ischemia.[3] Despite improvements in operative technique and postoperative patient care, more recent series continue to verify unacceptably high rates of morbidity. Jivegård and colleagues observed a 20% mortality rate in patients treated operatively.[4] Even the more recent prospective studies of selected patients with recent peripheral arterial occlusions observed rates of limb loss and death that exceed desired targets.[5-8]

Table 1. Early (in-hospital or 30-day) rates of amputation and death in selected series of patients with recent peripheral arterial occlusion, treated with primary open surgical intervention

Study	Year	Amputation rate	Mortality rate
Blaisdell	1978	25%	30%
Jivegård	1988	–	20%
Rochester	1994	14%	18%
STILE	1994	5%	6%
TOPAS	1998	2%	5%

Thus, the risk of morbidity and mortality following open surgical intervention remains at an unacceptably high level. What factors explain this finding? Clearly, the baseline medical status of the patients that present with acute peripheral arterial occlusion underlie the observation. Patients are frequently elderly, with a high rate of cardiac and other co-morbidities. They are ill equipped to tolerate the insult of ischaemia of an extremity, let alone an invasive surgical intervention to relieve the obstruction. A multivariable analysis of the data from the Rochester series uncovered several variables that were predictive of poor outcome, irrespective of the type of treatment instituted.[9] A summary of available literature would appear to confirm that individuals who present with acute, limb-threatening ischaemia comprise one of the sickest subgroup of patients that the peripheral vascular practitioner is asked to treat.[10]

Evidence

There is evidence to confirm the impression that a less invasive intervention is better tolerated in this very ill group of patients who develop acute limb ischaemia. Poor technique, inadequate devices and inferior agents coloured the initial experiences with catheter-directed thrombolytic therapy. For instance, the now well-accepted principle of ensuring infusion of the thrombolytic agent directly into the substance of the occluding thrombus was not always ardently adhered to. End-hole catheters were employed; it was not until the late 1980s that multisided-hole catheters were available. Lastly, streptokinase was the most frequently used agent until the landmark article of McNamara in 1985 documented improved results with locally administered high-dose urokinase.[11]

There have been three well-controlled, randomized comparisons of thrombolytic therapy versus primary operation in patients with recent peripheral arterial occlusion. From the start, one should realize that thrombolytic therapy must be followed by definitive therapy to address the underlying lesion that caused the occlusion. In some cases this may entail a percutaneous intervention such as balloon dilatation or intraluminal stenting. In others, a patch angioplasty or jump-graft may be necessary to create a bypass an unmasked stenotic lesion. When no culprit lesion can be found, the risk of early rethrombosis is unacceptably high.[12] Sullivan observed post-thrombolytic 2-year patency rates of 79% in bypass grafts with flow-limiting lesions identified and corrected by angioplasty or surgery versus only 9.8% in those without such lesions.

The first study, the Rochester series, compared urokinase with primary operation in 114 patients presenting with what has subsequently been called 'hyperacute ischaemia.' Enrolled patients in this trial all had severely threatened limbs (Rutherford Class IIb) with mean symptom duration of approximately 2 days. After 12 months of follow-up, 84% of patients randomized to urokinase were alive compared with only 58% of patients randomized to primary operation (Fig. 1). By contrast, the rate of limb salvage was identical at 80%.

A closer inspection of the raw data revealed that the defining variable for mortality differences was the development of cardiopulmonary complications during the periprocedural period. The rate of long-term mortality was high when such periprocedural complications occurred but was relatively low when they did not occur. It was only the fact that such complications occurred more commonly in patients taken directly to the operating theatre that explained the greater long-term mortality rate in the operative group.

The second prospective, randomized analysis of thrombolysis versus surgery was the Surgery or Thrombolysis for the Ischaemic Lower Extremity (STILE) trial.[7]

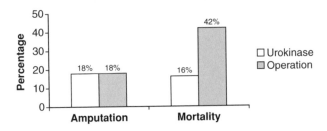

**Rochester Trial
12 Month Follow-up Data**

Figure 1. The rate of amputation was identical in the two treatment groups in the Rochester Trial, but the mortality rate was significantly lower in patients assigned to the thrombolytic arm.

Genentech (South San Francisco CA), the manufacturer of the Activase brand of rt-PA, funded the study. At its termination, 393 patients were randomized to one of three treatment groups, rt-PA, urokinase or primary operation. Subsequently, the two thrombolytic groups were combined for purposes of data analysis when the outcome was found to be similar. The primary publication of the STILE trial appeared in 1994 and encompassed the complete group of 393 patients with native artery or bypass graft occlusions. Overall, there were similar rates of mortality (4% thrombolytic, 5% surgery) and amputation (5% thrombolysis, 6% surgery) in the two groups. In 1996, Comerota published the results of the subset of 124 patients treated for bypass graft occlusions.[13] Despite the inability to place the catheter into the occluded graft in 39% of patients, the 1-year amputation rate was lower in patients with acute (<14 days) graft occlusions treated with thrombolysis (p = 0.026), suggesting that thrombolysis may be of greatest benefit in patients with acute bypass graft occlusion.

The third and final randomized comparison of thrombolysis and surgery was the Thrombolysis Or Peripheral Arterial Surgery (TOPAS) trial, funded by Abbott Laboratories (Abbott Park, IL). The primary objective of the study was to compare recombinant urokinase to operation as treatment for acute lower limb ischaemia. The trial was initiated with a dose-ranging trial in 213 subjects.[14] After an intermediate dose of 4000 IU/min was identified, 544 additional subjects were randomized to a recombinant form of urokinase or primary operative intervention. After a mean follow-up period of 1 year, the rate of amputation-free survival was identical in the two treatment groups, 68.2% and 68.8% in the urokinase and surgical patients, respectively (Table 2).

Table 2. Results of the TOPAS trial, demonstrating similar mortality rates and amputation-free survival rates in patients with acute bypass graft occlusion treated with recombinant urokinase or surgery

	Urokinase (N=150)	Surgery (N=152)	p Value
Increase in ABI	0.48±0.03	0.50±0.03	0.76
Mortality			
6 months	12.1%	9.4%	0.45
12 months	16.2%	15.0%	0.77
Amputation-free survival			
6 months	75.2%	73.9%	0.79
12 months	68.2%	68.8%	0.91

While this trial failed to document improvement in survival or limb salvage with thrombolysis, fully 31.5% of the thrombolytic patients were alive without amputation with nothing more than a percutaneous procedure after 6 months of follow-up. After 1 year, this number had decreased only slightly, with 25.7% alive, without amputation and with only percutaneous interventions.

Summary

- The rate of amputation and death is higher than expected when patients with acute limb ischaemia are treated by primary open surgical means in spite of technical improvements in the conduct of operative procedures and advances in perioperative patient care.

- The findings of prospective, randomized comparisons of thrombolytic therapy versus primary surgery are somewhat conflicting. Some observations appear valid, however:

  - Mortality may be lower in medically compromised patients with very severe ischaemia when treated with thrombolysis (Rochester Trial)

  - Patients with bypass graft thromboses fare better with thrombolysis than patients with native arterial occlusions (STILE Trial)

  - Thrombolysis offers the potential to achieve similar rates of mortality and limb salvage, avoiding the need for open surgical procedures in a significant proportion of patients (TOPAS Trial)

References

1. Jackson MR, Belott TP, Dickason T et al. The consequences of a failed femoropopliteal bypass grafting: comparison of saphenous vein and PTFE grafts. J Vasc Surg 2000; 32: 498–504.
2. Edwards JE, Taylor LM, Jr, Porter JM. Treatment of failed lower extremity bypass grafts with new autogenous vein bypass grafting. J Vasc Surg 1990; 11: 136–145.
3. Blaisdell F W, Steele M, Allen RE. Management of acute lower extremity arterial ischemia due to embolism and thrombosis. Surgery 1978; 84: 822–834.
4. Jivegård L, Holm J, Scherstén T. Acute limb ischemia due to arterial embolism or thrombosis: Influence of limb ischemia versus pre-existing cardiac disease on postoperative mortality rate. J Cardiovasc Surg 1988; 29: 32–36.
5. Ouriel K, Shortell CK, DeWeese JA et al. A comparison of thrombolytic therapy with operative revascularization in the initial treatment of acute peripheral arterial ischemia. J Vasc Surg 1994; 19: 1021–1030.
6. Ouriel K, Veith FJ, Sasahara AA. A comparison of recombinant urokinase with vascular surgery as initial treatment for acute arterial occlusion of the legs. N Engl J Med 1998; 338: 1105–1111.
7. Anonymous. Results of a prospective randomized trial evaluating surgery versus thrombolysis for ischemia of the lower extremity. The STILE trial. Ann Surg 1994; 1220: 251–266.
8. Ouriel K, Kandarpa K, Schuerr DM et al. Prourokinase versus urokinase for recanalization of peripheral occlusions, safety and efficacy: the PURPOSE trial. J Vasc Interv Radiol 1999; 10: 1083–1091.
9. Ouriel, K. and Veith, F. J. Acute lower limb ischemia: determinants of outcome. Surgery 1998; 124: 336–341.
10. Dormandy J, Heeck L, Vig S. Acute limb ischemia. Semin Vasc Surg 1999; 12: 148–153.
11. McNamara TO, Fischer JR. Thrombolysis of peripheral arterial and graft occlusions: improved results using high-dose urokinase. AJR 1985; 144: 769–775.

12. Sullivan KL, Gardiner GAJ, Kandarpa K *et al.* Efficacy of thrombolysis in infrainguinal bypass grafts. *Circulation* 1991; **83**(Supp 2): 99–105.
13. Comerota AJ, Weaver FA, Hosking JD *et al.* Results of a prospective, randomized trial of surgery versus thrombolysis for occluded lower extremity bypass grafts. *Am J Surg* 1996; **172**: 105–112.
14. Ouriel K, Veith FJ, Sasahara AA. Thrombolysis or peripheral arterial surgery: phase I results. TOPAS Investigators. *J Vasc Surg* 1996; **23**: 64–73.

Thrombolysis is irrelevant in the treatment of acute arterial graft occlusion

Charing Cross Editorial Comments towards Consensus

It never ceases to amaze the reader that data can be used to make an argument in two totally different directions and here we see this approach in its full glory!

Take the Stile Study; the proposers show the broken down data and stress the superiority of surgery over lytic therapy in terms of composite clinical outcome (adverse outcome), and also the significant superiority of surgery in terms of ongoing and recurrent ischaemia. This latter factor is given as 50% for surgery and 73% for lytic therapy, a significant difference with a p value of 0.01. Then the opposition states about the same study 'overall there were similar rates of mortality (4% thrombolytic, 5% surgery) and amputation (5% thrombolysis, 6% surgery) in the two groups'. What are we to believe?

Dr Ouriel comments 'from the start, one must realise that thrombolytic therapy must be followed by definitive therapy to address the underlying lesion that causes the occlusion. Clearly he is not saying that surgery and angioplasty play no role, but poses the motion that thrombolysis is irrelevant in the treatment of acute arterial graft occlusion.

He also draws attention to the different thrombolytic agents used over the years and it is clear that the price of thrombolytic agents such as urokinase vary considerably in different parts of the world, being apparently much cheaper in the United States than in parts of Europe. These issues are relevant.

Dr Ouriel placed great store in making certain that the catheter is placed right inside the clot. He implies very careful supervision of lytic therapy and clearly finds limited lytic therapy helpful as an adjunct.

It is possible that it matters in which centre lytic therapy is performed and under whose control. If it is performed by an unenthusiastic radiological group for example, then complications can easily occur. By the same token if a patient with thrombolysis is sent to a surgical ward and receives poor supervision during this lytic phase, this also invites complications. The implication is that thrombolysis, if used, should be targeted, low dose and injected right into the clot. This is to be followed by surgery or angioplasty for correction. Certainly this is not available at every vascular centre and clinical trials meta-analyses can only report what is in the literature at the present time and the proposers have done just that.

Roger M Greenhalgh
Editor

Saphenofemoral ligation and stripping is the method of choice for treating long saphenous varicose veins

For the motion
Bruce Campbell

Introduction

This debate is about the arguments for conventional surgery compared with a variety of new endovenous treatments for treating long saphenous vein (LSV) incompetence. The main new techniques are radiofrequency ablation (VNUS®*), laser ablation (for example EndoVenous Laser Treatment – EVLT®*), and the use of sclerosant foam (such as Varisolve®*).

Surgical removal of the LSV by flush saphenofemoral ligation and stripping (referred to in this chapter simply as 'stripping') is supported by many years of use and a considerable evidence base. When done thoroughly (usually with phlebectomies) it provides durable benefit for most patients,[1,2] better results than saphenofemoral ligation alone,[2,3] and better results than sclerotherapy.[4] Large numbers of patients are treated by stripping and their quality of life is demonstrably enhanced by the operation.[5]

All the new endovenous alternatives to stripping aim to avoid an incision in the groin and haematoma in the thigh, to reduce pain, and to speed recovery. Other possible advantages are less risk of nerve damage and other complications, and avoidance of neovascularization in the groin which might lessen recurrence. This chapter examines the evidence for each of these, and also considers which patients might benefit, at what cost, and with what implications for health services. It will show that surgical stripping remains the treatment of choice for the majority of patients.

The limited evidence base for endovenous treatments

The majority of studies are on radiofrequency ablation, and most are simply case series[6] or registries.[7] Published figures from the main multicentre registry[7] have been

---

* Registered trade marks:
VNUS: Medical Technologies Inc, Sunnyvale, California, USA.
EVLT: Diomed Limited, Cambridge, CB4 9TE, England.
Varisolve: Provensis Limited, South Harefield, UB9 6NS, England.

criticized for missing data.[8] There is just one recent randomized trial involving 28 patients.[9] The literature on laser treatment is more limited, and there are no properly controlled trials:[10] it is likely that longer term effects are a matter of conjecture based partly on extrapolation from the radiofrequency ablation studies. The evidence for sclerosant foam is also based on case series.[11,12] A particular problem is the fact that the endovenous treatments have been introduced by enthusiasts, largely in settings of private practice with substantial financial interests at stake, and in the context of publicity material which leads patients to expect less discomfort and quicker return to activity. Blinding is impossible in any comparative study.

Which patients might benefit from endoluminal treatment?

LSV surgery stripping can be done in any patient, regardless of their build, venous anatomy or the severity of their venous disease. By contrast, many patients are excluded from radiofrequency ablation – 85 of 121 screened for a randomized trial by Rautio et al.[9] (some simply because they had bilateral disease). Wide (>12mm) or tortuous LSVs are a relative contraindication, and the advantages are reduced in patients who need many phlebectomies for extensive varicose veins, which may be followed by extensive bruising and tenderness. These are important considerations, because big saphenous veins and extensive varicosities are common among patients with the strongest indications for treatment, such as severe symptoms or skin changes.

Slim patients with just a few varicosities and modest calibre LSVs who request treatment for cosmetic reasons are ideal candidates for endovenous ablation techniques. However, they also do well after surgical stripping, with a small groin wound, little haematoma or discomfort, and a rapid return to full activity.

In summary, endovenous treatment may not be applicable to those patients at most at risk of complications or those with greatest clinical need.

What is the evidence for reduction in pain and more rapid recovery?

A recent randomized study[9] has shown 'significantly less pain' after radiofrequency ablation (15 patients) than after surgical stripping (13 patients). Examining the results, however, the average pain scores were only 0.7 versus 1.7 at rest, and 1.8 versus 3.0 on walking - on an analogue scale up to 10 – all minor degrees of discomfort. The 'significantly less analgesia' was based on an average daily dose of 1.3 ibuprofen tablets in the surgical group – by any standards a minimal analgesic requirement. Return to work was quicker in the endovenous treatment group, but this might well have been biased by the expectations of patients and the attitude of their medical advisors. A number of patients had refused randomization because they wanted endovenous treatment, and this must call into question the expectations which patients were given about each treatment. It is interesting to note that the patients given laser treatment by Min et al.[10] had all been offered a choice of surgery, radiofrequency ablation or laser. What had these patients read before they attended for treatment and how were they advised?

The publicity surrounding the new endovenous treatments has had an important effect on the expectations of patients. Enthusiasts have fostered press reports and internet websites which have both extolled the possible advantages of endovenous treatments, and which have portrayed conventional surgery as invariably very painful and disabling. These have led patients to demand the new treatments when their benefits are uncertain and their long-term effects are unproven.

Complications of treatment

The publicity about endovenous treatment makes much of the advantages of avoiding a groin wound and the problems associated with stripping. However, in a consecutive series of 599 surgical patients from a UK district hospital Critchley *et al.*[13] observed wound complications in just 2.2% and minor neurological disturbance in 6.6%. Nerve damage and paraesthesia occurs after radiofrequency ablation with a similar incidence – multicentre registry data describe 15% at 1 week and 5% at 2 years for radiofrequency[7] – and occasional paraesthesiae after laser treatment.[6]

The technique used in stripping is important to consider when making comparisons with surgery. For example, the one randomized comparison between radiofrequency ablation and stripping involved use of a 9mm olive on the stripper.[9] This causes more trauma and bruising than the inversion method of stripping which is in common use among modern venous specialists. It is important to note that bruising and lumpy haematoma in the thigh is particularly common when the LSV is very large, and large LSVs may be unsuitable for endovenous ablation. The higher risks of saphenous nerve damage associated with stripping the LSV to the ankle[14] are no longer relevant in the modern era of stripping to knee level only; and it is also important to recognize that many cases of nerve damage are due to phlebectomies, which are commonly required as an adjunct to endovenous LSV ablation, just as for surgical stripping.

In the series by Critchley *et al.*[13] major complications were rare (0.5%) and only one was associated with stripping the LSV: this involved damage to femoral vein, which is also a potential complication of all the endovenous techniques. Skin damage due to thermal injury can occur after radiofrequency ablation,[7] and laser treatment can cause bruising.[10]

In summary, there is little good evidence for a substantially lower incidence of complications with the new endovenous treatments.

Durability of treatment

The risk of recurrence after varicose vein surgery is well recognized[1] and some of the possible reasons for this apply equally to surgery and endovenous treatments – incorrect assessment, and failure to recognize or deal with all incompetent major veins. Most surgeons believe that flush LSV ligation, with division of all tributaries in the groin beyond their first confluences, is important. The fact that endovenous treatments neither remove the LSV nor deal individually with tributaries therefore raises concerns about the thoroughness and durability of treatment. By contrast, proponents of endovenous methods suggest that avoiding dissection in the groin may prevent the neovascularization which can lead to recurrence.[2]

Current data suggest that radiofrequency ablation can achieve obliteration of the LSV as well as surgery up to 2 years.[7] Results of laser treatment are claimed to be similar although fewer data are available.[10] On balance, therefore, it seems that endovenous obliteration may be as effective as surgery at ablating the LSV in the longer term, but the best data extend only to a couple of years. Neovascularization probably occurs largely during the first year or two,[2] and so it seems most unlikely that longer term data could show any substantial advantage over surgical stripping.

Recurrent varicose veins

Recurrent varicose veins are perceived by many surgeons as a potentially attractive indication for endovascular treatment. When a residual LSV trunk is present in the thigh and there is recurrent reflux in the groin, then endovenous obliteration of the LSV might avoid reoperative surgery in the groin. It is, however, worth considering a common finding during groin re-exploration – an incompetent vein joining the femoral vein, but dense scar tissue just distal to this, with no clear single lumen for downward or upward passage of a stripper. Will endovenous methods often fail to obliterate incompetent tributaries right up to their junction with the femoral vein? What would be the long-term result of leaving neovascular recurrence close to the femoral vein, while simply obliterating the LSV trunk distally?

As with primary varicose veins, claims for the advantage of endovenous methods in treating recurrence will need to be substantiated by well controlled studies with good long-term follow-up.

Cost implications and general applicability

The equipment costs of endovenous treatment are substantially higher than those of surgery; extra personnel are required to operate the duplex scanner (although some surgeons do this themselves) and operating time is increased.[9] These additional costs have been documented very clearly by Rautio *et al.*[9] who also calculated 'societal costs' on the assumption that patients are in gainful employment, concluding that the overall costs of endovenous treatment are less than those of surgery, provided a sufficient number of patients is treated. However, the 'direct medical costs' of endovenous treatment in their study were more than double those of surgery, and this is likely to be the focus of hospitals and health services.

With regard to operating time Rautio *et al.*[9] reported an average of 92 minutes and 115 minutes respectively for stripping and radiofrequency treatment, either of which would be completely impractical in giving timely treatment to the numbers of patients presenting to the health service in the UK. Weiss *et al.*[6] have reported less prolonged operating times for radiofrequency ablation, but fewer than two-thirds of their patients required concomitant phlebectomies.

Availability of personnel skilled in duplex scanning is also an important logistic issue which argues against the use of endovenous methods in a busy health service setting. Skilled vascular technologists are in short supply in the UK, and time spent in the operating theatre removes them from diagnostic scanning.

In summary, radiofrequency and laser ablation cost more than surgery, take longer, and involve more personnel.

What about sclerosant foam?

This method sounds attractive, but published data[11,12] are limited to case series from a few experts: no comparative or randomized trials are available. Large LSVs can be treated, and foam sclerotherapy can also ablate quite extensive varicose veins. Three years after treatment about 20% LSVs are no longer obliterated[11] but proponents point out that even if veins do recur, further treatment is relatively straightforward. Cabrera et al.[12] described no important adverse effects in their series of 500 treated limbs, but in a smaller series Frullini et al.[12] reported occasional phlebitis, visual disturbance, deep vein thrombosis (one due to 'technical mistake') and skin necrosis. The risks of sclerosant entering deep veins in harmful amounts is a particular concern if this technique starts to disseminate into more widespread use for treating the LSV (rather than for minor varicosities). Lack of the need for general anaesthesia gives sclerosant foam treatment particular appeal for 'office' treatment in private practice, whence complications may well go unreported.

More data are needed from properly controlled studies before there can be serious debate about the place of foam sclerotherapy in clinical practice.

Summary

- The evidence for endovenous methods is based almost entirely on case series, and mostly relates to radiofrequency ablation.

- Patients whose clinical need for treatment is greatest may be least well suited to endovenous methods (those with large LSVs or extensive varicosities).

- Publicity has wrongly led patients to believe that LSV stripping is always very painful and that recovery is much quicker after endovenous treatment.

- The incidence of important complications after endovenous techniques differs little from stripping: unreported complication rates may increase as endovenous treatments disseminate in an uncontrolled way.

- The data on long-term effectiveness of endovenous treatments suggest they that will not be superior to surgery.

- Radiofrequency and laser ablation take longer than surgery, involve extra personnel, and cost substantially more.

References

1. Perrin MR, Guex JJ, Ruckley CV et al. and the REVAS group. Recurrent varices after surgery (REVAS), a consensus document. Cardiovasc Surg 2000; **8**: 233–245.
2. Dwerryhouse S, Davies B, Harradine K, Earnshaw JJ. Stripping the long saphenous vein reduces the rate of reoperation for varicose veins: five year results of a randomised trial. J Vasc Surg 1999; **29**: 589–592.
3. Sarin S, Scurr JH, Coleridge Smith PD. Stripping of the long saphenous vein in the treatment of primary varicose veins. Br J Surg 1996; **81**: 1455–1458.
4. Einarrson E, Eklof B. Sclerotherapy or surgery as treatment for varicose veins: a prospective randomised study. Phlebology 1993; **8**: 22–26.
5. MacKenzie RK, Paisley A, Allan PL et al. The effect of long saphenous vein stripping on quality of life. J Vasc Surg 2002; **35**: 1197–1203.
6. Weiss RA, Weiss MA. Controlled radiofrequency endovenous occlusion using a unique radiofrequency catheter under duplex guidance to eliminate saphenous vein reflux: a 2-year followup study. Dermatol Surg 2002; **28**: 38–42.

7. Merchant RF, DePalma RG, Kabnick LS. Endovascular obliteration of saphenous reflux: a multi-center study. *J Vasc Surg* 2002; 5: 1190–1196.

8. Harris EJ. Radiofrequency ablation of the long saphenous vein without high ligation versus high ligation and stripping for primary varicose veins. *Semin Vasc Surg* 2002; 15: 34–38.

9. Rautio T, Ohinmaa A, Perala J *et al*. Endovenous obliteration versus conventional stripping operation in the treatment of primary varicose veins: a randomised controlled trial with comparison of the costs. *J Vasc Surgery* 2002; 53: 958–965.

10. Min RJ, Zimmet SE, Isaacs MN, Forresta MD. Endovenous laser treatment of the incompetent greater saphenous vein. *J Vasc Intervent Radiol* 2001; 12: 1167–1171.

11. Cabrera J, Cabrera JJr, Garcia-Olmedo MA. Treatment of varicose long saphenous veins with sclerosant in microfoam form. *Phlebology* 2000; 15: 19–23.

12. Frullini A, Cavezzi A. Sclerosing foam in the treatment of varicose veins and telangiectases: history and analysis of safety and complications. *Dermatol Surg* 2002; 28: 11–15.

13. Critchley G, Handa A, Maw A *et al*. Complications of varicose vein surgery. Annl Roy Coll Surg Engl 1997; 79: 105–110.

14. Munn SR, Morton JB, Macbeth WAAG, McLeish AR. To strip or not to strip the long saphenous vein? A varicose veins trial. Br J Surg 1981; 68: 426–428.

Saphenofemoral ligation and stripping is the method of choice for treating long saphenous varicose veins

Against the motion
Charles N McCollum, Francis Dix

Introduction

Varicose veins are a frequent problem for patients, General Practitioners (GPs) and surgeons alike. They are also a challenge which is not currently being met by our National Health Service (NHS). Around 15–20% of the adult population have varicose veins with an annual incidence in adults of 2.5%.[1] This equates to 4–5 million patients with varicose veins in the UK of which approximately 600 000 approach their GPs each year for advice on treatment. Department of Health statistics show, however, that between 1998 and 2001 only 48 000 operations for varicose veins were performed by the NHS each year with perhaps another 15 000 done privately.[2,3]

Patients rightly expect an improvement in symptoms, limb function and appearance from varicose vein surgery but the quality of this surgery has been poor for many years with unacceptable recurrence rates varying from 7 to 65% with many patients requiring re-operation.[4,5] Recent studies have shown conclusively that for long saphenous varices, complete division of the saphenofemoral junction and all its tributaries combined with removal of the long saphenous vein by stripping or eversion has lower recurrence rates than simple division of the saphenofemoral junction alone without stripping.[6,7] This operation has become the gold standard against which all other treatments are judged.

From the available figures, each year ten times more patients approach their GPs with varicose veins than those who actually receive treatment. Of course, not all require treatment but the NHS has found it impossible to provide a fast, cost-effective, reliable and up-to-date service for those who do need treatment.[4,8] A major investment in surgery for varicose veins would be unattractive to the government as the health consequences for many patients with minor and moderate varicose veins are minimal. Not surprisingly, surgeons and health authorities have been attracted to alternative approaches to treatment such as injection sclerotherapy and ambulatory phlebectomy as these techniques can be done inexpensively under local anaesthesia with less bruising, less discomfort and a quicker return to normal activity. However, recurrence rates following these techniques are currently unacceptable. Novel approaches to long and short saphenous ablation are essential in order to gain economic savings for the NHS particularly in terms of bed occupancy and a long-term reduction in recurrence. Perhaps more importantly, our patients want an alternative to surgery: a single newspaper report on a less invasive treatment performed by our department as part of a clinical trial, generated thousands of enquiries blocking our telephone lines for more than a month.

Principles of varicose vein treatment

Long-term success in the treatment of primary varicose veins depends on: (i) **ligation or occlusion of the highest point of reflux**, (ii) **removal or ablation of the incompetent truncal vein** and (iii) **removal or ablation of the varicose veins**. These factors have been adequately, if invasively, addressed by surgical ligation of the saphenofemoral junction or saphenopopliteal junction combined with removal of the incompetent long saphenous vein by stripping or rod eversion. Comparative studies comparing stripping or not stripping the long saphenous vein have shown that the frequency of recurrent reflux is approximately halved by removing the long saphenous vein to the knee.[6,7] Clinical outcome is also improved, with lower varicose vein recurrence rates when the long saphenous vein is removed.

Figures from our varicose vein service suggest that venous incompetence may be through the long saphenous vein (62%), the short saphenous vein (16%), through perforators (2%) or a combination of these (20%). Accurate diagnosis of all sites of incompetence is essential to successful treatment. Hand-held Doppler is the most appropriate initial investigation for all patients with varicose veins in the Outpatient Department and colour duplex imaging is essential for complex cases, popliteal recurrence or where there is any doubt on clinical or Doppler examination.

Causes of recurrence

Inadequate diagnosis is perhaps the most frequent cause for recurrence as it leads to inappropriate surgery. In patients with calf varicose veins, saphenofemoral ligation ignoring saphenopopliteal incompetence will inevitably lead to rapid recurrence. **Inadequate surgery** is also regrettably common; all tributaries in the groin must be divided and the saphenofemoral junction ligated flush with the femoral vein. Misidentification of the anterior vein of the thigh as the long saphenous vein will leave incompetence of the vein and lead to rapid recurrence.

Failure to strip an incompetent long saphenous vein may also lead to recurrence, either through proximal or mid-thigh perforating veins or by incompetence through neovascularization in the groin wound.

Neovascularization, the growth of thin-walled incompetent veins in healing tissue is a potential cause of recurrence when the long saphenous vein is not stripped.[9] Originally proposed by Glass, and generally regarded as an extension of angiogenesis during wound healing, it has been suggested that covering the ligated saphenofemoral junction with a mersilene mesh or a polytetrafluoroethylene (PTFE) patch may prevent neovascularization.[10] However, there is little convincing evidence that these approaches are better than careful saphenofemoral junction division with removal of the incompetent long saphenous vein.

In an attempt to avoid invasive surgery, lesser procedures such as ambulatory phlebectomy have gained popularity particularly among non-surgeons. Phlebectomy alone without saphenofemoral junction or saphenopopliteal disconnection and long saphenous vein stripping for proximal venous incompetence inevitably leads to an early recurrence via incompetent truncal veins. The newer minimally invasive alternatives to surgery, such as microfoam sclerotherapy for the long and short saphenous veins are promising but need to be fully evaluated in randomized clinical trials. The potential is for equivalent results in terms of recurrence, from an outpatient procedure with substantial reductions in pain, recovery time, cost and NHS resources needed to meet the demand.

Can vascular surgeons meet the demand?

The Vascular Surgical Society of Great Britain and Ireland (VSS) currently lists 438 Consultants with an interest in vascular surgery. There is a general move towards specialization and most patients with varicose veins are now appropriately being referred to specialists, particularly for recurrent disease. Certainly teaching trainees competent varicose vein diagnosis and surgery should be the responsibility of vascular surgeons.

Even if only 48 000 NHS operations were performed each year by these 438 Consultant Surgeons, then each would need to perform a minimum of 110 varicose vein operations per year. The number of operations currently performed by the NHS each year is clearly a small fraction of those requested by 600 000 patients who see their GPs for varicose vein treatment – a demand that could not be met by Vascular Surgeons. Less invasive procedures performed as outpatient services in specialist units are clearly preferable to diagnosis and surgery performed by the trainee of a surgeon with no interest in varicose veins. There needs to be a clear strategic NHS plan regarding varicose vein referral and treatment if we are to provide the high standard of care that patients expect with low recurrence rates.[11,12]

What is the ideal varicose vein treatment?

Surgery is invasive for the patient and labour intensive for the NHS. Outpatient procedures allowing for the treatment of far greater numbers of patients must be developed and will be popular with patients. Slightly higher recurrence rates from less invasive techniques will be acceptable if patients receive a fast, painless outpatient procedure that at least cures the majority. The ideal treatment would offer the following:

1. single one-stop outpatient treatment;
2. pain-free procedure under local or no anaesthesia;
3. quick and simple to perform;
4. low complication rates;
5. early return to work, sport and leisure activities;
6. recurrence should be infrequent *and* easy to treat;
7. affordable set up and running costs.

Novel treatments for varicose veins

Minimally invasive techniques to ablate the incompetent long saphenous vein are being developed in an attempt to provide out-patient treatment under local anaesthesia with little discomfort and more rapid return to work. These less invasive methods aim to minimize recurrence, but if in the event of recurrence they can be easily repeated, then higher rates of recurrence than surgery would still be acceptable to patients. The most promising methods include radiofrequency ablation, endovenous laser and microfoam sclerotherapy. Proponents of these novel techniques initially claim results comparable to or better than surgery based on personal series; however, in designing a strategy for varicose vein treatment only evidence from randomized clinical trials should be accepted.

Radiofrequency ablation (RFA) or 'VNUS closure' (VNUS medical technologies, Sunnyvale, California) uses an endovenous radiofrequency probe to obliterate the vein by controlled thermal injury at 85° C. Sufficient temperature is sustained within the vein wall to cause collagen contraction and endothelial necrosis with spasm and fibrosis. Initially RFA was used to ablate the long saphenous vein following saphenofemoral disconnection but the procedure is now being promoted for saphenofemoral junction ablation. RFA can be done under local anaesthesia (tumescent, regional or both) with or without sedation. In a study by Merchant, at 2 years, 85% of 142 saphenous veins were reported to be completely occluded, 4% were near-occluded and 11% were recanalized although 95% of patients were pleased with the result.[13]

Complication rates were low but included deep vein thrombosis and pulmonary embolus in one patient. Skin burns became infrequent with experience and paraesthesia was reported in 5.6% which is comparable with conventional surgery. Similar results have been reported with less postoperative pain, and faster recoveries.[14,15] However, operating time and costs were higher than with conventional surgery and this procedure would be painful without full regional anaesthesia. RFA cannot obliterate saphenofemoral junction tributaries which we believe is an important principle in the prevention of recurrence. This procedure therefore fails to fulfil many of the ideal criteria for a novel varicose vein treatment.

Endovenous laser (EVL) can also be used to ablate truncal veins by thermal injury. It probably acts by indirect local heat injury of the inner vein wall caused by boiling blood.[16] Navarro reported closure of all of 40 long saphenous veins at 16 months with few complications.[17] It should be remembered however, that RFA and EVL treat the truncal incompetent vein but fail to treat other varices which will still need to be removed by conventional phlebectomy.

Sclerotherapy has been used in the treatment of varicose veins since introduction of the hypodermic needle in the mid nineteenth century. Compression sclerotherapy re-gained popularity in the 1960s but had poor results as the proximal source of incompetence could rarely be treated. In a rare randomized trial including 164 patients, recurrence at 5 years was 10% following surgery compared with 74% for sclerotherapy.[18]

Microfoam sclerotherapy

Microfoams were suggested for sclerotherapy by Orbach in the 1950s but not adequately investigated until recently. Microfoam displaces blood in the vein, minimizing the dose of sclerosant, its dilution by blood and thrombophlebitis.

Microbubble echogenicity makes it highly visible on ultrasound so that the spread of foam can be controlled. Duplex imaging during injection into the long or short saphenous vein prevents spread of foam into the femoral or popliteal veins, although the flow of blood in the deep veins rapidly disperses microbubbles in the foam. Sclerosant foam may also fill incompetent tributaries around the saphenofemoral junction. Cabrera demonstrated that this technique may be used on large veins such as the incompetent long saphenous vein with good results and few complications.[19] More recently, the production of polidocanol microfoam (Provensis Ltd) which interferes with cell surface lipids promoting intense spasm and thrombosis has been investigated in the treatment of varicose veins.

Microfoam sclerotherapy: a pilot study

In collaboration with Mr Harper in Aberdeen, we conducted a pilot study investigating microfoam sclerotherapy in primary varicose veins due to severe long saphenous vein incompetence with reflux times of less than 6 seconds and a long saphenous vein diameter of more than 7mm. Forty one patients median age 43, range 25–64 years, 23 women and 18 men) were assessed clinically, by duplex imaging and digital photography, preoperatively and at 1, 2, 6, 12 and 52 weeks.

Following local anaesthesia, a cannula was introduced into the long saphenous vein in the mid-thigh under duplex guidance (Figs 1a, b). With the leg elevated, Polidocanol microfoam was injected and its passage proximally along the long saphenous vein imaged by duplex until it reached the saphenofemoral junction (Fig. 2). This junction was then compressed while further foam was injected, refluxing down the incompetent long saphenous vein to fill calf varices. The leg was elevated for 5–10 minutes before a class II full length elastic stocking was applied. The patient was then mobilized and allowed to go home immediately. The elastic stocking was worn day and night for the first week and then throughout the day for a further 3 weeks.

At 3 months follow-up, 27 patients (66%) had complete occlusion of the long saphenous vein and saphenofemoral junction, six (14%) an occluded saphenofemoral junction alone and eight (20%) had recanalized (Fig. 3a). One year after sclerotherapy, duplex imaging in the 38 limbs of patients who attended for review revealed that 27 (71%) had complete occlusion of the long saphenous vein and saphenofemoral junction, four (11%) had an occluded saphenofemoral junction with a competent long saphenous vein and seven (18%) had an incompetent recanalized long saphenous vein (Fig. 3b).

Overall this implies an 82% clinical success rate. The procedure was almost entirely pain–free; only 14 patients (34%) took any form of analgesia, usually a non-steroidal anti-inflammatory drug and only seven (17%) patients continued analgesia after the first postoperative day. Two patients had asymptomatic short segment occlusions of the posterior tibial vein demonstrated on duplex imaging but there were no other complications. Appearance was graded independently as improved or excellent in all limbs, visible varicosities as none or improved in all limbs with good cosmetic results (Figs 4a, 4b). A randomized clinical trial comparing polidocanol microfoam sclerotherapy with standard surgical techniques for long saphenous and short saphenous varicose veins is now underway. This novel approach has the advantage that the long saphenous vein can be ablated up to the saphenofemoral junction without inhibiting the subsequent use of microfoam sclerotherapy or even surgery for recurrence.

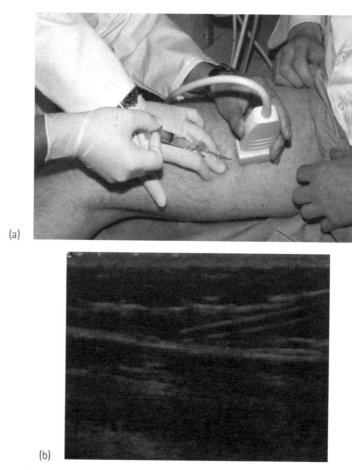

(a)

(b)

Figure 1. The long saphenous vein is canulated under duplex imaging (a) with clear views of the canula in the vein (b)

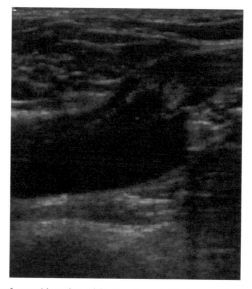

Figure 2. The saphenofemoral junction with microfoam in the long saphenous vein.

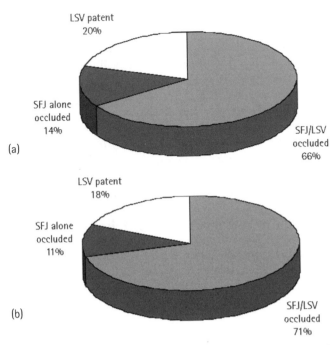

(a)

(b)

Figure 3. Occlusion rates by polidocanol microfoam sclerosant of the long saphenous vein (LSV) and saphenofemoral junction (SFJ) assessed by duplex imaging at 3 months (n=41) (a) and at 12 months (n=38) (b).

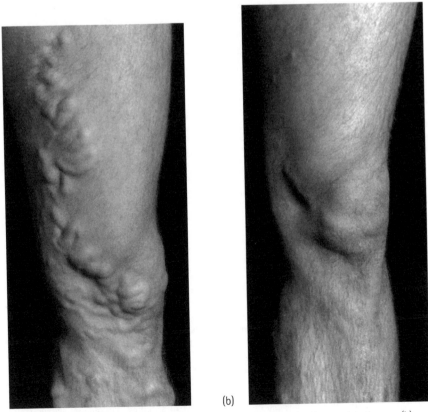

(a)

(b)

Figure 4. Varicose veins before treatment (a) and 1 year following microfoam sclerotherapy (b).

Conclusions

The principles of treatment are: (i) ablation of the most proximal sources of incompetence, (ii) ablation of incompetent truncal veins and (iii) removal or ablation of varicose veins. Accurate diagnosis of all sites of incompetence by hand-held Doppler or duplex imaging is essential before treatment. Accurate surgery performed by experienced surgeons currently achieves the best results with the lowest recurrence rates but surgery is invasive and the demand for varicose vein treatment outweighs the ability of the NHS to provide a specialist service. Novel treatments have become a necessary but also realistic and economic option.

Radiofrequency ablation and endovenous laser act by burning the inner vein which would be painful without full regional anaesthesia. They are slow, expensive and require access to operating facilities. Randomized controlled trials with long-term follow-up comparing microfoam sclerotherapy with surgery may demonstrate that this novel approach has the potential to offer a comprehensive and yet affordable varicose vein service for our population. More importantly, it will be our patients who will ultimately choose the treatment they want.

Summary

- Recurrence rates after varicose vein surgery are unacceptably high due to inaccurate preoperative diagnosis, inadequate surgery and neovascularization

- Both varicose vein surgery and newer less invasive techniques require accurate diagnosis by hand-held Doppler. Duplex imaging may be required for recurrent veins, difficult veins and saphenopopliteal incompetence.

- Surgery, which has traditionally been the gold standard, requires precise division of all sites of incompetence. It is invasive and painful requiring recovery of 10–15 days.

- Recurrence following surgery is difficult to treat.

- Radiofrequency ablation and laser treatment for long saphenous incompetence are slow and expensive requiring similar regional anaesthesia to the equivalent surgery.

- By popular demand microfoam sclerotherapy may replace surgery within a few years providing treatment to many more patients than is currently possible.

References

1. Brand FN, Dannenberg AL, Abbott RD, Kannel WB. The epidemiology of varicose veins: The Framingham study. *Am J Prev Med* 1988; **4**: 96–101.
2. Bradbury A, Evans CJ, Allan P *et al.* The relationship between lower limb symptoms and superficial and deep venous reflux on duplex ultrasonography: The Edinburgh vein study. *J Vasc Surg* 2000; **32**: 921–931.
3. Department of Health website: www.doh.gov.uk/hes/tables
4. Negus D. Recurrent varicose veins: a national problem. *Br J Surg* 1993; **80**: 823–824.
5. Royle JP. Recurrent varicose veins. *World J Surg* 1986; **10**: 944–953.
6. Sarin S, Scurr JH, Coleridge Smith PD. Assessment of stripping the long saphenous vein in the treatment of primary varicose veins. *Br J Surg* 1992; **79**: 889–893.

7. McCollum CN, Dix FP. Phlebectomy is the treatment of choice for varicose veins: against the motion. In: *The Evidence for Vascular or Endovascular Reconstruction.* Greenhalgh RM (ed). London: Saunders, 2002: 409–417.

8. Davies GC. The Lothian surgical audit. *Medical Audit News* 1991; 1: 26–27.

9. Jones L, Braithwaite BD, Selwyn D *et al.* Neovascularisation is the principal cause of varicose vein recurrence: results of a randomised trial of stripping the long saphenous vein. *Eur J Vasc Endovasc Surg* 1996; 12: 442–445.

10. Earnshaw JJ, Davies B, Harradine K, Heather BP. Preliminary results of PTFE patch saphenoplasty to prevent neovascularisation leading to recurrent varicose veins. *Phlebology* 1998; 13: 10–13.

11. Budd JS, Reid A, Thompson M *et al.* The changing workload of a surgical workload with a vascular interest. *Eur J Vasc Endovasc Surg* 1995; 9: 176–180.

12. Wolfe JHN. The future of vascular services: the need for a strategy. *BMJ* 1997; 315: 695–696.

13. Merchant RF, DePalma RG, Kabnick LS. Endovascular obliteration of saphenous reflux: a multicenter study. *J Vasc Surg* 2002; 35: 1190–1196.

14. Rautio T, Ohinmaa A, Perala *et al.* Endovenous obliteration versus conventional stripping operation in the treatment of primary varicose veins: a randomized controlled trial with comparison of the costs. *J Vasc Surg* 2002; 35: 958–965.

15. Chandler JG, Pichot O, Sessa C *et al.* Treatment of primary venous insufficiency by endovenous saphenous vein obliteration. *Vasc Surg* 2000; 34: 201–214.

16. Proebstle TM, Lehr HA, Kargl A *et al.* Endovenous treatment of the greater saphenous vein with a 940nm diode laser: thrombotic occlusion after endoluminal thermal damage by laser-generated steam bubbles. *J Vasc Surg* 2002; 35,4: 729–736.

17. Navarro L, Min RJ, Bone C. Endovenous laser : a new minimally invasive method of treatment for varicose veins – preliminary observations using an 810nm diode laser. *Dermatol Surg* 2001; 27: 117–122.

18. Einarsson E, Eklof B, Neglen P. Sclerotherapy or surgery as treatment for varicose veins: a prospective randomized study. *Phlebology* 1993; 8: 22–26.

19. Cabrera J, Cabrera J (Jr), Garcia-Olmeda MA. Sclerosants in microfoam: a new approach in angiology. *Int Angiol* 2001; 20: 322–329.

Saphenofemoral ligation and stripping is the method of choice for treating long saphenous varicose veins

Charing Cross Editorial Comments towards Consensus

The opposers of this motion indicate that conventional varicose vein surgery can be performed badly and they say that the recurrence rate is unacceptably high because of inadequate preoperative diagnosis, poor surgery and neovascularization. They predict that novel techniques will almost certainly replace surgery within a few years. They regard this as of great importance to the NHS.

However, the proposers of the motion say that the evidence for endovenous methods is based almost entirely on case series and most relate to radiofrequency ablation. They say that publicity has wrongly led patients to believe that long saphenous vein stripping is always very painful and that recovery is much quicker after endovenous treatment. It will be an interesting debate.

Roger M Greenhalgh
Editor

Deep vein thrombosis risk during flying is exaggerated

For the motion

Michael Horrocks

Introduction

Over the past 5 years there have been increasing number of reports in the daily newspapers highlighting concern about the incidence of deep vein thrombosis during flying, the so called 'Economy Class Syndrome'. This has led to a huge increase in anxiety amongst the travelling population and a call for less cramped seating, particularly for long-haul flights. The problem has been further compounded by fear of terrorism raising anxiety levels in passengers and this in itself allegedly may increase the risk of deep vein thrombosis and possible pulmonary embolism

Although the first cases of deep venous thrombosis and pulmonary embolism were reported in 1940 in members of the public who were crammed into air raid shelters and found to have unexpectedly died from pulmonary embolism, it seemed remarkable that there have been so few reported cases of deep vein thrombosis or pulmonary embolism following long-haul flights until the last few years.

During the last 30 years aircraft have become larger and larger with aircraft seats better designed and available space for passengers gradually improved. Planes from the 1960s and 1970s were much slower, cabins were less well pressurized and seating space was much smaller, yet very few cases of deep vein thrombosis were suspected and there are no reports of sudden death from pulmonary embolism following long-haul flights in the literature at that time. In the first major series trying to link deep vein thrombosis and long-haul flying, 44 passengers with deep vein thrombosis following air travel in 1996 were studied and most were found to have significant predisposing factors which may have contributed to the cause of the deep vein thrombosis.[4]

In a randomized trial published[1] in *the Lancet* in May 2001 an attempt was made to determine the frequency of deep vein thrombosis in the lower limb during long-haul economy class air travel and the efficacy of graduated compression stockings on its prevention.

The trial recruited 89 men and 142 women all over 50 years of age with no history of thromboembolic problems. The passengers were randomly allocated to two groups. The first group wore Class I below-knee graduated compression stockings and the other group did not. All the passengers made journeys lasting more than 8 hours (median total duration was 24 hours), all returned to the UK within 6 weeks. Duplex ultrasound was used to assess the deep veins before and after travel. Blood samples were also taken and analysed for two specific gene mutations, Factor V Leiden and prothrombin G20210A, both of which predispose to venous thrombosis.

A D-dimer assay was used to detect evidence of a recent thrombosis. Twelve of 116 passengers developed an asymptomatic deep vein thrombosis in the calf and none of these passengers wore elastic compression stockings. Two were heterozygous for Factor V Leiden. Four other passengers who wore elastic compression stockings and who had varicose veins developed superficial thrombophlebitis. One of these passengers was heterozygous for both Factor V Leiden and prothrombin G20210A. None of the passengers who wore Class I Compression stockings developed deep vein thrombosis. The authors concluded that symptom-less deep vein thrombosis might occur in up to 10% of long-haul airline travellers and that this risk was reduced by wearing elastic compression stockings. There were, however, many passengers excluded from this study and results of the D-dimer test were not significant. The suggestion that 10% of long-haul airline passengers may develop deep vein thrombosis is clearly much too high as this would suggest that up to 40 passengers on every long haul Boeing 747 flight would have a deep vein thrombosis. It would have been helpful if passengers in this study had had a full thrombophylia screen to exclude other predisposing causes.

In another study[2] on South African Airlines, 900 passengers, 700 in economy and 200 in business class, were screened by D-dimer assay and duplex scanning before and after flying. Only one passenger of the 900 developed a deep vein thrombosis, and this passenger already had thrombophlebitis. This perhaps gives a more accurate estimate of the true incidence of deep vein thrombosis associated with long-haul flying.

One group of the population who fly the most are the airline crew. A study from Johannesburg[6] in 2002 looked at 27 cockpit crew who were due to fly two or more international flights per day. The study group were subjected to venesection at the beginning and end of the study period looking specifically at full blood count, differential and D-dimer levels. All participants completed a detailed questionnaire to include age, alcohol consumption in the previous 24 hours, the amount of liquid consumed during flying time, the number of times they went to the lavatory and the amount of time spent sitting during the flight. Whilst there were minimal changes in their blood tests there was no suggestion of any clinical or subclinical thrombotic event and the changes in the full blood count were not thought to be significant.

Although it has been suggested that hypobaric hypoxia as encountered within aeroplane cabins may produce an increase in markers of activated coagulation, the rise is only transient and moderate with no proven association with deep vein thrombosis. In a letter to *the Lancet* in 2002, Bendz and colleagues[3] suggested that such transient hypoxia in association with dehydration and being sedentary may cause an increase risk of venous thrombosis, but produced no hard data as evidence.

The impact of obesity on immobility, leg oedema and deep vein thrombosis particularly for economy class passengers has recently been highlighted. There seems little doubt that grossly overweight passengers may have difficulty actually sitting in an economy sized seat, and once in place may be rigidly fixed and unable to move. Despite this immobility there is little evidence of an increased risk of deep vein thrombosis in these passengers even though some airlines now insist that such overweight passengers should buy two seats rather than one.

In an overview of long-haul flights and deep vein thrombosis, Levi[5] concludes that the combined observational and case-controlled studies available up to 2001 do not indicate an increased incidence of thromboembolism amongst air travellers. The report goes on to conclude that many of the published studies may be biased by incomplete data, poor follow-up, a lack of use of objective tests to establish thrombosis and difficulty with selecting control patients with different travel behaviour.

In a study of 86 patients who developed deep vein thrombosis within 28 days of flying, Kesteven and Robinson[7] found that 72% of these patients had at least one recognized risk factor for venous thromboembolism. They concluded that the majority of venous thromboembolic events occurring within 28 days of flying were associated with identifiable risk factors present prior to the flight.

Conclusion

In conclusion despite numerous leading articles in newspapers[8-10] raising anxiety amongst the travelling population there is little objective data showing that clinical deep vein thrombosis or pulmonary embolism is anything but a rare occurrence in association with long-haul flights. In those rare cases where deep vein thrombosis appears to follow a long-haul flight, there is usually a predisposing factor. In personal communications with hospitals around major airports there is no objective or anecdotal evidence of significant numbers of airline passengers presenting with deep vein thrombosis following long-haul flights. It would seem therefore that the deep vein thrombosis risk during flying has been grossly exaggerated, and the anxiety raised in the travelling public has been unnecessary.

Summary

- A large number of newspaper articles describe an apparent high incidence of deep vein thrombosis following long-haul flights.

- There are few prospective studies looking at the true incidence of deep vein thrombosis.

- One study suggesting a 10% incidence of deep vein thrombosis remains uncorroborated and does not reflect clinical experience. When deep vein thrombosis occurs within 28 days of a long-haul flight the majority of passengers are found to have pre-existing risk factors prior to the flight.

- Observational studies suggest the incidence of deep vein thrombosis is very low following long-haul flight and appears to be grossly exaggerated.

References

1. Scurr JH, Machin SJ, Bailey-King S et al. Frequency and prevention of symptomless deep vein thrombosis in long-haul flights; a randomised trial. Lancet 2001 357: 1485–1489.
2. Scurr JH. Travellers' thrombosis. J R Soc Health 2002; 122: 11–13.
3. Bendz B, Rostrup M, Sevre K et al. Association between acute hypobaric hypoxia and activation of coagulation in human beings. Lancet 2000; 356: 1657–1658.
4. Brundrett G. Comfort and health in commercial aircraft: a literature review. J R Soc Health 2001; 121: 29–37.
5. Levi M, Kraaijenhagen RA. Long flights and the risk of venous thrombosis. Ned Tijdschr Geneeskd 2001; 145: 292–294.

6. Jacobson BF, Philippides M, Malherbe M, Becker P. Risk factors for deep vein thrombosis in short haul cockpit crews: a prospective study. *Aviat Space Environ Med* 2002; **73**: 481–484.

7. Kesteven PJ, Robinson BJ. Clinical risk factors for venous thrombosis associated with air travel. *Aviat Space Environ Med* 2001; **72**: 125–128.

8. *Sunday Times* 29 June 1997.

9. *The Independent* Thursday 24 January 2002.

10. *The Daily Telegraph* Thursday 24 January 2002.

Deep vein thrombosis risk during flying is exaggerated

Against the motion
Inge Fourneau, André Nevelsteen

'One out of every thirty air travellers will develop blood clots in the lower limbs.'
Het Laatste Nieuws, November 2002

Introduction

The subject of air travel and thrombosis has been a topic of much debate in both the lay and medical press recently, although the possible link has already been widely suspected for many years.

Venous thromboembolism associated with extended quiet sitting has been described since World War II, when pulmonary embolism was found to be the occasional cause of sudden death in people sleeping overnight in deck chairs in London air raid shelters.[1]

The first cases of air flight-related venous thromboembolism were reported by John Homans in 1954.[2] He reported two cases with clinical calf deep vein thrombosis after about 15 hours air flight and wrote that 'prolonged dependency stasis, a state imposed by airplane flights, automobile trips and even attendance at the theatre, is able, unpredictably, to bring on thrombosis'. He suggested 'the advisability of making movements of the toes, feet, and lower legs when one is sitting for long periods and of getting up and exercising when opportunity offers.'

The best-known case of deep vein thrombosis related to air travel was that of President RM Nixon who had suffered a deep vein thrombosis of his left leg in 1965. In 1974, during a long trip to Europe, the Middle East, and the Soviet Union, he developed swelling and pain in the left leg. His personal physician diagnosed a deep vein thrombosis and started anticoagulation therapy.

Evidence

Does air travel pre-destine to venous thromboembolism?

The evidence linking venous thromboembolism with flying is mainly circumstantial. Numerous reports have appeared on this issue but most are very small series or case reports.[3-6] With a population incidence of 1–2 per 1000 per annum and no apparent symptoms in up to 50% of events, venous thromboembolism is a common disorder and given the high prevalence of long-distance travel by air, it is not possible to judge from case reports alone if recent travel contributes to the risk of venous thromboembolism. [7]

Stronger evidence that prolonged air travel predisposes to thrombosis comes from the travel history of patients presenting with venous thromboembolism. This is the way Symington and Stack launched the term 'economy-class syndrome'.[8] From a cohort of 182 patients with pulmonary embolism, they identified eight patients in whom the embolism had developed soon after prolonged travel in the coach-class section of an airplane. The first detailed clinical study of venous thromboembolism associated with prolonged air travel was published by Eklof *et al.* in 1996.[5] This retrospective study of 254 patients admitted under the diagnosis of deep vein thrombosis and/or pulmonary embolism identified 44 patients who developed symptoms during or after air flight.

In the absence of large controlled prospective studies, the strongest evidence is based on case-control studies. Ferrari *et al.* scrupulously investigated the history, in particular the history of recent travel, of 160 patients presenting in the department with venous thromboembolism.[9] All journeys undertaken during the preceding 4 weeks and lasting longer than 4 hours by whatever means of transport were considered. The same questionnaire was submitted to a control group. When the two groups of patients were compared, a history of recent travel was found almost four times more frequently in the venous thromboembolism group (p<0.0001). However, only nine were related to flying while 28 followed a trip by car and two by train. A case-control study by Samama *et al.* had similar findings.[10]

The consensus at a meeting of experts convened in March 2001 by the World Health Organisation was that, based on the available circumstantial evidence, there is 'probably' a link.[11] Large prospective studies are on the way.

How common is flight-related venous thromboembolism?

It is commonly thought that people are at increased risk of venous thrombosis during air flights, but the magnitude of the risk is largely unknown. Some data are available about the incidence of pulmonary embolism associated with air travel. In a study of 61 cases of sudden death in airline passengers on flights arriving at Heathrow airport in London between 1979 and 1982, pulmonary embolism was identified as the cause at autopsy in 11 (18%) cases.[12] Ten cases had involved flights of longer than 12 hours. In contrast, only one of 28 (3.5%) cases in passengers waiting to embark and none of 15 deaths among spectators and staff deaths were due to pulmonary embolism. The Emergency Medical Services of the Paris airports have reported a total of 109 cases of pulmonary embolism since 1990.[13] The overall incidence of pulmonary embolism among airline passengers was estimated to be 0.5/million passengers, but this is likely to be an underestimate as the data only refer to passengers seen at the airport. Indeed, it is hard to quantify pulmonary embolism in airline passengers, since the embolus may not manifest itself until some time after disembarkation. Neither the passenger nor general practitioner may link the incident with the flight and, even if the link is made, there seems to be no method of reporting and collating the information. Moreover, cases of symptomatic pulmonary embolism clearly only represent the 'tip of the iceberg' of cases of deep vein thrombosis.

More recently, Lapostolle *et al.* reported an association between duration of travel and risk of pulmonary embolism based on 56 confirmed cases of pulmonary embolism among 135.3 million passengers passing through one airport in the period

1993–2000.[14] The incidence of pulmonary embolism was significantly higher (1.5 cases per million) for passengers travelling more than 5000km when compared with a risk of only 0.01 cases per million among passengers travelling less than 5000km. For those travelling more than 10000 km the incidence of pulmonary embolism was 4.8 cases per million.

Scurr *et al.* were the first to determine the frequency of deep vein thrombosis in the lower limb during long-haul economy class air travel in a prospective way.[15] Of 116 passengers making journeys lasting more than 8 hours without history of thromboembolic problems and not wearing elastic compression stockings, 10% developed symptomless deep vein thrombosis of the calf. The diagnosis was made by duplex ultrasonography and confirmed by a sensitive D-dimer assay.

In the LONFLIT 1 study 355 subjects at low-risk for deep vein thrombosis and 389 at high-risk were studied prospectively.[16] The diagnosis was made by ultrasound scans within 24 hours after the flights. In low-risk subjects no events were recorded while in high-risk subjects 11 had deep vein thrombosis (2.8%) with 13 thromboses in 11 subjects and six superficial thromboses (total of 19 thrombotic events in 389 patients (4.9%)).

However, much larger prospective studies are required to establish the incidence of flight-related deep vein thrombosis with some degree of precision. A truly prospective study would start before the flight, with colour duplex Doppler screening of a large number of patients, and the examination would then be repeated after the flight. Ideally, this examination would be repeated some time later to identify patients with late-onset venous thromboembolism. Such a study would be extremely difficult to conduct.

What causes flight-related venous thromboembolism? What are the risk factors? (Fig. 1)

It has since long been understood that, according to the Virchow's triad, deep vein thrombosis can be associated with reduction of blood flow, changes in blood viscosity and damage or abnormality in the vessel wall.[17]

Stasis in the venous circulation of the lower limbs is undoubtedly the major factor in promoting development of deep vein thrombosis associated with travel. The potential danger of confinement in cramped conditions has been recognized for some years and led to the term 'Economy class syndrome'.[3,4,8] That immobility contributes is suggested by the observation that only three of 45 long-distance air passengers with subsequent pulmonary embolism claimed to have left their seat during prolonged flight while the other 42 remained seated throughout, and by the finding that in de LONFLIT study most subclinical deep vein thrombosis were detected in subjects sitting in window or central seats.[14,16]

Moreover, using cadavers, Schmitt and Mihatsch demonstrated that when in the seated position, the popliteal vein develops transverse rippling.[18] This may be sufficiently damaging to the endothelium, or cause sufficient alteration to flow, as to trigger the initial thrombus formation (in accordance with Virchow's triad).

Apart from immobilization there might be additional cabin-related factors associated with air travel in particular that further predispose air travellers to thrombosis. Whether the combination of low cabin humidity, the diuretic effect of alcohol ingested during flight, and insufficient non-alcoholic fluid intake, can dehydrate passengers enough to cause significant hyperviscosity and haemoconcentration is still point of debate.[19–21] Bendz *et al.* studied the association between hypobaric hypoxia

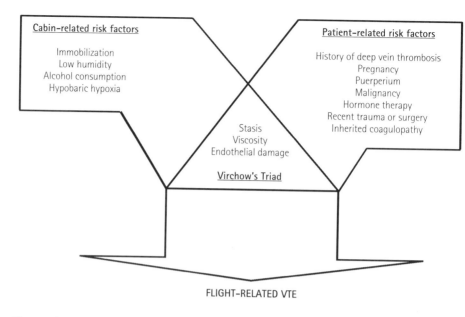

Figure1. Pathophysiology of flight-related venous thromboembolism.

and activation of coagulation.[22] No link with thrombogenesis was obvious, unless an increase in activated blood coagulation markers observed during 8 hours of hypobaric hypoxia. These changes were prevented by a high prophylactic dose of low molecular weight heparin.[23]

However, in most cases, travel-related thrombosis affects people who have other risk factors for deep vein thrombosis. For instance, Kesteven and Robinson examined clinical data from a large cohort of patients with traveller's thrombosis.[24] Of the patients, 72% had at least one risk factor for venous thromboembolism prior to their flight. The prospective LONFLIT 1 study came to the same findings.[16] In low-risk subjects no events were recorded while in high-risk subjects thrombotic events were seen in 4.9% of the patients. These data support Rosendaal's 'multiple-hit' theories of venous thromboembolism.[25]

It is useful to think of deep vein thrombosis as the result of a cumulative series of risk factors, which eventually exceed some 'threshold' for the thrombotic event to occur. The risk factors act through the classical triad proposed by Virchow . As known from the experience in the setting of surgery, risk factors for venous thromboembolism include previous or strong family history of venous thromboembolism, pregnancy and the puerperium, malignancy, hormone therapy, trauma and, more recently, an expanding array of inherited blood disorders.

Prevention of flight-related venous thromboembolism

As in travellers with patient-related risk factors, the cabin-related risk factors are superimposed, the risk for air travel-related acute venous thromboembolism is considerably increased. Most authors agree that air travellers should be advised about hazards and precautions, at least until formal study validates some other approach, especially because this potentially fatal syndrome may be entirely preventable by simple means based on the experience in the setting of surgery.[2-5,28]

Perhaps the most important step is to consider at the outset whether the patient is actually fit to fly. For example, it is probably wise to defer long-haul travel after recent major orthopaedic surgery. Passengers should be encouraged to carry out leg exercises from time to time while seated. Passengers should also take advantage of refuelling stops on long-haul flights to get off the plane and walk round for a while. Baggage under the seat should be avoided to have more leg space. Also the wearing of constrictive clothes should be avoided. Adequate hydratation should be ensured during the flight.

For people at risk of thrombosis, the wearing of below-knee elasticated stockings on both legs may be helpful. Scurr *et al.* were the first to evaluate the efficacy of graduated elastic compression stockings in the prevention of air travel related deep vein thrombosis.[15]

None of the passengers who wore class I compression stockings developed deep vein thrombosis whereas 10% of those not wearing compression stockings did.

In the LONFLIT 2 study the authors studied 833 high-risk for deep vein thrombosis subjects (randomized into 422 control subjects and 411 using below-knee stockings).[16] In the control group there were 4.5% of subjects with deep vein thrombosis while only 0.24% in the stockings group.

Aspirin has been advocated by some in the general prophylaxis of thrombosis associated with travel, although this is not based on compelling clinical data and, thus, remains the subject of considerable debate. A meta-analysis of several surgical studies concluded that aspirin does offer limited protection.[26] This was confirmed in a large prospective study which demonstrated that aspirin reduced the risk of both venous thrombosis and pulmonary embolism by at least one-third in the setting of hip fracture or major orthopaedic surgery.[27] However, the consensus at the WHO meeting referred to above was that indiscriminate use of pharmacological agents such as aspirin should not be encouraged in view of potential side-effects such as allergic reactions or gastrointestinal bleeding.[11]

The use of heparin may be considered in the relatively few passengers considered to be at particularly high risk of thrombosis, although many such subjects are already likely to be on long-term oral anticoagulation anyway. The LONFLIT 3 study aimed to evaluate methods of prevention in high-risk subjects.[28] Three hundred high-risk for deep vein thrombosis passengers were randomized after informed consent into three groups:

1. a control group that had no prophylaxis;
2. an aspirin treatment group, in which patients were treated with 400mg;
3. a low-molecular-weight heparin group in which one dose of enoxaparine was injected between 2 and 4 hours before the flight.

The dose was weight-adjusted; 249 subjects completed the study. Of the 82 subjects in the control group, there were 4.82% of subjects with two superficial thromboses. Of 84 subjects in the aspirin treatment group, there were 3.6% of patients with deep vein thrombosis and three superficial thromboses. In the low-molecular-weight heparin group (82 subjects), there were no cases of deep vein thrombosis. One superficial thrombosis was documented. One dose of low-molecular-weight heparin is an important option to consider in high-risk subjects during long-haul flights. These findings were confirmed by Bendz *et al.* who examined the ability of low molecular weight heparin to prevent thrombotic activation in 12 healthy male volunteers who were given 40mg enoxaparin as a single subcutaneous injection 1 hour prior to exposure.[23] They found no activation of coagulation as judged by F1+2 or TAT. Anti-activated factor X activity levels and release of tissue factor pathway inhibitor was normal.

Summary

- The evidence for flight-related venous thromboembolism is largely circumstantial but an association is likely.

- In travellers with patient-related risk factors for deep vein thrombosis, cabin-related risk factors are superimposed.

- Considering the number of people travelling by air, the incidence of the condition is significant.

- This potentially fatal syndrome may be entirely preventable by simple means.

- People 'at risk' should be advised about hazards and precautions.

References

1. Simpson K. Shelter deaths from pulmonary embolism. *Lancet* 1940; ii: 744.
2. Homans J. Thrombosis of the deep leg veins due to prolonged sitting. *N Engl J Med* 1954; **250**: 148–149.
3. Cruickshank JM, Gorlin R, Jennett B. Air travel and thrombotic episodes: the economy class syndrome. *Lancet* 1988; 2: 497–498.
4. Sahiar F, Mohler S. Economy class syndrome. *Aviat Space Environ Med* 1994; 10: 957–960.
5. Eklof B, Kistner RL, Masuda EM *et al.* Venous thromboembolism in association with prolonged air travel. *Dermatol Surg* 1996; 22: 637–641.
6. Geroulakos G, Hossain J, Tran T. Economy-class syndrome presenting as phlegmasia caerulea dolens. *Eur J Vasc Endovasc Surg* 2000; **20**: 102–104.
7. Hansson PO, Werlin L, Tibblin G *et al.* Deep vein thrombosis and pulmonary embolism in the general population. *Arch Intern Med* 1997; **157**: 1665–1670.
8. Symington IS, Stack BH. Pulmonary thromboembolism after travel. *Br J Dis Chest* 1977; **71**: 138–40.
9. Ferrrari E, Chevallier T, Chapelier A, Baudouy M. Travel as a risk factor for venous thromboembolic disease. A case-control study. *Chest* 1999; **115**: 440–444.
10. Samama MM. An epidemiological study of risk factors for deep vein thrombosis in medical outpatients. *Arch Mt Med* 2000; **160**: 3415–3420.
11. World Health Organisation (WHO). Consultation on air travel and thromboembolism: Geneva, 12–13 March 2001. http://www.who.int/ncd/cvd/dvt.htm
12. Sarvesvaran R. Sudden natural deaths associated with commercial air travel. *Med Sci Lax* 1986; 1: 35–38.
13. Caillard G, Clerel M. Travel and risk of venous thrombosis. *Lancet* 2001; **357**: 554–555.
14. Lapostolle F, Surget V, Borron SW *et al.* Severe pulmonary embolism associated with air travel. *N Engl J Med* 2001; **345**: 779–783.
15. Scurr JH, Machin SJ, Bailey-King S *et al.* Frequency and prevention of a symptomless deep-vein thrombosis in long-haul flights: a randomised trial. *Lancet* 2001; **357**: 1485–1489.
16. Belcaro G, Geroulakos G, Nicolaides AN *et al.*Venous thromboembolism from air travel. The LONFLIT study. *Angiology* 2001; **52**: 369–374.
17. Virchow R. Gesammelte Abhandlungen zur Wissenschaftlichen Medizin. Frankfurt: Meidinger, 1856.
18. Schmitt HE, Mihatsch MJ. Thrombosis of the popliteal vein. *Cardiovasc Intervent Radiol* 1992; **15**: 234–239.
19. Carruters M, Arguelles AE, Mosovich A. Man in transit: biochemical and physiological changes during intercontinental flights. *Lancet* 1976; 8: 977–980.
20. Simons R, Krol J. Jet lag, pulmonary embolism, and hypoxia. *Lancet* 1996; **348**: 416.
21. Landgraf H, Vanselow B, Schulte-Huermann D *et al.* Economy class syndrome: rheology, fluid balance, and lower leg edema during a simulated 12-hour long distance flight. *Aviat Space Environ Med* 1994; 65: 930–935.
22. Bendz B, Rostrup M, Sevre K *et al.* Association between acute hypobaric hypoxia and activation of coagulation in human beings. *Lancet* 2000; **356**: 1657–1658.

23. Bendz B, Sevre K, Andersen TO, Sandset PM. Low molecular weight heparin prevents activation of coagulation in a hypobaric environment. *Blood Coagul Fibrinolysis* 2001; **12**: 371–374.
24. Kesteven PJL, Robinson BJ. Clinical risk factors for venous thrombosis associated with air travel. *Aviat Space Environ Med* 2001; **72**: 125–128.
25. Rosendaal FR. Venous thrombosis: a multicausal disease. *Lancet* 1999; **353**: 1167–1173.
26. Antiplatelet Trialist's Collaboration. Collaborative overview of randomised trials of antiplatelet therapy III. Reduction in venous thrombosis and pulmonary embolism by antiplatelet prophylaxis against surgical and medical patients. *Brit Med J* 1994; **308**: 235–246.
27. The Pulmonary Embolism Prevention (PEP) Trial Collaborative Group. Prevention of pulmonary embolism and deep vein thrombosis with low dose aspirin: the Pulmonary Embolism Prevention (PEP) trial. *Lancet* 2000; **355**: 1295–1302.
28. Cesarone MR, Belcaro G, Nicolaides AN *et al*. Venous thrombosis from air travel: the LONFLIT 3 study. Prevention with aspirin versus low-molecular-weight heparin in high-risk subjects: a randomized trial. *Angiology* 2002; **53**: 1–6.

Deep vein thrombosis risk during flying is exaggerated

Charing Cross Editorial Comments towards Consensus

Michael Horrocks supports this motion and acknowledges that even though there are a large number of newspaper articles describing an apparently high incidence of deep vein thrombosis following flying, there are few prospective studies to establish the true incidence. He says that true deep vein thrombosis incidence is grossly over-exaggerated.

The opposition acknowledges that the evidence for flight-related venous thromboembolism is largely circumstantial but believes that the incidence is significant. They stress that this potentially fatal syndrome can be prevented by simple means.

All would agree that at-risk flyers should be advised against hazards.

Roger M Greenhalgh
Editor

Anticoagulant therapy remains the gold standard for the management of lower limb deep vein thrombosis

For the motion
Sudip Ray

Introduction

Acute deep vein thrombosis is a serious and potentially fatal disorder which occurs with an incidence of between one and two cases per 1000 population per annum.[1-3] Although the incidence is probably falling due to the introduction of thromboprophylaxis within hospitals, pulmonary embolism is still thought to be the primary cause of death in 100 000 patients per annum in the USA.[4] The pathophysiology of deep vein thrombosis formation is well documented in relation to Virchow's triad of vessel wall damage, stasis and increased coagulability of the blood. Whilst the first two are often acquired conditions, hypercoagulability is increasingly recognized as an inherited condition, particularly the factor V Leiden mutation which is found in 10-20% of patients with venous thrombosis.[5]

Complications of deep vein thrombosis

In the short-term the most serious systemic complication of lower limb deep vein thrombosis is pulmonary embolism, which is far more likely with proximal (iliofemoral) than distal (calf) thromboses. Untreated, around 50% of iliofemoral deep vein thromboses will produce pulmonary emboli, of which 20-40% will be fatal.[6] Proximal deep vein thromboses are also more likely than calf deep vein thromboses to produce the post-thrombotic syndrome.[7] This develops as a result of valvular damage, deep and superficial venous hypertension, and calf muscle pump dysfunction,[8] and is characterized by pain, swelling, dermatitis and ulceration. Abnormalities in venous reflux can be detected within 3 months of the deep vein thrombosis[8] and post-thrombotic syndrome is often clinically apparent within 2 years.[9]

The strongest risk-factor for post-thrombotic syndrome is recurrent venous thrombosis whilst the extent of initial thrombosis does not appear to be important.[5] Over a

10-year period the majority of patients with proximal deep vein thrombosis will suffer from post-thrombotic syndrome,[10,11] up to 10% will develop leg ulcers, and a small number will require amputation.[12] By contrast, although haemodynamic impairment may be detected in 20% of patients with calf deep vein thrombosis,[13] post-thrombotic syndrome is rare and ulceration almost negligible.[14]

The most dramatic local effect of deep vein thrombosis occurs when extensive iliofemoral thrombosis produces significant venous and lymphatic outflow obstruction, resulting in phlegmasia. With or without subsequent arterial compromise the leg may develop compartment syndrome and sensorimotor damage, and eventually gangrene or massive pulmonary embolus may follow. Amputation is necessary in 20–50% of cases whilst in-hospital mortality is as high as 40% in some series, especially as 20–40% of these patients have underlying malignancies.[15]

Goals of treatment of deep vein thrombosis

The aims of treatment of deep vein thrombosis are, in the short-term, to control pain and swelling, to prevent extension of deep vein thrombosis or pulmonary embolism, and to avoid amputation from venous gangrene. In the long term the aims are to prevent recurrent thromboembolism and reduce the incidence of post-thrombotic syndrome.

All patients should be offered simple measures such as wearing elastic compression stockings which reduces swelling as well as the subsequent development of post-thrombotic syndrome.[9,16] There is controversy over whether patients should be confined to bed with leg elevation, or encouraged to walk. However, in a randomized trial, Partsch demonstrated that patients with proximal deep vein thrombosis who were given thigh-length stockings and encouraged to mobilize were in less pain and had less leg swelling than those who were prescribed bedrest only, and there was no increase in thromboembolic events on ambulation.[17] However, where there is gross limb swelling or a high thrombotic load it may be prudent to apply high limb elevation until the swelling resolves.[18]

In addition to these measures most patients with deep vein thrombosis undergo therapeutic anticoagulation in the absence of contraindications such as active bleeding. The following sections will concentrate on the published evidence on the rationale, efficacy, methods and duration of such treatment, and present a brief comparison with the evidence for alternative, more invasive, therapies of pharmacological thrombolysis and surgical thrombectomy.

Evidence

Initiation of anticoagulation

The efficacy of intravenous heparin followed by oral anticoagulation in preventing thromboembolic complications in patients with popliteal or iliofemoral deep vein thrombosis is well established. In untreated or inadequately treated thromboembolic disease the incidence of recurrence is approximately 25–50% which is reduced to less than 10% during treatment with anticoagulation.[10,19]

There is now evidence that initial heparinization can be effectively achieved using a single daily subcutaneous injection of low-molecular weight heparin (LMWH) rather than continuous intravenous infusion.[20] This allows outpatient management of the whole episode in approximately 80% of patients, with the remaining 20% requiring admission because of massive thrombosis, pulmonary embolism, other medical conditions, or difficulties complying with the regime.[21] LMWH may even replace warfarin as the long-term agent of anticoagulation. In a randomised study Gonzalez-Fajardo showed that 3 months treatment with LMWH for deep vein thrombosis was associated with enhanced venographic resolution of deep vein thrombosis, lower recurrence rates (9.5% vs 23.7%) as well as reduced haemorrhagic complications (1.1% vs 10%) compared with warfarin.[22]

Other advantages of LMWH include decreased mortality in patients with cancer and a decreased risk of heparin-induced thrombocytopaenia.[20,23] It is less certain whether patients with uncomplicated calf-vein thrombosis should receive anticoagulation, especially as only 20% of these propagate proximally, and overt pulmonary emboli are rare even without treatment.[14,24]

Duration of anticoagulation

Heparin is usually the first anticoagulant to be given in the treatment of deep vein thrombosis because of its immediate action. The importance of heparin in the management of deep vein thrombosis has been shown in a randomized clinical trial which showed fewer recurrent thromboembolic events if heparin was added to oral anticoagulants[25].

If heparin is to be given as an intravenous infusion the dose must be adjusted to maintain a partial thromboplastin time of between 1.5 and 2.5 times control values, a range which reduces recurrence without unduly increasing haemorrhagic complications.[26] Warfarin is normally started immediately, at a dose determined by algorithm, and a target international normalized ratio (INR) of between 2.0 and 2.5,[26] with an INR of 2.2–2.3 being optimal.[27] Once this is achieved the heparin can be stopped as prolonged heparin therapy merely increases the risk of bleeding and thrombocytopaenia.[26]

The optimum duration of anticoagulation for deep vein thrombosis is controversial, and depends on a balance between recurrent thrombosis and haemorrhagic complications. The annual cumulative incidence of recurrent thrombosis after a first untreated deep vein thrombosis declines from around 40% immediately to around 5-8% per annum.[26,28] Overall, about 20–25% of patients will suffer recurrence within 5 years.[29,30] Younger patients, those with a history of previous deep vein thrombosis or cancer, and patients with idiopathic deep vein thrombosis have a higher risk of recurrence, whilst older patients, those with postoperative deep vein thrombosis and patients taking a long course of anticoagulants have a smaller risk.[28,30,31] The annual incidence of haemorrhagic complications varies from 7.6 to 16.5%, of which 1.1–2.7% are major haemorrhages and 0.25–0.64% fatal.[32,33] For every unit increase in INR above 2.5 the risk of haemorrhagic death more than doubles.[27]

The currently recommended duration of anticoagulation following a first episode of venous thrombosis has been addressed in a review of several studies comparing short- and long-term anticoagulation.[34] One of the largest studies showed a decrease in recurrent deep vein thrombosis at 1 year from 7.8% to 4.0% if patients were anticoagulated for 3 months instead of 4 weeks,[35] whilst Schulman found that 6 months treatment was better than 6 weeks.[28] Subgroup analysis showed that recurrent deep vein thrombosis was rare following postoperative deep vein thrombosis, and therefore this group needed a shorter anticoagulant course than those with permanent risk factors for deep vein thrombosis, or idiopathic thrombosis. If patients with isolated calf deep vein thrombosis are to be anticoagulated, there does not appear to be any benefit of extending the period past 6 weeks, during which there is only a 2% risk of recurrence.[36]

Patients with recurrent thromboembolism are at highest risk of further deep vein thrombosis. For example, 21% of such patients developed recurrent disease over a 4-year period despite an initial 6-month period of anticoagulation, whilst only 3% developed recurrent disease if anticoagulation was indefinite.[37] This benefit comes at the expense of a three-fold increase in haemorrhagic complications (8.6% vs 2.7%).

In practice, therefore, it would appear that 6 weeks anticoagulation is sufficient for distal (calf) deep vein thrombosis, 3 months is sufficient for proximal (iliofemoral) deep vein thrombosis with temporary risk factors (surgery, immobilization, puerperium), 6 months for proximal deep vein thrombosis with permanent risk factors or of idiopathic origin, and up to 12 months in those with recurrent deep vein thrombosis. Almost as important as the duration of anticoagulation is the maintenance of a therapeutic INR, as Caprini has shown that patients with incompletely resolving deep vein thromboses are more likely to have subtherapeutic INR levels than those with deep vein thrombosis resolution.[38]

Rationale for thrombolysis or surgical thrombectomy for acute deep vein thrombosis

Although anticoagulation is a simple and effective method of reducing recurrent thromboembolism following deep vein thrombosis, the majority of patients with proximal deep vein thrombosis will develop post-thrombotic syndrome as a result of the destruction of venous valves by the initial thrombosis,[39] and only around 20% will achieve recanalization.[40] Since the rate of recanalization appears to be an important determinant of valvular competence,[41] it seems logical to propose that early removal of thrombus may delay or prevent the development of post-thrombotic syndrome. In practice this can be achieved surgically, by thrombectomy, or by pharmacological lysis.

Thrombectomy

The surgical removal of deep vein thrombosis was first attempted in the 1920s but required the development of phlebography and then the Fogarty catheter before being widely adopted. Most of the literature regarding these procedures is anecdotal and associated with high rates of rethrombosis in the postoperative period.[42] However, these patients usually have phlegmasia and sometimes venous gangrene so it has proved difficult to obtain comparative results with anticoagulation only.

In selected series improvement following thrombectomy may be found in 40–80% of patients,[43,44] although Stirnemann noted that clinical relief in the majority of 37 patients undergoing thrombectomy was nevertheless associated with venographic rethrombosis in 63% of cases.[45]

Although reocclusion may be reduced by the addition of an arteriovenous fistula to maintain high flow through the cleared segment,[46] long-term follow-up following surgical thrombectomy suggests residual oedema and stasis requiring stockings in over 90% of patients.[47] Operative morbidity is also an issue, since many of the patients are not fit for general anaesthesia. Surgery tends to be associated with significant blood loss, prolonged hospitalization and high mortality, with two-thirds of deaths due to pulmonary emboli.[47]

Since thrombectomy does not address thrombus within distal veins the results are generally poor in venous gangrene and valvular incompetence is not reversed.[15] For that reason thrombectomy is generally restricted to patients presenting with massive iliofemoral thrombosis and a threatened limb, although Patel has noted that aggressive limb elevation, hydration and anticoagulation still has a role in these critically ill patients.[48]

Thrombolysis

There is good evidence that fibrinolytic therapy accelerates the lysis of venous thrombi, especially in patients with symptoms of recent onset.[49-51] However, the evidence that this approach improves clinical outcomes, especially in terms of recurrent thromboembolism and post-thrombotic syndrome, is poor. Although streptokinase was the first agent used, it became clear that the haemorrhagic complications were unacceptable in the context of the natural history of deep vein thrombosis,[52] and recombinant tissue plasminogen activator has subsequently become the agent of choice.

Forster and Wells reviewed four randomized trials of recombinant tissue plasminogen activator and intravenous heparin versus heparin alone in patients with deep vein thromboses diagnosed within 10 days of symptoms.[53] They noted that satisfactory (greater than 50%) venographic lysis was achieved far more frequently with thrombolysis (mean 29.8% vs 3.7%) but at the expense of increased complications (27.7% vs 3.3%) and increased major haemorrhage rates (8.4% vs 3.3%). Whether the improved rates of lysis result in decreased incidence of long-term post-thrombotic syndrome was not studied objectively. Forster and Wells concluded that their systematic review 'does not support routine use of recombinant plasminogen activator for deep vein thrombosis of the lower extremities' as the increased complication rate was not balanced by improvement in important clinical outcomes, and that higher doses of thrombolytic were no more efficacious.

It has to be added that many patients presenting with deep vein thrombosis are not suitable for thrombolysis. For example, in a recently published randomized trial of thrombolysis a total of 207 patients with deep vein thrombosis were diagnosed but only 35 (17%) were eligible for entry due to exclusion criteria such as recent surgery, duration of symptoms over 10 days, history of gastrointestinal bleeding, age over 70 years and terminal illness.[54] Hold has noted a similar figure of ineligibility, only performing thrombolysis in 25 (16%) patients from a total of 158 presenting with deep vein thrombosis.[55]

Multidisciplinary approach

The three treatment regimes discussed above have specific and often exclusive advantages over one another. Anticoagulation prevents rethrombosis with minimal morbidity, thrombectomy effects rapid restoration of patency, and thrombolysis allows controlled removal of fresh thrombus with the possibility of uncovering a residual web or stenosis which can be further treated by endovascular means.

It is therefore unsurprising that Comerota advocates a multimodality method of addressing venous thrombosis.[56] This is based on the principles of complete proximal clot removal, removal of as much distal thrombus as possible, venographic assessment of the iliofemoral venous system for residual thrombus or anatomical abnormalities, and the creation of an arteriovenous fistula or a crosspubic bypass together with anticoagulation to maintain patency. Using such an approach in 12 patients whose thromboses had not responded to anticoagulation, improvement was seen in nine, but large numbers have not been subjected to prospective, randomized comparisons with any single modality.

Conclusions

For the majority of patients who present with deep vein thrombosis without phlegmasia surgical thrombectomy is probably unnecessarily invasive, and appears to be complicated by high rates of rethrombosis unless adjuvant surgical procedures are performed. A trial of surgery versus anticoagulation for phlegmasia would be difficult due to the relative infrequency of the complication, as well as the patients' poor general prognosis, so indications for surgery are yet to be clearly determined.

Whilst there is undoubtedly impressive evidence for the rapid clearance of venous thrombosis using thrombolytic agents, their role is undermined by ineligibility in over 80% of patients presenting with deep vein thrombosis, haemorrhagic complications in up to 10% of patients of those treated, and little evidence that short-term clearance of thrombus translates into long-term avoidance of the post-thrombotic syndrome. By contrast, conventional anticoagulation is applicable to the majority of patients with venous thrombosis, often on an outpatient basis, with acceptably low morbidity.

Whilst thrombolysis may ultimately prove to be superior in selected patient groups such as those with short duration of symptoms, significant iliofemoral thrombosis or underlying venous abnormalities amenable to angioplasty or stenting, there is no published, randomized evidence in support for this. For the time being, therefore, anticoagulation must remain the treatment of choice for lower limb deep vein thrombosis.

Summary

- Anticoagulation reduces the incidence of recurrent thrombosis following iliofemoral deep vein thrombosis but a large number of these patients still develop post-thrombotic syndrome

- Surgical thrombectomy and thrombolysis may achieve rapid restoration of venous flow following deep vein thrombosis but this has not yet been proven to reduce the incidence of post-thrombotic syndrome.

- Thrombectomy and thrombolysis are only suitable for a minority of patients with deep vein thrombosis and have procedure-related complication rates far higher than anticoagulation alone.

Acknowledgement

The author would like to acknowledge the help of Mr Aziz Anjum FRCS in the collection of reports for this chapter.

References

1. Kierkegaard A. Incidence of acute deep vein thrombosis in two districts. A phlebographic study. *Acta Chir Scand* 1980; **146**: 267–269.
2. Nordstrom M, Lindblad B, Bergqvist D, Kjellstrom T. A prospective study of the incidence of deep-vein thrombosis within a defined urban population. *J Intern Med* 1992; **232**: 155–160.
3. Hansson PO, Werlin L, Tibblin G, Eriksson H. Deep vein thrombosis and pulmonary embolism in the general population. *Arch Intern Med* 1997; **157**: 1665–1670.
4. Adams JG, Silver D. Deep venous thrombosis and pulmonary embolism. In: *Current Diagnosis and Treatment in Vascular Surgery*. Yao JST, Brewster DC (eds). Norwalk: Appleton and Lange, 1995: 375.
5. Lensing AWA, Pradoni P, Prins MH, Buller HR. Deep-vein thrombosis. *Lancet* 1999; **353**: 479–485.
6. Lyerly HK, Sabiston DC. Deep vein thrombosis and pulmonary embolism. In: Morris PJ, Malt RA (eds). *Oxford Textbook of Surgery*. Oxford: Oxford University Press, 1994: 597–607.
7. Saracen J, Kale T, Lento M *et al*. The occurrence of the post-thrombotic changes after an acute deep vein thrombosis. A prospective two year follow-up study. *Ann Vasc Surg* 1999; **13**: 436–438.
8. Haenen JH, Janssen CH, Wollersheim H *et al*. The development of postthrombotic syndrome in relationship to venous reflux and calf muscle pump dysfunction at 2 years after the onset of deep vein thrombosis. *J Vasc Surg* 2002; **35**: 1184–1189.
9. Brandjes DPM, Buller HR, Heijboer H *et al*. Randomised trial of the effect of compression stockings in patients with symptomatic proximal-vein thrombosis. *Lancet* 1997; **349**: 759–762.
10. Lagerstedt CI, Olsson CG, Fagher BO *et al*. Need for long term anticoagulant treatment in symptomatic calf vein thrombosis. *Lancet* 1985; **ii**: 515–518.
11. Bauer G. A roentgenological and clinical study of the sequels of thrombosis. *Acta Chir Scand* 1942; **86**: 1.
12. Nelzen O, Bergqvist D, Lindhagen A. Long-term prognosis for patients with chronic leg ulcers: a prospective cohort study. *Eur J Vasc Endovasc Surg* 1997; **13**: 500–508.
13. Kakkar VV, Lawrence D. Haemodynamic and clinical assessment after therapy for acute deep vein thrombosis. A prospective study. *Am J Surg* 1985; **150**: 54–63.
14. Masuda EM, Kessler DM, Kistner R *et al*. The natural history of calf vein thrombosis: lysis of thrombi and development of reflux. *J Vasc Surg* 1998; **28**: 67–74.
15. Perkins JM, Magee TR, Galland RB. Phlegmasia caerulea dolens and venous gangrene. *Br J Surg* 1996; **83**: 1160–1161.
16. Milne AA, Ruckley CV. The clinical course of patients following extensive deep vein thrombosis. *Eur J Vasc Surg* 1994; **8**: 56–59.
17. Partsch H, Blattler W. Compression and walking versus bedrest in the treatment of proximal deep venous thrombosis with low molecular weight heparin. *J Vasc Surg* 2000; **32**: 861–869.
18. McCollum C. Avoiding the consequences of deep vein thrombosis. *Br Med J* 1998; **317**: 696.
19. Hull RD, Delmore T, Genton E *et al*. Warfarin sodium versus low-dose heparin in the long-term treatment of venous thrombosis. *N Engl J Med* 1979; **301**: 855–859.
20. Van Den Belt AG, Prins MH, Lensing AW *et al*. Fixed dose subcutaneous low molecular weight heparins versus adjusted dose unfractionated heparin for venous thromboembolism. *Cochrane Database Syst Rev* 2000; **2**: CD001100.
21. Eikelboom J, Baker R. Routine home treatment of deep vein thrombosis. *Br Med J* 2001; **322**: 1192–1193.
22. Gonzalez-Fajardo JA, Arreba E, CAstrodeza J *et al*. Venographic comparison of subcutaneous low-molecular weight heparin with oral anticoagulant therapy in the long-term treatment of deep vein thrombosis. 1999; *J Vasc Surg* **30**: 283–292.
23. Warkentin TE, Levine MN, Hirsh J *et al*. Heparin-induced thrombocytopaenia in patients treated with low molecular weight heparin or unfractionated heparin. *N Engl J Med* 1995; **332**: 1330–1335.
24. Schwarz T, Schmidt B, Beyer J, Schellong SM. Therapy of isolated calf muscle vein thrombosis with low molecular weight heparin. *Blood Coagul Fibrinolysis* 2001; **12**: 597–599.
25. Brandjes DPM, Heijboer H, Buller HR *et al*. Acenocoumarol and heparin compared with acenocoumarol alone in the initial treatment of proximal vein thrombosis. *N Engl J Med* 1992; **327**: 1485–1489.
26. Fennerty A, Campbell IA, Routledge PA. Anticoagulants in venous thromboembolism. *Br Med J* 1988; **297**: 1285–1288.
27. Oden A, Fahlen M. Oral anticoagulation and risk of death: a medical record linkage study. *Br Med J* 2002; **325**: 1073–1075.
28. Schulman S, Rhedin AS, Lindmarker P. A comparison of six weeks with six months of oral antico-

agulant therapy after a first episode of venous thromboembolism. *N Engl J Med* 1995; **332**: 1661–1665.

29. Pradoni P, Lensing AW, Cogo A *et al.* The long term clinical course of acute deep vein thrombosis. *Ann Intern Med* 1996; **125**: 1–7.

30. Hansson PO, Sorbo J, Eriksson H. Recurrent venous thromboembolism after deep vein thrombosis. *Arch Intern Med* 2000; **160**: 769–774.

31. Beyth RJ, Cohen AM, Landefeld S. Long term outcomes of deep vein thrombosis. *Arch Intern Med* 1995; **155**: 1031–1037.

32. Palareti G, Leali N, Coccheri S *et al.* Bleeding complications of oral anticoagulant treatment. *Lancet* 1996; **348**: 423–428.

33. Landefeld CS, Beyth RJ. Anticoagulant related bleeding:clinical epidemiology, predictionand prevention. *Am J Med* 1993; **95**: 315–328.

34. Pinede L, Cucherat M, Duhaut P *et al.* Optimal duration of anticoagulant therapy after an episode of venous thromboembolism. *Blood Coagul Fibrin* 2000; **11**: 701–707.

35. Research Committee of the British Thoracic Society. Optimum duration of anticoagulation for deep-vein thrombosis and pulmonary embolism and pulmonary embolism. *Lancet* 1992; **340**: 873–876.

36. Pinede L, Ninet J, Duhaut P *et al.* Comparison of three and six months of oral anticoagulant therapy after a first episode of proximal were or pulmonary embolism and comparison of six and twelve weeks of therapy after isolated calf deep vein thrombosis. *Circulation* 2001; **103**: 2453–2460.

37. Schulman S, Granqvist S, Holmstrom M *et al.* The duration of oral anticoagulant therapy after a second episode of venous thromboembolism. *N Engl J Med* 1997; **336**: 393–398.

38. Caprini JA, Arcelus JI, Reyna JJ *et al.* Deep vein thrombosis outcome and the level of anticoagulation therapy. *J Vasc Surg* 1999; **30**: 805–811.

39. Edwards EA, Edwards JE. Effects of thrombophlebitis on venous valves. *Surg Gynec Obstet* 1937; **65**: 310.

40. Mavor GE, Galloway JMD. Iliofeoral venous thrombosis: pathological considerations and surgical management. *Br J Surg* 1969; **56**: 43–59.

41. Markel A, Manzo RA, Bergelin RO *et al.* Valvular reflux after deep venous thrombosis: incidence and time of occurrence. *J Vasc Surg* 1992; **15**: 377.

42. Karp RB, Wylie EJ. Recurrent thrombosis after iliofemoral venous thrombectomy. *Surg Forum* 1966; **17**: 147.

43. Lindhagen J, Haglund M, Haglund U *et al.* Ileofemoral venous thrombectomy. *J Cardiovasc Surg* 1978; **19**: 319–327.

44. Roder OC, Lorentzen JE, Hansen HJ. Venous thrombectomy for iliofemoral thrombosis. Early and long-term results in 46 consecutive cases. *Acta Chir Scand* 1984; **150**: 31–34.

45. Stirnemann P, Althaus U, Kirchhof B *et al.* Early phlebographic results after iliofemoral venous thrombectomy. *Thorac Cardiovasc Surg* 1984; **32**: 299–303.

46. Plate G, Einarsson E, Ohlin P *et al.* Thrombectomy with temporary arteriovenous fistula: the treatment of choice in acute iliofemoral venous thrombosis. *J Vasc Surg* 1984; **1**: 867–876.

47. Lansing AM, Davis WM. Five-year follow-up study of iliofemoral venous thrombectomy. *Ann Surg* 1968; **168**: 620–628.

48. Patel KR, Paidas CN. Phlegmasia caerulea dolens: the role of non-operative therapy. *Cardiovasc Surg* 1993; **1**: 518–523.

49. Comerota AJ, Aldridge SC. Thrombolytic therapy for deep venous thrombosis: a clinical review *Can J Surg* 1993; **36**: 359–364.

50. Lensing AWA, Hirsh J. Rationale and results of thrombolytic therapy for deep vein thrombosis. In: EF Bernstein (ed) *Vascular Diagnosis* 4th edn. St Louis: Mosby, 1993: 875–879.

51. Hirsh J, Bates S. Clinical trials that have influenced the treatment of venous thromboembolism: a historical perspective. *Ann Intern Med* 2001; **134**: 409–417.

52. O'Meara J, McNutt R, Evans A *et al.* A decision analysis of streptokinase plus heparin as compared with heparin alone for deep vein thrombosis. *N Engl J Med* 1994; **330**: 1864–1869.

53. Forster A, Wells P. Tissue plasminogen activator for the treatment of deep venous thrombosis of the lower extremity: a systematic review. *Chest* 2001; **19**: 572–579.

54. Elsharawy M, Elzayat E. Early results of thrombolysis vs anticoagulation in iliofemoral venous thrombosis. A randomised clinical trial. *Eur J Vasc Endovasc Surg* 2002; **24**: 209–214.

55. Hold M, Bull PG, Raynoschek H, Denck H. Deep venous thrombosis: results of thrombectomy versus medical therapy. *Vasa* 1992; **21**: 181–187.

56. Comerota AJ, Aldridge SC, Cohen G *et al.* A strategy of aggressive regional therapy for acute iliofemoral venous thrombosis with contemporary venous thrombectomy or catheter directed thrombolysis. *J Vasc Surg* 1994; **20**: 244–254.

Anticoagulant therapy remains the gold standard for the management of lower limb deep vein thrombosis

Against the motion
Trevor Cleveland

Introduction

Anticoagulation for the treatment of lower limb deep venous thrombosis has been regarded by many physicians as the strategy which is used as the sole therapy, for a large majority of patients who present with acute deep venous thrombosis. In practical terms this treatment strategy is composed of immediate placement of the patient on a programme of heparin (either unfractionated or the low molecular weight version) supplemented by oral warfarin for a relatively poorly defined period of time.

For a treatment plan to be regarded as a 'gold standard', it is necessary to define the term. According to the *Concise Oxford Dictionary*[1] a gold standard is 'the system by which the value of a currency was defined in terms of gold, for which the currency could be exchanged'. However, in common medical practice the term is used more as a definition of the best practice, and one which other treatment modalities must try to match. In essence to be regarded as the gold standard implies a management plan which is at the pinnacle of achievement. Other treatments must aim to achieve this high standard, without the realistic likelihood of surpassing the treatment regarded as the gold standard.

The size of the problem

Whilst it is well recognized that deep venous thrombosis is a common clinical problem, which is frequently encountered in daily practice, a variety of population-based surveys have been undertaken, aiming to quantify the incidence, all of which have limitations. A major flaw in such surveys is that the clinical diagnosis of deep venous thrombosis is inaccurate when assessing the prevalence of the disorder in the population, and if the endpoint of pulmonary embolus is used the data available from death certification is again inaccurate. Studies which have been performed on the living population, have all focused on geographical areas, within which there may be relative under-representation of certain groups of the population, such as the elderly. However, allowing for such limitations, the Tecumseh Community Health Study[2] performed in 1973 would suggest that the prevalence of deep venous thrombosis in the

399

population of the USA was in the region of 122/100 000 per year, with 23/100 000 per year experiencing pulmonary emboli. This equated with an annual incidence in the USA of approximately 250 000 new clinically recognized deep venous thromboses per year.

It was possible to identify a number of risk factors from this and other studies[3,4] of people with newly diagnosed deep venous thrombosis. For example, if patients under the age of 46 were considered, the prevalence was three to four times higher in females. This was thought to be attributable in approximately half of cases to complications of pregnancy. In terms of the total population, those under 46 with deep venous thrombosis represent a relatively small number. If patients aged 60–70 years were considered there was a great increase in the prevalence of deep venous thrombosis, attributable to the increasing prevalence of cancer and the need for surgical intervention, particularly orthopaedic surgery.

If the incidence of deep venous thrombosis is compared between the Tecumseh Study[2] and the Worcester Study,[3] then a fall in projected deep venous thrombosis incidence is seen from 250 000 new cases per year to 170 000 per year. It seems likely that this apparent fall represents a change in practice between 1973 and 1991, and is a reflection on the success of routine anti-deep venous thrombosis prophylaxis.

Spectrum of lower limb thromboembolic disease

The term 'lower limb deep venous thrombosis' encompasses a wide range of clinical disease, the extent of which dictates the primary and long-term outcome for the disease. At one end of the spectrum is minor calf vein deep venous thromboses, many of which appear to produce no clinical symptoms or signs, and therefore go unnoticed. This disease entity may extend to more extensive calf vein thrombosis, which may extend above the level of the knee joint to involve the deep veins of the thigh. More extensive disease involves thrombus in the iliac veins and may result in the clinical entities of phlegmasia alba dolens, phlegmasia cerulea dolens and ultimately lead to venous gangrene. At any stage along this range, the disease may be complicated by the detachment of a small or large piece of this thrombus, which will embolize to the lungs resulting in pulmonary embolus.

The diagnosis of deep venous thrombosis may be both difficult and inaccurate, indeed it has been shown that if clinical diagnosis is relied upon then it is no more accurate than tossing a coin with a 50% chance of false positive or false negative diagnosis.[5,6] This particularly relates to the minor, localized thromboses, which are confined to the calf. At the other end of the clinical spectrum are the obvious states of phlegmasia. In phlegmasia alba dolens the leg is turgid, white and painful. There is usually tenderness over the common femoral vein which indicates iliofemoral deep venous thrombosis. As this was most commonly seen in years gone by in the puerperium, it was mistakenly ascribed by eighteenth century physicians to the accumulation of milk in the leg. In phlegmasia cerulea dolens the leg is also turgid and painful, but in these circumstances the limb is deeply cyanotic and much more painful. This cluster of clinical signs and symptoms indicate an even more extensive venous involvement in the thrombotic process, with both the deep and superficial systems thrombosed. This is a life-threatening situation, with significant blood lost in the thrombosed segments, with loss of fluid into the severely swollen interstitial compartment. As a result patients are often in clinical shock, and as the disorder progresses, haemorrhagic bullae may appear and venous gangrene ensues.

Natural history and consequencies of deep venous thrombosis

Whilst deep venous thrombosis itself may very widely in its presentation as detailed above, in the majority of cases it is the complications of the thrombosis which are of most consequence to the individual. The acute complication of deep venous thrombosis is pulmonary embolus, the late complications are recurrent thromboembolism and the post-thrombotic syndrome.

It is widely believed that calf deep venous thrombosis is uncommonly associated with pulmonary embolus, a supposition which leads many clinicians to believe that this entity does not require active treatment other than graded compression hosiery. However, it has been shown that thrombi may be associated with pulmonary emboli, which are detectable on lung perfusion scanning in 20–30% of patients who have a positive leg scan of the calf veins.[7,8] Despite treatment with anticoagulation a 29% rate of symptomatic extension into the popliteal veins has been shown if the level of anticoagulation has been suboptimal.[9] It is to be expected that isolated calf deep venous thrombosis, which is left untreated, will have a higher rate of extension into the popliteal, and above, veins and have a resultant increased risk of pulmonary emboli.

The long-term risk of recurrent thromboembolism depends upon the persistence of a significant risk factor for pulmonary emboli, if a temporary risk is identifiable then the chances of recurrent deep venous thrombosis are approximately one-third of that where a permanent risk factor can be identified.[10] However, overall it is significant to note that in a large randomized clinical trial comparing 6 weeks of anticoagulant therapy with 6 months of therapy, patients with symptomatic deep venous thrombosis were followed for 2 years for recurrences or death.[10] Whilst this showed a significant reduction in the risk for recurrent thromboembolism among the patients in the 6-month group, there was no difference in the recurrent events in the two groups from 6 to 24 months after the initial episode. In both groups there was a cumulative risk of 5–6% per year of recurrence, once anticoagulation had been stopped.

Post-thrombotic syndrome is caused by venous hypertension, which is the result of the combination of venous outflow obstruction and venous valve damage. The syndrome consists of:

1. Oedema.
2. Lipodermatosclerosis.
3. 'Bursting' pain on exercise (venous claudication).
4. Ulceration (indeed if a patient has an oedematous leg 1 year after a deep venous thrombosis, then he or she has a 50% risk of lower limb ulceration in 10 years[11]).

Goals of treatment for deep venous thrombosis

When treating any patients it is important to be clear as to the goals of the therapeutic regime. For patients with lower limb deep venous thrombosis these are:

1. Healing of the acute inflammatory and oedematous clinical picture.
2. Prophylaxis against recurrent deep vein thrombosis.
3. Prophylaxis against thrombus propagation.
4. Prophylaxis against pulmonary embolus.
5. Prevention of post-thrombotic syndrome.

Post-thrombotic syndrome

The precise incidence of post-thrombotic syndrome following confirmed deep venous thrombosis has been shown to vary between 20 and 100%.[12-22] Difficulties with the precise definition and objective criteria for this condition may explain the widely reported variation. A Dutch prospective randomized trial on the prevention of post-thrombotic syndrome was published in 1997.[23] This studied 194 consecutive patients with confirmed proximal deep venous thrombosis and randomly allocated elastic compression stockings in addition to anticoagulation. A scoring system was utilized to classify patients into mild-to-moderate or severe post-thrombotic syndrome. Median follow-up was 76 months, and in this period of time 20% of the patients using stockings and 47% of those without developed mild–to-moderate post-thrombotic syndrome. Severe post-thrombotic syndrome developed in 11.5% of the stocking group and 23.5% of the non-stocking group. In both groups the syndrome was identified within the first 2 years of the initial episode of deep venous thrombosis.

In 1996 long-term follow-up data from 355 patients with symptomatic, venographically proven deep venous thrombosis was reported.[24] All of the patients were fully anticoagulated and instructed to wear compression stockings for 3 years following discharge from hospital. The cumulative incidence of post-thrombotic syndrome was 18% at 1 year and 24.5% at 2 years. After that time the incidence of post-thrombotic syndrome increased to 29.6% at 5 years, but did not increase after that time. Approximately one-quarter of the patients with post-thrombotic syndrome at 5 years was considered severe.

Post-thrombotic syndrome is therefore a distressing condition for patients, which has considerable economic consequences for both the patient and the healthcare system.[25] The above studies show that if a patient has a proven deep venous thrombosis and is treated with anticoagulation, they can expect to run a risk of a 1:2 chance of developing mild-to-moderate symptoms of post-thrombotic syndrome and approximately half of these can look forward to severe symptoms. These symptoms are also not too far in the future as they are likely to develop within 2–5 years of their deep venous thrombosis.

Pathophysiology of PTS

The underlying causes of venous hypertension following deep venous thrombosis are:

1. Outflow obstruction.
2. Venous valve dysfunction.

Following deep venous thrombosis the body mounts an acute inflammatory response with organization and recanalization of the thrombus. However, this process is incomplete for two reasons. Firstly resorption and recanalization may be only partial, if it occurs at all. For example Killewich *et al.* showed that following deep venous thrombosis recanalization will occur in only 50% of limbs by 90 days,[26] and there is no specific evidence that full anticoagulation will improve this recanalization rate. Even if recanalization occurs, with venographic evidence of unobstructed flow in the affected segment, a cross-section of the vein demonstrates that there are multiple channels, which are the result of the recanalization process, but a large percentage of the normal lumen remains obstructed.[27]

The function and structure of the valves in the leg veins are vital to the maintenance of a low pressure within the venous compartment. Without the integrity of these structures, the 'muscle pump' is unable to function efficiently, venous pressure rises and the post-thrombotic syndrome develops. It has been demonstrated that there is a progressive development of valvular reflux as time elapses from the onset of the deep venous thrombosis. Markel et al.[28] followed 268 patients with deep venous thrombosis and performed duplex imaging at presentation, 1 week, 1 month and 3 months. At presentation, 14% of patients demonstrated reflux; this had increased to 17% by the end of the first week. At 1 month this figure had risen to 40% and by 1 year 66% had valvular reflux. This should be compared with a cohort of 1000 patients who had symptoms but did not have deep venous thrombosis; only 6% demonstrated reflux at 1 year. Also of interest was that of those patients who did not develop reflux, the majority had complete recanalization of their thrombus within 30 days.

In addition to the direct effect of thrombus and organization causing valve destruction there are indirect effects of the venous obstruction. The blood which would normally return through the deep veins, is directed around the obstruction via collaterals. The subsequent distension of these collateral channels results in the malfunction of the valve leaflets which further exacerbates the venous hypertension.

In terms of treatment for deep venous thrombosis, designed to reduce the incidence of post-thrombotic syndrome, the distribution of the valves in the venous system is of importance. The evidence above would indicate that it is important to relieve the valves of the thrombus, which will lead to their destruction during the organization process. It would appear that there are few valves located in the deep venous system above the knee, with the majority confined to the infrapopliteal segments. It also appears that these are the most important to the correct functioning of the 'muscle pump' and that those located above have a lesser role in ensuring effective venous return to the heart.[29,30] This is supported by data demonstrating that 40% of legs with distal valvular incompetence develop abnormal pigmentation,[31] and that two-thirds of limbs with severe stasis changes have incompetent valves below the knee. Patients who have active or healed venous ulceration demonstrate incompetence of the popliteal or posterior tibial veins in 84% of limbs,[32] and the relationship between proximal venous reflux and ulceration was weak compared with the relationship of ulceration and calf incompetence.

The evidence is, therefore, clear that anticoagulation which aims to prevent propagation of thrombus and does not accelerate clearance will not contribute to the prevention of the development of PTS.

Problems with anticoagulation

Anticoagulant regimes are not without problems and complications. A conflict exists between the need to fully anticoagulate for a significant period of time and the tendency to bleeding complications of this treatment. The probability of bleeding correlates closely with the level of anticoagulation, and monitoring is essential. Most haemorrhagic complications occur early in the treatment, with an overall risk of major bleeding of 2–3% in the first month.[33] Thereafter in subsequent months the risk falls to 0.8% per month for up to 1 year. This equates with a risk of major bleeding of 3.6–4.6% in the first 3 months and 6–7% in the first 6 months. This is the period of time for which most patients with deep venous thrombosis are anticoagulated.

Whilst anticoagulants do reduce the risk of pulmonary emboli in patients with deep venous thrombosis, they do not prevent it. If a patient does suffer with a pulmonary embolus whilst taking heparin, then the rate of recurrent pulomonary embolus or death within the next 2 weeks is greater than 10%.[34] The PIOPED study[34] also excluded all patients considered too ill to undergo pulmonary angiography, and therefore the rate of death and pulmonary emboli is likely to be even higher.

The commonly used anticoagulants are heparin (either low molecular weight versions or unfractionated) or warfarin. The low molecular weight heparins have a more reliable bioavailability profile than their unfractionated relations; however, should monitoring be required Anti-Factor Xa assay is required, which is not commonly available and difficult to obtain. These heparins also have a long half-life, which may be convenient some of the time, but should any interventional procedure be required (such as surgery, caval filter placement, pulmonary angiography etc) then the monitoring and reversal is complex, and may delay potentially lifesaving procedures. Unfractionated heparin requires continuous infusion and the reliability of anticoagulation can be very variable.

Warfarin on the other hand is administered orally, which is much more convenient for the patient, but monitoring of the effective dose requires repeated testing, frequently early in the treatment, and adequate control may be difficult or impossible. In addition the *British National Formulary*[35] lists no less than 26 classes of drugs which interact with warfarin altering the effective dose. This makes management of patients difficult and may be life- threatening.

Thrombolysis for deep venous thrombosis

The data presented above makes it clear that anticoagulation can only hope to reduce the propagation of thrombus, it does not aim to accelerate the clearance of thrombus; endogenous lytic agents are relied upon to achieve this. The figures above show that recanalization is patchy and incomplete in these circumstances and the risk of development of post-thrombotic syndrome remains unacceptably high. The restoration of vein patency, with valve function preservation should be the aim of treatment for deep venous thrombosis. This can only be achieved by the use of pharmacological or mechanical methods of thrombectomy.

Reports demonstrate that lysis can be achieved and patency restored with thrombolytic therapy, and that the long-term post-thrombotic sequelae can be reduced if there has been successful clearing of the deep vein thrombus.[36] Those who oppose the use of thrombolysis express concern over the risks of the treatment, cost, the fact that it is not suitable for all patients with deep venous thrombosis and the relatively low success rate in some studies.

The converse of this is that the contraindications to lytic agents have become clearer over time and that the complications have been reduced with more careful patient selection and refinement of the doses and drugs used. In addition the advent of thrombectomy devices has made the technique more widely applicable by either reducing or eliminating the need for adjuvent thrombolysis. The cost of the lytic drugs are immediately obvious; however, the costs of not preventing the very costly post-thrombotic syndrome over years are largely hidden to the health provider,[37] but not to the patient. No treatment regime for deep venous thrombosis is applicable to all patients, least of all anticoagulants for which there are a long list of contraindications. Whilst a number of patients with acute deep venous thrombosis are not candidates for thrombolysis, many of those who are eligible are young and therefore have the most to gain from prevention of post-thrombotic syndrome.

Between 1968 and 1990, 13 studies were reported comparing anticoagulant and thrombolytic therapy for acute deep venous thrombosis. These were pooled by Comerota,[27] and this revealed that only 4% of patients treated with anticoagulants had significant or complete lysis and an additional 14% had partial lysis. The majority (82%) had no objective clearing, or extension, of their thrombus. When treated with systemic thrombolysis, 45% had significant or complete clearing of the clot and 18% had partial clearing. Only 37% failed to improve or worsened. Jeffrey et al.[38] showed that this translated into a significant functional benefit 5–10 years after therapy if the lysis had been successful. Some of the failures of systemic lysis relates to patient selection. In most studies patients with the most extensive deep venous thromboses were included and systemic thrombolysis is likely to fail because the iliofemoral system was completely occluded and so the lytic agent would not have reached these areas. The bleeding complications were high because high doses of thrombolytic agents are necessary to achieve the systemic effect.

Catheter-directed thrombolysis overcomes the majority of these problems. In this technique the thrombolytic agent is delivered directly into the thrombus via a catheter embedded in the clot. Significantly reduced doses of the thrombolytic agent are needed to achieve much more reliable and rapid dissolution of the thrombus. In addition in the most severe form of deep venous thrombosis (phlegmasia) intra-arterial catheter-administered thrombolytics may be given which rapidly clear the capillary and venular thrombus, alleviating the impending venous gangrene. A recent randomized trial comparing catheter-directed thrombolysis and anticoagulation [39] showed that with the catheter-lysed patients 72% patency was achieved compared with 12% in the anticoagulated group and that venous reflux was found in 41% of the anticoagulant group and only 11% of those treated by catheter-directed lysis. There was no major bleeding and no deaths in this group and only one pulmonary embolus, which was in a patient in the anticoagulation-only group.

Data are therefore available which show that in patients in whom there is not a contraindication to thrombolysis, there is a significantly improved short- and long-term outcome to be achieved by the use of thrombolysis. It would seem that a higher success and lower complication rate can be expected if catheter-directed techniques are used, and that the population in whom this is indicated is widened by the use of local therapy.

Mechanical thrombectomy

Mechanical thrombectomy devices are relatively new, and have been more widely applied to dialysis fistula thrombosis than to deep venous thrombosis. However, these may be used alone, or as a method of reducing the need for thrombolytic agents. They have the advantage of not being associated with the same level of haemorrhagic complications and are more rapid for both treatment and resolution of symptoms. There are two basic principles used in the devices available, one type utilizes a rotating propeller to macerate the clot, the other uses hydrodynamics (Venturi effect) for clot destruction.

These devices are available with CE [European standard] marking for dialysis fistulae and are thought to be safe and effective in these structures. Thrombosed iliac veins tend to have a larger diameter, which may limit the usefulness in lower leg deep venous thrombosis, and at present there are no randomized trials comparing the different devices.

Caval filtration

Surgical interruption to treat deep venous thrombosis dates back to 1784, when John Hunter performed the first femoral vein ligation, but operative mortality rates in the region of 12% lead to searches for more acceptable ways to prevent the embolization of deep venous thrombosis. In modern practice inferior vena caval filters are placed percutaneously, through 7–8F introducer systems. In this manner inferior vena caval filters of three basic types may be deployed:

1. Permanent filters
2. Permanent filters with the option of retrieval
3. Temporary filters

These devices do not treat the thrombus directly, and so do not improve the outcome of the deep venous thrombosis in terms of prevention of recurrence and post-thrombotic syndrome, but they are designed to reduce the problems of pulmonary emboli. A randomized clinic trial in 1998[40] studied 400 patients with proximal deep venous thrombosis and who were anticoagulated. The patients were randomized to receiving an inferior vena caval filter or not. Within 12 days there were significantly fewer pulmonary emboli in those patients who received an inferior vena caval filter (1.1%) compared with those who did not (4.8%). At 2-year follow-up nearly twice as many recurrent pulmonary emboli were seen in the group without filtration. Inferior vena caval filters therefore seem to have an additional function in the treatment of deep venous thrombosis, particularly in the short term, and are extremely useful in patients who cannot tolerate anticoagulation. These devices have also been used as a short-term measure to prevent pulmonary emboli during thrombolysis of deep venous thrombosis.

Summary

The motion states that anticoagulation is the gold standard treatment for lower limb deep venous thrombosis. But:

- A significant proportion of patients have a contraindication to, or complications from anticoagulation.

- Pulmonary emboli occur despite optimal anticoagulation.

- Recurrent deep venous thrombosis, or thrombus propagation occur despite optimal anticoagulation.

- Post-thrombotic syndrome is common after deep venous thrombosis despite anticoagulation.

- Thrombolysis clears clot.

- Catheter-directed thrombolysis is applicable to many patients.

- Prompt thrombolysis prevents the post-thrombotic syndrome.

- Mechanical thrombectomy may be as effective as chemical lysis, or may reduce the dose required.

- Caval filtration significantly reduces pulmonary emboli, even if used in conjunction with anticoagulation

- Anticoagulation is not the 'Gold Standard' it is the 'Bog Standard' and other treatment options may offer a much improved outcome compared with anticoagulation.

References

1. *Concise Oxford Dictionary* 10th Edition. Oxford: Oxford University Press, 1999.
2. Coon WW, Willis PW, Keller JB. Venous thrombosis and other venous diseases in the Tecumseh Community Health Study. *Circulation* 1973; **48**: 839.
3. Anderson FA, Wheeler HB, Goldberg RJ *et al*. A population-based perspective of the hospital incidence and case-fatality rates of deep vein thrombosis and pulmonary embolism. The Worcester DVT Study. *Arch Intern Med* 1991; **151**: 933.
4. Rossman I. True incidence of pulmonary embolisation and vital statistics. *JAMA* 1974; **230**: 1677.
5. Cranley JJ, Canos AJ, Sull WJ. The diagnosis of deep vein thrombosis. *Arch Surg* 1976; **111**: 34.
6. JohnsonWC. Evaulation of newer techniques for the diagnosis of venous thrombosis. *J Surg Res* 1974; **16**: 473.
7. Browse NL, Thomas M. Source of non-lethal pulmonary emboli. *Lancet* 1974; **i**: 258–259.
8. Doyle DJ, Turpie AGG, Hirsh J *et al*. Adjusted subcutaneous heparin or continuous intravenous heparin in patients with acute deep vein thrombosis. *Ann Intern Med* 1987; **107**: 441–445.
9. Lagerstedt CJ, Olsson CG, Fagher BO *et al*. Need for long-term anticoagulant treatment in symptomatic calf-vein thrombosis. *Lancet* 1985; **ii**: 515–518.
10. Schulman S, Rhedin AS, Lindmaarker P *et al*. A comparison of six weeks with six months or oral anticoagulant therapy after a first episode of venous thromboembolism. *N Engl J Med* 1995; **332**: 1661–1665.
11. Bauer G. A roentgenological and clinical study of the sequels of thrombosis. *Acta Chir Scand* 1942; **86**(Suppl 74): 1.
12. Bauer G: A roentgenological and clinical study of the sequels of thrombosis. *Acta Chir Scand* 1942; **86**(Suppl 74): 1–110.
13. Gjores J. The incidence of venous thrombosis and its sequelae in certain districts of Sweden. *Acta Chir Scand* 1956; **206**(Suppl 1): 1–88.
14. O'Donnell FF, Brose NL, Burnand KG, Lea Thomas M. The socio-economic effects of an ilio-femoral venous thrombosis. *J Surg Res* 1977; **22**: 483–488.
15. Strandness DE, Langlois Y, Cramer M *et al*. Long-term sequelae of acute venous thrombosis. *JAMA* 1983; **250**: 1289–1292.
16. Widmer LK, Zemp E, Widmer MTH *et al*. Late results in deep-vein thrombosis of the lower extremities. *Vasa* 1985; **14**: 264–268.
17. Lindner DJ, Edwards JM, Phinney ES *et al*. Long-term hemodynamic and clinical sequelae of lower extremity deep-vein thrombosis. *J Vasc Surg* 1986; **4**: 436–442.
18. Heldal M, Seem E, Snadset PM, Abildgaard U. Deep-vein thrombosis: a 7-year follow-up study. *J Intern Med* 1993; **234**: 71–75.
19. Monreal M, Martorell A, Callejas JM *et al*. Venographic assessment of deep-vein thrombosis and risk of developing post-thrombotic syndrome: a prospective study. *J Intern Med* 1993; **233**: 854–859.
20. Milne AA, Ruckley CV. The clinical course of patients following extensive deep venous thrombosis. *Eur J Vasc Surg* 1994; **8**: 56–59.

21. Saarinen J, Sisto T, Laurikka J *et al.* Late sequelae of acute deep venous throbosis: evaluation five and ten years after. *Phlebology* 1995; 10: 106–109.

22. Beyth RJ, Cohen AM, Landfeld S. Long-term outcomes of deep-vein thrombosis. *Arch Intern Med* 1995; 155: 1031–1037.

23. Brandjes DPM, Büller, Heijboer H *et al.* Radnomised trial of effect of compression stockings in patients with somtomatic proximal-vein thrombosis. *Lancet* 1997; 349: 759–762.

24. Prandoni P, Lensing AWA, Cogo A *et al.* The long-term clinical course of acute deep venous thrombosis. *Ann Intern Med* 1996; 125: 1–7.

25. Bergqvist D, Jendteg S, Johansen L *et al.* Cost of long-term complications of deep venous thrombosis of the lower extremities: an analysis of a defined patient population in Sweden. *Ann Intern Med* 1997; 26: 454–457.

26. Killewich LA, Bedford GR, Beach KW *et al.* Spontaneous lysis of deep venous thrombi: rate and outcome. *J Vasc Surg* 1989; 9: 89–97.

27. Comerota AJ. Venous thromboembolism. In: *Vascular Surgery*, 4th Edition, Rutherford (ed), Vol II, 1995; 134: 1785–1810.

28. Markel A, Manzo R, Bergelin R, Strandness DE. Valvular reflux after deep vein thrombosis: Incidence and time of occurrence. *J Vasc Surg* 1992; 15: 377.

29. Arnoldi CC, Linderholm H. Venous pressures in patients with valvular incompetence of the veins of the lower limb. *Acta Chir Scand* 1966; 132: 628.

30. Höjensgård IC, Stürup H. Static and dymaic pressures in superficial and deep veins of the lower extremity in man. *Acta Physiol Scand* 1953; 27: 49.

31. Strandness DE Jr, Langlois Y, Cramer M *et al:* Long-term sequelae of acute venous thrombosis. *JAMA* 1983; 250: 1289.

32. van Bemmelen PS, Bedford G, Beach K, Strandness DE Jr. Status of the valves in the superficial and deep venous system in chronic venous disease. *Surgery* 1991; 109: 730.

33. Becker RC, Ansell J. *Oral Anticoagulants (Antithrombotic Agents) for Cardiovascular Disorders. Disorders of Thrombosis.* London, Philadelphia:Saunders. 1996; Ch 7, 75-87.

34. Carson JL, Kelley MA, Duff A *et al:* The clinical course of pulmonary embolism. *N Engl J Med* 1992; 326: 1240–1245.

35. *British National Formulary,* Appendix I – Drug Interactions. London: British Medical Association Publications, 2002.

36. Comerota AJ. Thrombolytic therapy for acute deep vein thrombosis. *Semin Vasc Surg* 1992; 5: 76.

37. O'Donnell TF, Browse NL, Burnand KG, Lea TM. The socioecomomic effects of an ilio-femoral venous thrombosis. *J Surg Res* 1977; 22: 483.

38. Jeffry P, Immelman E, Amoore J. Treatment of deep vein thrombosis with heparin or streptokinase: Long-term venous function assessment. In: *Proceedings of the Second International Vascular Symposium.* London, 1986: abstr S20.3.

39. Elsharaway M, Elzayat E. Early results of thrombolysis vs anticoagulation in iliofemoral venous thrombosis: a randomised clinical trial. *Eur J Vasc Endovasc Surg* 2002; 24: 209–214.

40. Decousus H, Leizorovicz A, Parent F *et al.* A clinical trial of vena caval filters in the prevention of pulmonary embolism in patients with proximal deep vein thrombosis. *N Engl J Med* 1998; 338: 409–415.

Anticoagulant therapy remains the gold standard for the management of lower limb deep vein thrombosis

Charing Cross Editorial Comments towards Consensus

Sudip Ray makes the case for conventional anticoagulant therapy and quotes the references, but essentially Trevor Cleveland develops the theme that conventional anticoagulant therapy is standard, but certainly not the gold standard. He stresses that pulmonary emboli can occur despite optimal anticoagulation, and thrombolysis is required to clear the clot. He feels that catheter-directed thrombolysis is applicable to many patients, and the long-term outcomes in terms of post-thrombotic syndrome are superior if lysis is used.

Roger M Greenhalgh
Editor